HOMEOPATHIC
GUIDE TO STRESS

Also by Miranda Castro

The Complete Homeopathy Handbook

Homeopathy for Pregnancy, Birth, and Your Baby's First Year

HOMEOPATHIC GUIDE TO STRESS

Miranda Castro, F.S. Hom.

St. Martin's Griffin 🕮 New York

IMPORTANT NOTE TO THE READER:

It is advisable to seek the guidance of a physician before implementing the approach to health suggested in this book. It is essential that any reader who has any reason to suspect that he or she suffers from illness check with his or her doctor before attempting to treat it with this method. Neither this nor any other book should be used as a substitute for professional medical care or treatment.

HOMEOPATHIC GUIDE TO STRESS. Copyright © 1996 by Miranda Castro. All rights reserved. Printed in the United States of America. No part of this book may be used or reproduced in any manner whatsoever without written permission except in the case of brief quotations embodied in critical articles or reviews. For information, address St. Martin's Press, 175 Fifth Avenue, New York, N.Y. 10010.

Library of Congress Cataloging-in-Publication Data

Castro, Miranda.
    Homeopathic guide to stress : safe and effective natural ways to treat physical, emotional, work-related, and personal stress / Miranda Castro.
        p.   cm.
    ISBN 0-312-29180-9
    1. Stress (Psychology)—Homeopathic treatment.
    2. Stress (Physiology)—Homeopathic treatment.   3. Stress management.
    I. Title.
    RX590.S75C37   1997
    155.9′042—dc21   96-37350
                                                                           CIP

First published in Great Britain by Pan Books, an imprint of Macmillan Publishers Ltd.

First U.S. Edition: May 1997

10 9 8 7 6 5 4 3 2 1

For Jeremy

Contents

Physical Stresses

Homeopathic Remedies

Acknowledgements

The stress of writing books in addition to being a homeopath, a single parent and human being have stretched me, at times, to my limits. I joined a town choir and found that singing twice a week released some of that strain, and created more physical relaxation, more inner joy and more peace than ten hot baths or a day on the Yorkshire moors. It took me forty-two years to find a way to sing the notes that rattled around in my head! Because my life is (willingly) rather stressful, singing is the first place I look to when I become over-stressed or need a massage for my body *and* my soul.

I would like to thank the following friends, family and colleagues for their encouragement, feedback, input, support (moral and otherwise!) . . . and, of course, for their part in alleviating the stress of writing this book: Barbara Levy, Daniel, Ellen Goldman, Joy Chang, Hazel Orme, John Morgan, Mary Clarke, Jeanne Ellin, Jeremy Castro, Maggi Sikking, Mike Jackson, Miranda Walsh, Rachel Packer, Rob Barker, Rosie, Sue Morrison, all at the Society of Homeopaths' office, Victoria Pryor, and finally, all at Macmillan UK.

Seattle, Washington, USA
February 1996

How to Use This Book

The goal of this book is to enable you to use homeopathic medicines safely and effectively so that you can treat some common stresses and stress-related complaints after consulting with your medical professional. I hope it will also encourage you to enter into a lively, on-going relationship with your own stress responses, by understanding them within a holistic, homeopathic framework.

Understanding stress
This section discusses some common stress responses, suggests ways to identify stressful areas in your life and outlines steps to take in order to deal with them.

Understanding homeopathy
This chapter looks at the history and principles of homeopathy, and ends with twenty cases from my practice which bring the theory to life.

Emotional and physical stresses
These sections focus on specific stresses, including practical advice for avoiding a particular stress and/or working with it, as well as a brief discussion of homeopathic solutions.

Homeopathic remedies
This part describes forty-three common homeopathic remedies for acute or recent stresses. Each one describes the emotional and general state, as well as some common physical symptoms.

Stress indexes
You can use these as a short cut once you become familiar with the pictures outlined above. Or you may want to look up a particular stress or symptom in order to see which remedies are appropriate.

Appendices
Here you will find stress charts to help you work out how stressed you may be, as well as a glossary of terms and a list of books and organizations.

Introduction

When I first 'discovered' homeopathy I felt as if I had 'come home'. One of the main reasons for this feeling was that my homeopath took a wide view of stress, one I hadn't experienced or heard of in any other medical discipline. It was such a relief to know that there was a place where medical professionals not only saw that each individual was unique, with particular strengths and weaknesses, but that each person was potentially vulnerable to different stresses, or would at least respond in their own way to different stresses – whether they were physical, mental or emotional. This made tremendous sense to me.

In my early years in practice, however, I found myself somewhat perplexed when patients would tell me at the beginning of a consultation that they had come to see me because they were stressed, or because their doctors had diagnosed them as having stress. I would ask them to tell me more and I would also ask what they meant by the word 'stress'. Some of these patients would look at me somewhat suspiciously, even irritably, as if to say: 'What kind of homeopath are you? Don't you know what stress is?' And they would repeat their original statement, but speaking a little slower this time, as if they were talking to someone whose first language was not English. Some patients would go into a lengthy explanation about stress, in a genuine attempt to educate me. Others would shrug their shoulders and look at me baffled as if to say: 'Well, if you don't know what I mean then I certainly don't.'

In the past, doctors who were having difficulty helping certain patients would often, if all tests came back negative, make a diagnosis of psychosomatic illness. They might add that the patient had to learn to live with their complaint, that there was nothing they could do. This has always seemed to me to be a rather cruel blow to deal to those who may be running out of hope anyway.

Then there came a time when the diagnosis changed to 'stress'. It was an easier word to say (and spell!) and tripped off everyone's tongues without any trouble whatsoever. Doctors now added that the patient had to learn to live with their complaint, that there was little advice they could offer except, maybe, to learn to relax.

The trouble is that stress, like psychosomatic illness, is almost completely meaningless as a diagnosis. It is like taking your beloved car to the garage, saying that it has a worrying knocking sound every time you brake hard, and that you have noticed some other peculiar symptoms as well. Your mechanic takes a close look and performs many sensible tests but is not able to find what ails it. He then hands it back to you saying that he cannot therefore treat it, and you will have to live with it. You *know* that it is just a question of time before something goes wrong. Your mechanic knows it too, but neither of you say anything. You don't want to make your mechanic feel bad, especially since he has done his best to uncover the cause of the problem.

It has been suggested that the human body is like a car. That we have to attend to it with the same degree of loving care and attention. If only it were that simple! We cannot take it apart, lay all the parts out on the garage floor, clean them and put them back together again. We cannot easily replace parts that have become damaged. And we do not run on fuel alone. Our vitality and our energetic processes are not fully understood. The sheer complexity of the human body should be listed as one of the seven wonders of the world.

Any system of medicine that seeks to treat the human body as a mechanical object is going to be limited in terms of its ability to offer serious healing. Patients have learned to rely on doctors more as mechanics than anything else . . . presenting a straightforward complaint and expecting and getting a simple solution which treats the complaint (a prescription). The problems start when the complaints become more complicated and do not respond to standard drug treatment.

A car is mostly a three-dimensional object, operating within fairly comprehensible boundaries. A body is multi-dimensional, multi-faceted. And so is life. My task as a homeopath is to make a four-dimensional jigsaw puzzle out of the mass of information that each patient presents, one that makes sense to both of us, one that I can prescribe on, that takes these many facets into account.

I have learnt to ask my patients about the stresses they have experienced and to describe the effect they have had. As they tell their story I listen carefully, in order to pick up clues about their emotional responses to a stressful situation, to build up a picture I can understand and work with. For many people, everyday stresses include those which are mundane (like poor diet, commuting or lack of exercise); unpleasant (living with an abusive partner or a sulky, angry adolescent); or severe (the death of a close friend or relative or redundancy). For some people traumatic stress is a tragic reality, either as a one-off (a disabling accident or sexual abuse) or in an ongoing way (those caught up in war-torn areas or nursing staff on an accident and injury unit). The stress of being shot at in Bosnia or Northern Ireland is very different to that of being stuck in a traffic jam on a motorway.

Alternative medicine in general, and homeopathy in particular, can offer much to patients who have been encouraged to dismiss or ignore their complaint because it has been diagnosed as 'psychosomatic' or 'stress-related'. There is almost unlimited help available in the homeopathic medicine chest, whether the stress is physical (headaches caused by a head injury, a cough caused by teething, or an earache after a chill); emotional (depression due to a difficult relationship or resentment due to an unpleasant work situation); or mental (exhaustion and inability to make decisions after an exam, or a period of overworking). A well chosen homeopathic remedy can heal emotional pain as well as physical symptoms, and enable people to recover their vitality and sense of well-being.

This book is intended as an introduction to homeopathy with a specific focus on stress. It isn't a comprehensive guide to either stress or homeopathy. I hope that you will use this book to begin to build a healthy relationship with stress: to identify your own unique responses to particular stresses, to understand what affects you and when, to check out ways to balance out those stresses, and to explore the part that homeopathy may play in helping you on your path to health.

UNDERSTANDING STRESS

What is Stress?

Stress is an integral part of life's rich tapestry. It is an on-going, ever-present ebb and flow in all our lives. We need to understand its place in our lives and work *with* it rather than sink hopelessly into it, or worse, see it only as something to eliminate.

I hope to provide a wider, holistic view of stress that acknowledges the many forms it can take: physical, mental, emotional and even spiritual; healthy and unhealthy; chronic and acute; everyday and traumatic.

Working with everyday stress is about how we interact with life and express ourselves in all our relationships and at all levels. We need to understand that it is neither a good nor a bad thing – necessarily – it is our response to it that makes it healthy or unhealthy, energizing or draining.

Health is more than simply the absence of disease. It involves a sense of well-being, of feeling good, of being in balance and in harmony, that is hard to dislodge. It is, above all, the ability to respond appropriately to stress.

Under stress we each react according to our strengths and weaknesses. We all have different Achilles' heels – and these weaknesses may be our greatest assets. Some people only know they have been under pressure when they get a migraine or have difficulty sleeping. We need to respond to these calls for help and not ignore them. That way we can begin to see them as a resource for preserving our health rather than as a nuisance, which seeks to undermine us when we least expect it. We can look on illness as a warning sign that there may be some stress or stresses in our lives that need attending to or balancing out: to make choices about which healthy stresses to add in, which unhealthy stresses to cut down on or even cut out; or what additional support or practical measures (including medical treatments if appropriate) are necessary to help us through this particular time.

The homeopath largely ignores the label of a disease, being more interested in how each individual experiences it, and what stress or stresses led up to their becoming ill. No two people with a cough, for example, will have the same symptoms and neither will the stresses that precipitated the cough necessarily be the same. Where one person may develop it after the emotional stress of, say, feeling betrayed by a good friend, another can develop it after a physical stress such as getting chilled in a cold wind.

I hope that you will use this book to identify areas where homeopathy can help you, where you can easily, safely and swiftly treat yourself, and where and when you need to seek professional advice. If self-prescribing isn't appropriate and the stresses in your life are affecting your health, then I hope that the information in this book will encourage you to seek out constitutional treatment from a professional homeopath.

My goal is to provide a model for understanding stress within a framework that takes into account the whole person, so that you can identify your own responses to it and begin to build a healthy relationship with stress on a daily basis – to harness it as a positive enlivening force in your own life.

STRESS RESPONSES

A healthy response to the many stresses of life enables us to be alert, to have plenty of energy and feel fully alive, to be creative, adaptable, approachable and to express ourselves appropriately: physically, emotionally, mentally and spiritually. Stress can be enlivening, exciting, stimulating – providing us with challenge and stretching us.

Or it can be a pressure, a strain. At times we may be *understressed* – feeling unchallenged, or unmotivated, tired, apathetic or even depressed; and at others *overstressed* – feeling tense, tired, anxious, irritable. Once we are overstressed it becomes harder to relax. Conversely, if we are understressed, it becomes harder to get going. Either way, we are not able to deal with stress as effectively and appropriately as when we are more relaxed and in balance.

Every cell in our body contracts and expands continuously throughout our life. All our bodily processes pulsate, have their own ebbing and flowing – as do our feelings and our thinking processes. To live in a healthy relationship with stress we *have* to be able to relax: mentally, emotionally and physically. Stress stimulates (causing contraction), after which we need to relax (causing expansion), after which we can contract again. This natural rhythm involves a constant movement between tension and relaxation.

We are perhaps most familiar with the stress reaction known as the 'fight-or-flight' response which gets switched on when we are frightened, shocked or need to perform at a higher level than normal. This response involves all of the body's systems, all organs, all cells, and interrupts our natural rhythms. Chemicals (neurotransmitters via nerve impulses and hormones via the blood) are triggered by, say, the stress of a shock, causing measurable physical reactions: the heart rate and respiration increase in anticipation of action, hormones (especially adrenaline) are released, which in turn trigger the release of stored body sugar to provide a surge of energy – in other words, our body goes on 'red alert'. In a dangerous, difficult or life-threatening situation this response is vital, because it gives us a heightened awareness and extra energy.

Problems arise when this fight-or-flight response becomes habitual, when everyday events (getting stuck in traffic, waiting in a supermarket checkout, going for a job interview) evoke it regularly, because the body is constantly flooded with adrenaline. A constant state of tension develops and it becomes difficult, and eventually impossible, to relax. Jaw clenching, tooth grinding (especially when asleep), a chronic stiff neck are all typical physical symptoms of this type of overstress.

When the demands, which can be either physical or emotional, exceed our available resources, our system gears up to deal with the challenge. This is when the overstress can tip us over into distress. It is only when we are *distressed*, when our stress levels exceed our ability to cope with them, that we can become completely exhausted and even burnt out.

'Burnt out' is the term often given to people who are seriously worn out. It is an emotive term which gives the impression that everything has fused inside! Which, of course, it hasn't. We have simply become run down and our battery needs recharging. The term 'breakdown' would be more accurate. Once we have reached this state we often need a complete rest for as long as it takes for our vitality to return.

6

Understanding Stress

You take a risk with your health if you don't listen to your own
warning signs telling you that you are overstressed, or heading for
distressed. You can take precautions to avoid becoming distressed
or even burnt out. But first you need to be familiar with your own
symptoms.

If you can answer yes to most of the following questions it is
unlikely that you are suffering from either under- or overstress.

- Do you feel good and on top of your life?
- Do you feel full of vitality?
- Are you eating well and regularly?
- Are your energy levels high without the use of tea and/or coffee?
- Do you sleep well and easily at night and wake feeling refreshed?
- Are you happy with your friendships and relationships?
- Is your work satisfying?
- Are the following a regular part of your life: fun; exercise;
  creativity; rest; relaxation?

If you answered 'no' to many of the above questions then you may
want to use this book to help you reassess how stress fits into your life.

The immediate effects of stress and strain are that people often
feel tired and tense and compensate by overusing caffeine, sugar,
cigarettes, alcohol and other 'drugs' (including prescribed drugs
such as the minor tranquillizers often given to people suffering from
anxiety and/or insomnia). Chemical stimulants boost our hormones
artificially if our natural energy levels drop. Chemical sedatives
force us into an artificial sleep. Overstressed, and some understressed people, tend to mix these, either daily or with occasional
binges, using caffeine to get going, sugar to keep going and alcohol
to switch off. They may also be making things worse by missing
meals or eating badly. This creates a shaky equilibrium, an internal
roller coaster, as people balance stresses by using this form of over-
the-counter self-medication instead of taking practical, health-
preserving steps to deal with the stresses.

Prolonged abuse of stimulants and sedatives simply stresses the
body further. The long term effect of having the body flooded with
chemical stimulants is damaging, especially for those who are
sedentary. Adrenaline, for example, needs burning off, needs
physical activity for it to be used up productively otherwise it
leaves acidic residues.

If the body needs rest and instead the hormones are artificially stimulated to respond, then the whole system will eventually destabilize, will become more and more run down. Our natural chemicals are an emergency resource, not something we should be stimulating on a daily basis.

If we become overstressed when we are awake, we generate stress chemicals which will prevent us from sleeping well at night, chemicals that are designed to promote alertness and combat sleep. We prepare for sleep during the day and so we need to weave rest into our waking hours, so that by the time we get to bed we *can* switch off. Otherwise we can set up a vicious cycle that is hard to break, where a bad night's sleep leads to waking tired so we use more stimulants to keep our energy levels high and have difficulty sleeping.

Rest isn't the only answer, the 'addictions' need dealing with, the patterns of overstress or understress need facing, the automatic response of the body to flood with stress hormones needs help to switch off. Exercise, diet, rest and relaxation, as well as fun and play time, adjustments to work schedules to create a healthy balance between work and rest – these all need dealing with for the sake of our long-term health.

Our brains operate a complicated juggling act with hormones, or chemical messengers, sending and receiving trillions of messages daily that deal with all the functions of the body – physical and emotional. When we are under stress, it is our hormones that are responsible for the initial warning symptoms – the lack of energy and enthusiasm, inexplicable aches and pains, sleep difficulties, changes in appetite and mood swings.

Typical symptoms of overstress include: headaches, back pain, stiff neck, nausea, physical tension and/or stiffness anywhere, dizziness, indigestion, constipation and/or diarrhoea, skin rashes, hair falling out, difficulties with menstrual periods, piles, stomach upsets, nosebleeds, cystitis, problems with teeth and gums, sweating, palpitations, cramps, twitchy legs, difficulty swallowing (a sensation of a lump in the throat), difficulty breathing (a sensation of not being able to get enough air), anxiety, irritability, poor concentration, memory loss, indecisiveness, 'gramophone' thoughts (going round and around), a general slowing down or even an overwhelming lethargy. In addition, we can become more suscep-tible to infections such as coughs, colds, sore throats and flus etc.

When symptoms surface at one level, other levels are often affected. For example, a head injury (physical) can initially cause shock (emotional) and amnesia (mental) as well as pain (physical). A difficult, aggressive boss may create an emotionally stressful environment for his or her staff, who may produce physical ailments such as headaches, indigestion or neck pain as a response to un-expressed emotions.

People are sometimes told that little or nothing can be done about the complaints that accompany or follow emotional stress. These may be termed psychosomatic, which implies that the patient has made him or herself ill. It is an outmoded view of disease that needs questioning. Nobody should be led to believe that they have made themselves ill on purpose. Or it may be suggested that the 'correct' mental attitude (or positive thought) is necessary for healing to take place. The message received by the patient if healing doesn't take place, is that again, they are responsible or even that they may be incurable.

Those who don't feel *physically* unwell as a result of emotional or even physical stress need to be especially careful, and may indeed need to balance out the stress in their lives more routinely since they won't be receiving warning signals when something is wrong.

If the relatively minor symptoms of under- or overstress are ignored and/or if people do not make some basic but essential lifestyle changes, then more serious chronic illness can develop. Disease is not necessarily a bad thing. It simply may be the body letting us know that we need to attend to some housekeeping. Any approach to dealing with disease that involves treating the under-lying stress or stresses will be of greater benefit in the long term than treating the symptoms alone.

Working with Stress

Life is stress-full. We need to stop and assess our stress load on a regular basis if we are to work with it effectively.

We need to understand where tension comes from in order to be able to relax. In stressful situations we have a tendency to react in the same old (stressful) ways over and over again – ways that we may have learnt as children. And when we grow up, in spite of knowing that these ways of responding are unhealthy, we can find it difficult to react differently.

It can be hard to change old habits. It isn't possible to change simply by wanting to. There are a number of steps to take, just as with learning any new skill. Use the following steps to help you to do this.

KEEPING A LOG

Start by keeping a diary of all your activities, and inactivities! Over a week, log in everything you do and how long it takes. If you have a complicated life, with changing schedules, you may need to plot your activities for longer than a week in order to get an overall picture.

You can use the charts or make up a system of your own. Classify your activities into work, school, home (household chores including shopping, cooking, cleaning, tidying, etc.), family time, travelling, eating, rest and relaxation, sleep, exercise, time off or fun (social) time, time spent watching television and anything else that matters to you.

At the end of the week add up the hours. What does it look like? What patterns do you notice? Understanding where stress fits into your life is an important first step in being able to deal with it. Are you surprised to find that you are working a thirty-two hour week when it felt like fifty? Why? Is it because you aren't getting enough sleep or exercise and are tired all the time? Or are you shocked to

To help you ascertain how you are spending your time each day, put a mark in each half-hourly box, then transfer the totals to the weekly chart.

DAILY CHART	Morning						Afternoon						Evening						Night						TOTAL
	7	8	9	10	11	12	1	2	3	4	5	6	7	8	9	10	11	12	1	2	3	4	5	6	
Work																									
School																									
Eating																									
Sleep																									
Rest / Relaxation																									
Exercise																									
Fun/Time with friends, etc.																									
Travel																									
Family time																									
Household chores																									
Television																									

WEEKLY CHART	Monday	Tuesday	Wednesday	Thursday	Friday	Saturday	Sunday	TOTAL
Work								
School								
Eating								
Sleep								
Rest/Relaxation								
Exercise								
Fun/Time with friends, etc.								
Travel								
Family time								
Household chores								
Television								

find that you have been working sixty hours a week without realizing it?

If you are unemployed it may be just as important to find out how you are spending your time. I know one man who was shocked to discover that he was watching television every day for between six and twelve hours. He wasn't taking any exercise either. It was hardly surprising he felt depressed. Children of all ages may also find it enlightening to learn how many hours they are spending in front of a television and/or computer screen. Those caring for elderly parents or disabled children or the sick will find it sobering to see how little time is left over, especially if they are caring around the clock seven days a week.

Those who are keeping many balls in the air may feel mystified about how they fit it all in. This is one way to find out. What are you cutting back on in order to be Superman or Superwoman? Working parents find that after a forty hour week at work, ten hours travelling, sixteen hours housework and shopping, twenty hours cooking and eating, forty-two hours sleeping, there aren't many hours left in the week to spend with their children, partners, friends or just by themselves. If they don't plan carefully, they are going to slip into feeling overstressed without any difficulty whatsoever.

ADD UP YOUR STRESSES

Use headings to help you identify stress in different areas of your life, work or school, home, relationships, time off. As you list each stress also write down your *uncensored* response to how this stress has affected or is affecting you. Is it acute (a one-off) or chronic (ongoing)? Is it preventing you from doing something you want to do? Is it affecting your health? How stressed are you really? How long is your list? Are your day-do-day stresses manageable or do they feel like hard work? Is it difficult to imagine how you have coped or have you sailed through some choppy waters with relative ease?

On a separate piece of paper, think over the past year and list the stressful situations you can remember – the traumatic or extraordinary stresses. Use the Holmes and Rahe charts on p. 383 to help you, or talk it through with a friend – someone close to you may well remember things you had forgotten. Make a note of whether each stress was physical, mental or emotional; mild, moderate or severe; a one-off or on-going; and whether it was an everyday or a traumatic stress. How many of these stresses are still present in your life?

Compare them with previous years. Have you had one stress-filled year after another? Stresses that have come and gone may still be having an effect. Maybe your beloved pet died four years ago and you still feel bereft but are ashamed about feeling so sad about an animal and have no one to confide in. Now look forward and list any imminent stresses.

Become an interested observer of your everyday life and notice how you react in different situations. What makes you feel tense, pressured, anxious, frustrated, frightened, and, conversely, what relaxes and energizes you or makes you feel good? Collect this information, without being judgemental or critical. Start noticing your patterns, the sorts of stresses that are familiar as well as your responses to them.

ADD UP YOUR PERSONAL ASSETS

An awareness and appreciation of your strengths and your fine qualities will see you through tough times and make the good times more enjoyable. Start with your strengths: for example, a strong constitution (good health/vitality); a sense of humour; a strong will; common sense and so on. Many people have learnt to be most aware of their weak points, to the exclusion of their assets. Part of your success with handling stress will be accepting your strengths along with your limitations. They are neither good nor bad but are the cornerstones of your individuality.

List your resources: people who will help out when you need them – friends, family, neighbours, etc., a friendly bank manager! It is all too easy to forget that you are not alone in stressful times.

List your skills: your areas of expertise which enable you to do with relative ease the tasks with which others might struggle. You may have learnt them on a course or at work. Many people do not count the cost to themselves of not having, for example, basic administration skills when it comes to dealing with paperwork, or basic accounting skills for book keeping in a small business. Neither budgeting nor filing comes naturally – any more than breastfeeding, parenting, communicating, cooking, driving or gardening!

LIFE SKILLS

Some skills are worth learning to help you cope more effectively with stress. People who lack assertiveness, and/or are bad at managing their time, and/or have never been encouraged to listen to their intuition, can find themselves muddling along, becoming increasingly frustrated or upset, not coping as well as they would like to and not getting what they want – or getting it, but at a high price.

Assertiveness training, time management, planning and problem-solving work hand-in-hand and you might consider taking a stress management course if you want to look at these areas of your life in a more structured way.

ASSERTIVENESS TRAINING

Our interactions with others can be a source of stress. Assertiveness is a learnt skill that comes more naturally to some than others: some learn it from their families, mainly by example, but many don't. Many people are now learning about human behaviour, often unconsciously, from the television. Unfortunately, 'assertive' characters in adverts, films or soap operas often perpetuate unhelpful, stereotypical behaviour. For example, when women get angry they may say nothing and storm out of a room, sometimes slamming the door; when men get angry they may become physically violent. Both of these are stressful ways of expressing anger in the real world.

Assertiveness training can reduce stress by helping people learn to stand up for their rights without being aggressive but without being bullied. Being assertive means having respect for one's own needs and rights as well as those of others; expressing thoughts, feelings, beliefs, likes, wishes, disagreements or confusions in a direct, honest and appropriate way, which is respectful of others and their feelings – without taking responsibility for them. Above all, an assertive person can laugh at him or herself, can keep stressful experiences in perspective and deal with them so that no one is damaged in the process.

MANAGING TIME

Be aware of time and how it fits into your life. Balance the time you spend at work with the time you devote to your family, friends and yourself. If you know you are working ridiculously long hours then start by cutting back half an hour a day. Spend it doing something that recharges you.

If you have become stuck and bored, are either unemployed, retired or doing a repetitive job, make time in the day to do something that will get you going again, that will stimulate your creative juices: an exercise or evening class, voluntary work, anything to give you some energy.

If you are a person who habitually rushes, develop rituals that slow you down: take things one at a time – you will find everything easier to remember. People who lose their keys are often people who do one thing while thinking of something else. Get up earlier in the morning so that you can have a leisurely breakfast; take a minute (or even two) just to sit before leaving home – it takes several minutes to go back and get the things you have forgotten in the stressful rush to get on your way. Make lists and always have them at hand to add to when you suddenly remember things. Build idling time into your daily routines, allow extra time for all journeys, be philosophical about delays – see them as a 'gift of time' and use them to think, relax, meditate or daydream.

Television has become a huge time-killer. Be ruthless with your planning and only watch the programmes you're really interested in. Avoid spending too much time on trying to get things perfect: make peace with yourself and agree that the housework, your job or whatever, is going to be done 'well enough' for now – especially if your priorities lie elsewhere. To have more fun, for example.

PROBLEM SOLVING

Your next step is to plan how you might handle your stresses – less stressfully. Your stress scales aren't static, neither will they ever be equally balanced.

When it comes to problem-solving with a particular stress you may get stuck with the idea that there are only two solutions – neither of which seems satisfactory. This is rarely true, but may be a measure of how stressed you are. Once you end up thinking that there isn't a satisfactory way out of a difficult situation it is easy to want to blame others or yourself for what is happening in an attempt to deal with feeling helpless. Be kind and considerate towards yourself and interested in how stress is affecting you and how you are going to deal with it.

Start by thinking through the situation, taking your feelings into account. Ask yourself what you *really* want, and what outcome you would ideally like. Is it different from what you need or think you need, or what others want from you?

Scribble down alternative solutions, without censoring the weird and the silly as well as the sensible. Then sleep on it and/or talk it through with people you trust. Ask a friend, someone who knows you well or who deals well with the sort of stress you are facing to share their solutions. But remember that *your* stresses and *your* solutions may be different from theirs.

A vast untapped resource for solving difficulties is intuition or mental creativity, hunches that come spontaneously, sometimes in seemingly disconnected thoughts or in pictures, feelings or even your dreams (during the day or at night!). Gut reactions can be brilliant and should always be listened to – just in case!

At some point you will begin to see possibilities for action and will then be in a position to plan your next step. But until then, keep scribbling and talking and thinking.

TAKING ACTION

Remind yourself that it is your ability to adapt and flow with stress that will help you to maintain your equilibrium and balance it out as you go along: take some exercise if you have sat at a desk for ten hours or take an extra day off work if your return journey from holiday was horribly delayed and spanned two nights in airports. If you struggle to return to work you may have to take off more than a day to deal with whatever complaint your body comes up with in order to get a rest. If you have been used to living with a lot of pressure and your health is beginning to suffer, you will need to consider changing a 'bad' habit, such as going to bed at midnight when you have a baby that wakes at 5.30 a.m.

Taking action can involve something as simple as saying 'no' instead of agreeing to something that you don't want to do, or saying 'yes' to something that you would love to do. Learn to offload and delegate. Learn also to recognize when you have reached your limits and to get support. It can be sobering to remind yourself that you are rarely indispensable, that your stresses count, and so do you.

Keep your strategies up your sleeve for when you need them. As you implement them be patient and don't force yourself to go too far too soon – you may feel you have failed if you don't manage it. Above all, don't give up if your strategies don't work. You may have to go back to the drawing board more than once!

Set yourself realistic goals and aims, at work and at home, and keep change to a minimum if you are overstressed. You need to plan strategies that won't simply add another burden. A house move, for example, can be a huge source of stress to somebody who needs the security of a home base, and who hasn't moved in many years; somebody who is a regular house mover and who finds all the newness exciting, may take the upheaval in their stride. However, if your current living situation is stressful because of, say, noisy neighbours, then when you weigh up the pros and cons of staying put against moving – and being able to sleep at night – you may decide to move. Or you may decide to postpone the move anyway (and get earplugs) because you have just taken on a new job and know your limits and will leave it to a year with fewer stresses.

PLANNING

Planning in the widest sense of the word is an essential
component of a healthy, relatively stress-free life, *and* it is a learnt
skill. We take planning into all areas of our life, both at home and
at school or work. If we don't plan, if we leave things to chance or,
worse, fate then we are vulnerable to life living us not the other
way round.

Decide what really matters and how flexible you are prepared to
be. Look at the larger picture, at your life plan, as well as the day-to-
day pictures. Are you happy with the quality of your life? Do you
need to reassess where you are going and what you are doing? The
stress of being in an unsatisfying job or a deteriorating relationship
can be huge.

But before you make any plans, be realistic about your priorities
and goals. Realistic expectations are a vital component of successful
planning. Having realistic expectations of both yourself *and* others
will greatly reduce your stress levels.

Establish a hierarchy of tasks on a daily basis (as well as with
your longer term goals) and be realistic about how long each task is
going to take. Overestimate if you know that things always take
longer than you think they will (and vice versa). Ask yourself
whether housework is really more important than taking your best
friend's baby swimming or having an early night.

Plan your life at work separately to your life at home but make
sure that you take both parts into account when doing so. Plan your
time off, whether it comes in tiny parcels at the end of a long and
exhausting week, or whether you have suddenly been given a huge
wodge of it by retiring. In an increasingly busy world many people
are finding that if they don't plan carefully then those who shout
loudest get the most attention, or more unimportant areas (like the
kitchen floor) get more attention than they deserve, or worse, that
valuable time just gets frittered away and nothing that you wanted
to do gets done.

Putting things off is stressful. Planning will help you prioritize
the important things in your life so that you don't fill your time with
trivia. Completing important tasks is part of what nourishes our

self-esteem and energizes us. Having them lurking can eat away at our self-confidence.

You might consider blocking out chunks of time to complete certain tasks, making sure that nothing interrupts you. Reading a bedtime story to a child can be a great pleasure for both the reader and the child. The interruptions of other members of the family, the telephone, the doorbell call all erode that pleasure, that special time. You might decide not to respond to demands – to the telephone (they can ring back if it is important), to the door (they can leave a note or call back), to anyone else (they can wait!).

Planning time to yourself may be the most difficult task if you live with others. Some people get up earlier to 'potter' and give themselves the luxury of a long bath or a cup of tea and a read of the paper. Conversely, if you live alone you will need to work harder to find time to spend with friends. If you are in a relationship you may need to plan to spend time together if you are both busy working and have a family to raise in addition. And so on.

Of course, we should never be too rigid. There are times when the best-laid plans etc., and other times when to plan ahead feels boring or stupid. We all have moments when we want to go with the flow, forget our plans and just have an adventure – be spontaneous for a change!

GETTING HELP

Remind yourself that others usually feel honoured to be asked for help. If you are struggling with a stressful situation and feel stuck, then swallow your pride, break out of a life-time's bad habit, especially if you are someone who soldiers on until they collapse, and ask for help.

Friends or relatives can be a rich source of support *because* they know you well. However, for that reason you may not want to talk to them. It is sometimes easier to confide in a stranger, or relative stranger, such as a health-care professional. A careers counsellor can help with work problems, a marriage guidance counsellor with relationships, a family therapist with family problems, an accountant with finances. A stress management consultant is trained to help with problem-solving at work. Remember, it's a sign of strength and not a sign of weakness to ask for help. You can get help from others by learning new skills; by looking at your weak areas and planning strategies for working with them.

A personal recommendation is the best way to find a therapist, but if this isn't available ask for a referral from your doctor. The organizations that represent the different therapies will be able to recommend registered practitioners in your area. It is a good idea to check the following: their training and background; their professional affiliation; how long they have been in practice; whether they are supervised; how often you would have to visit and for how long. Different therapists have different styles of working (including doctors) and you have every right to ask your health care professionals how they work.

After your first visit to any practitioner it is important to follow your instincts about whether to continue. You need to feel accepted, respected, cared-for and listened to. You need a therapist who is not over-concerned, patronizing or dismissive. In other words, you need to feel confident that this person can help you and that he or she is competent in their field.

If you are very stressed you won't necessarily feel good after your first visit, but you *must* feel good about the therapist and their integrity. For a psychotherapist or counsellor to help, it is sometimes necessary to evaluate or re-evaluate old hurts by examining them. This is an important part of the healing process. You may discover that your present stress is only the tip of an iceberg and that you are carrying around unexpressed hurts and emotional stresses from your past.

LEARNING FROM EXPERIENCE

Whether you are overstressed or understressed, do make a note of the ways in which you *are* coping; on a day-to-day basis your achievements, however apparently small or insignificant, do count. Make lists to help you gain a sense of achievement. Cross every task off your list with a flourish and allow yourself to feel pleased with what you have accomplished. Even if you have lots more to do.

Keep a note of what works to cement your success and create a positive feedback loop. Make a resolution to learn from your experience, to use mistakes and difficulties, stressful situations and opportunities to learn something about yourself – and others. To become more skilled at dealing with stress.

UNDERSTANDING
AND USING
HOMEOPATHY

What is Homeopathy?

THE HISTORY

Homeopathy is an increasingly popular alternative system of medicine whose basic philosophy has attracted much scepticism from the orthodox medical profession because it has been difficult to prove 'scientifically'. But its success with patients has meant that it has continued to grow and develop over the past two hundred years and has enjoyed a resurgence over the past ten years mainly owing to an increasing sense of disillusionment with the side effects of modern medicines.

It is based on the principle or law of similars, or *similia similibus curentur* which means 'let like be cured with like'. In other words, any substance that makes you ill can also cure you: anything that can produce symptoms of disease in a healthy person can cure a sick person with similar symptoms.

It was a German doctor by the name of Samuel Hahnemann who discovered this basic principle in an experiment he conducted on himself, in an attempt to understand *how* some medicines worked. He had, in fact, given up his practice because he was dissatisfied with the cruel and ineffective treatments of his time – leeches, blood-letting and the administration of medicines whose side effects were so often far worse than the disease itself.

He made a meagre living translating medical texts and it was through translating a text on the treatment of quinine for malaria that he began to question the basis on which these treatments had been prescribed. He took some *Cinchona* bark from which quinine was, and still is, derived in order to find out how it would affect a healthy person. After a number of days he started to experience the symptoms of malaria, which cleared up once he stopped taking the medicine. When he tried this out on others (his family and friends!) he had similar results, which led him to experiment with many other substances to find out what particular symptoms of illness they could produce in healthy individuals. He called these tests 'provings' and took meticulous notes of how each person reacted to each substance, noting in particular the common themes or patterns of illness that each substance produced. He then confirmed this theory in practice by giving the same substance to a sick patient with similar symptoms or symptom patterns, and seeing it act curatively.

Hippocrates in the fifth century BC and country people throughout the world had understood and used this principle of healing with 'similars', but it wasn't until Hahnemann stumbled on it that it was developed further. The standard medical assumption had always been that if the body produced a symptom, the appropriate treatment would be an antidote, an opposite medicine to that symptom. For example, constipation is treated with laxatives, which produce diarrhoea. Hahnemann's provings formed the basis of a new system of healing which he called homeopathy, from the Greek *homoios* (similar) and *pathos* (suffering or disease), in order to differentiate it from orthodox medicine, which he called 'allopathy', meaning 'opposite suffering'.

Hahnemann set up in practice again, this time using the symptom pictures from the provings as the basis for his prescriptions. He gave a single medicine at a time as opposed to the medical practice of asking the apothecaries to mix many medicines in one prescription. His departure from the 'accepted' medical practice of his time attracted much derision, especially from the apothecaries, but his success with his patients verified his theory and he carried on developing his system.

He experimented with diluting his medicines to minimize side effects but found that simple dilution (with stirring) caused the medicine to lose its efficacy altogether so he developed a new method of dilution whereby he diluted the substance in carefully measured steps, shaking it vigorously in between each dilution. This shaking he called 'succussion' and the resultant liquid a 'potentized remedy'. He found that this new remedy lacked side effects and had a stronger curative reaction. In fact, he found that the more he diluted and succussed it the stronger it became.

This process of dilution incurred further derision from the medical establishment, who could not explain, and therefore could not accept, how anything so dilute could have any effect. Despite opposition, homeopathy survived and spread quickly because it was remarkably effective.

The results spoke for themselves and many doctors trained under Hahnemann and then took his teachings out into the world: to South and North America, to India and to Europe, where homeopathy is still growing in popularity today.

Homeopathy has been compared to vaccination but they both have very different practices. Vaccines stimulate the immune system directly to produce specific antibodies *as if* that person had contracted a particular disease; in so doing they stress the immune system. They are tested on animals and then on humans to verify their safety, and even then children and adults can suffer serious side effects. Most vaccinations are introduced directly into the bloodstream, thereby bypassing the body's natural defence system and stressing it in a way that is not fully understood. Homeopathic medicines are administered orally in a safe, diluted dose; they are tested on healthy humans (not on animals) and when used correctly do not have side effects. They work on an individual's energy patterns, by stimulating the immune system generally.

THE PRINCIPLES

The principles of homeopathy are crucial to successful prescribing, and that includes successful home prescribing. They are as follows:

● **Simillimum**
The remedy is most similar to that which has caused similar symptoms in a healthy person.

● **Single remedy**
Remedies are tested (proven) one at a time and likewise prescribed on an individual basis.

● **Minimum dose**
Dilution with succussion releases the strength or 'potency' of any substance and makes it a more effective medicine whilst eliminating potential side effects.

● **Whole person**

The homeopath takes the emotional as well as the physical and the general symptoms into account when prescribing. Treating a part of the body without reference to the whole person is always going to be a hit-or-miss affair as far as holistic medicine is concerned.

THE REMEDIES

Homeopathic medicines are made from a wide variety of substances, from the plant world as well as from metals, minerals, poisons and acids. Because a homeopathic remedy is diluted beyond the point where there is anything measurable of the original substance – at a molecular level – absolutely anything can be used. The more noxious the original substance, the more power it may have to heal deep-seated diseases.

There are two scales for diluting substances: the decimal and the centesimal. The starting remedy – a 'tincture' or 'mother tincture' – is made by steeping soluble substances in alcohol and then straining them.

For the decimal scale, one-tenth of the tincture is added to nine-tenths alcohol and shaken vigorously; this first dilution is called a 1X. The number of a homeopathic remedy reflects the number of times it has been diluted and succussed: for example, *Sulphur* 6X has been diluted and succussed six times.

The centesimal scale is diluted using one part in a hundred of the tincture (as opposed to ten) and the letter C is added after the number (although in practice the C is often omitted). Paradoxically, a 6X is called a low potency and 200 (C) a high potency – the greater the dilution, the greater the potency, the stronger the medicine.

Homeopathy has been difficult to understand within established scientific frameworks, mainly because of this dilution process, and because of that has been labelled mysterious and unscientific. Critics maintain that it is little more than faith healing, that you have to believe in it for it to work, but homeopathic medicines are particularly effective on babies and animals, neither of whom are susceptible to the placebo effect. Research trials have shown over and over again that homeopathy *does* work, but there is a stumbling block for the scientifically trained mind with coming to terms with the fact that a medicine can be effective at a 'sub-molecular' level, i.e. where there are no molecules (measurable) of the original substance.

Many recent research trials using plants, animals and humans as controls have repeatedly proven the effectiveness of homeopathic medicines. Homeopathic medicines are prepared in a pharmacy or a laboratory, involving a technique subject to precise and clearly stated controls. Preparation does not involve mysterious and secret processes!

The most commonly used potency in the decimal scale is the 6X, although the 9X, 12X, 24X and 30X are used by some. In the centesimal scale those low potencies most commonly used are the 6, 12 and 30. The higher potencies – 200, 1M (diluted one thousand times), 10M (ten thousand times) and CM (one hundred thousand times) – are not for home use.

THE CONSTITUTION

Some people drink, smoke and work too much and don't eat or sleep enough – and never get ill. Others need to be careful about drinking any alcohol, need ten hours sleep a night and regular meals and still find themselves battling with poor health. Why? The answer lies in the constitution. The first person has a strong constitution, but may well be wasting his 'inheritance', because there *will* come a time when even they will get sick. A strong constitution can withstand considerable pressure before falling ill; a weak constitution is more susceptible to illness.

Susceptibility is simply the degree to which a person is vulnerable to an outside influence. Not everyone who goes for a walk in a cold wind will be affected, but those who are we call 'susceptible'. Their predisposition is due to an underlying constitutional weakness, which is either inherited or due to past and/or current stress (mental, emotional or physical).

If your grandparents all died of old age and your parents have been healthy all their lives, if your birth was planned and your mother was healthy throughout her pregnancy, if your parents' marriage is happy and your birth was uneventful, then your constitution should be of the strongest.

If, on the other hand, all your grandparents died at early ages of cancer or heart disease, one of your parents had tuberculosis as a child and the other suffered from asthma and eczema, then your chances of inheriting a weak constitution are greater. You can still escape the worst of a poor inheritance if your parents' marriage is happy, if they have taken care of their own health and brought you up with plenty of love and a good diet.

And that is where alternative medicine comes in. Many people come to a homeopath for 'constitutional treatment', to improve their general health rather than wait until they fall ill. The value of constitutional treatment is that it boosts the weak constitution and decreases its susceptibility to disease, by treating the whole person on a physical, mental and emotional level.

Illness does not exist in isolation, but is a reflection of how the whole person is coping with stress. Homeopaths look beyond the label of the disease (for example, 'tonsillitis', 'migraines' or 'food poisoning') to the whole person, including the stress or stresses that preceded the development of the symptoms. Each prescription is individualized to fit the whole person picture. Constitutional treatment strengthens the body's vitality and its ability to respond to stress without recourse to other medicines.

As far as home prescribing is concerned, you can prescribe on a single stress symptom such as head injury or complaints that start after being out in the cold wind, but the more symptoms you can build in that 'fit' the whole remedy picture, the more sure you can be that it will work well.

THE VITAL FORCE

Homeopaths believe that a balancing mechanism keeps us in health, provided that the stresses on our constitution are neither too prolonged nor too great. Hahnemann called it the 'vital force' and he believed it to be that energetic substance, independent of physical and chemical forces, that gives us life and is absent at our death.

The human organism, indeed any living thing, has a unique

relationship with its environment, which biologists refer to as 'homeostasis'. This means that a healthy living being is self-regulating, with an innate (protective) tendency to maintain its equilibrium and compensate for disruptive changes. Homeopaths believe that the vital force produces symptoms to counteract stresses and makes adjustments, moment by moment throughout our lives, to keep us healthy and balanced. These symptoms, then, are simply the body's way of telling us how it is coping with stress. Obvious examples are shivering when cold, perspiring when overheated and eating or drinking when hungry or thirsty, reactions which help to ensure the regulation of a constant, life-preserving environment within the body.

Homeopathic medicines act as a catalyst, stimulating the inner healer. They do not weaken the defence mechanism by suppressing it as do many orthodox medicines. The correct homeopathic treatment not only alleviates the symptoms but enables the patient to feel that life is once again flowing harmoniously.

You can't 'poison' yourself with a homeopathic medicine (because the dose is entirely non-toxic), but you can take it for too long and conduct an unintentional proving with either getting symptoms you never had before, or experiencing an aggravation of your current complaint that gets worse and worse (see page 26). Also, if you take one remedy after another that helps one symptom after another, without taking the whole person into account, you can end up confusing your 'symptom picture' and make it difficult to find the *simillimum*.

LAWS OF CURE AND SUPPRESSION

The Laws of Cure state that with successful homeopathic treatment symptoms move from within to without (from the innermost organs of the body, for example the heart, to the more superficial, such as the bowels or even the skin), and will also disappear from above to below, moving down the body.

If a disease or symptom of disease clears up but another develops which is more deep-seated or serious, this is known as suppression. For example, many children whose eczema has been 'successfully' treated with steroids may suffer from asthma at a later date. These two events are seen by the orthodox medical profession as having only a casual connection, whereas the homeopath believes that the suppression of the eczema ('pushing the disease' into the body) has caused the asthma. Successful homeopathic treatment involves the eczema reappearing at some point because the Laws of Cure also state that symptoms that have been formerly suppressed will recur in the reverse order from whence they came. It is also possible to suppress with homeopathic medicines – especially by treating a single symptom that doesn't take the whole person into account.

Homeopaths use the Laws of Cure to make sure that treatment is going in the 'right' direction. As far as home prescribing is concerned, occasionally a well-selected remedy will push to the surface an old symptom that may have been forgotten. This is a good thing and it will clear up without further treatment. It is important not to take another remedy, and by so doing suppress that symptom again.

Prescribing

If you fall ill and wish to prescribe for yourself (after consulting with a medical professional) do bear in mind that it may be difficult to be objective about your own symptoms, especially if you are feeling emotionally stressed. For example, you may feel low and depressed while those around you have experienced you as irritable and touchy; or you may already have forgotten the drenching you had the day before you fell ill. It can be useful to talk through your symptoms with someone close to you before you self-prescribe. Some people are competent at knowing exactly what is wrong and are clear about the stresses that led up to their feeling unwell; others need more help.

Never rush into recommending homeopathic remedies for someone else. It's all too easy to enthusiastically suggest a homeopathic solution to all your friends, once you have found it to work for you. Over-zealousness can be off-putting; you may want to offer to help but don't be fooled into thinking that you can cure anybody and everybody of their complaints, or impinge on other people's right to look after their own health in their own way.

Equally, don't think that you have to recommend a remedy just because you have the book and someone wants you to. If you don't feel right about recommending a remedy for someone you don't know very well, or are unsure about what remedy to suggest, then don't do it. Suggest that they go to a professional homeopath or to their GP.

It is essential that you write down your symptoms, and that you record the remedy with notes to explain your reasons for taking it, as well as its result. Even if you write only a few key words plus the date, name and potency of the remedy, that will remind you should the same problem recur. If you decide to do nothing and your body heals itself then make sure you write that down too. I suggest you open a loose-leaf file marked 'Health' and use it for keeping interesting articles as well as notes on your home prescribing.

Although it is hard to imagine, it is the easiest thing in the world to forget the one brilliant remedy you took after, say, a dental trauma, and here you are a year later, with a similar situation to prescribe for and you can't remember what you took the last time.

If you are interested in learning more about homeopathy then consider enrolling for a short homeopathic first-aid course. Many adult education colleges run courses and most homeopathic practitioners also run their own on a private basis. Do also consider taking a first-aid course with the St John Ambulance Brigade or the Red Cross to learn the mechanics of first-aid.

CHOOSING A REMEDY

Having identified your stress (emotional or physical), and read through the relevant section, look at the remedies that are listed at the end of that section. Check out those that fit particularly well by looking up any that have expanded pictures in the Remedies Chapter (see pages 255–354). You can use the indexes on pages 359–74 as a short cut at any time.

You may find yourself vascillating between two remedies (or more). The art of homeopathy resides in this place where we choose the remedy. Prescribing for yourself can have mixed results as it is mostly quite difficult to be objective about one's own symptoms, especially the emotional symptoms. You may find it helpful to ask a friend to help you in this process, and they may have noticed things (about yourself) that you had missed or discounted.

The remedy that is most likely to help is the one that most closely matches your symptoms. For a homeopathic remedy to work well, you need at least two of the following: a clear stress symptom, a strong emotional symptom, a general symptom and a physical symptom. The more symptoms you have the more confident you can be in your choice of remedy.

The case histories on pages 47–71 will help you to understand better this process of remedy selection, and of course, your own experience will enable you to understand the remedies and what they can do for you. Once you have used them successfully they become like old friends – ones that are hard to forget!

Some stresses, some effects and therefore some remedies will be straightforward – and others more complicated. For example, shock after surgery, or diarrhoea as a result of food poisoning have relatively few remedies and choosing between them will be quite a simple matter. But if you have experienced the loss of someone close to you, then you will need to think carefully about how that stress affected you, and then choose a remedy that reflects both the stress and your response. This can involve a more creative process than the mechanical matching of remedies with symptoms.

It is really important that you keep notes: of how you feel (emotionally); of your physical symptoms; and that you record the remedy you take as well as the result. Even if you write only a few words about your symptoms, the date (and year!), the name and the potency of the remedy. This will suffice to remind you should a similar problem recur.

If you cannot find a remedy to match your picture then look at related stresses as this can open the door to other remedy possibilities. If you still cannot work out what to take and especially if your stresses are chronic and long term, or if you have taken a remedy that hasn't helped, then you will need to consult a homeopath who has a larger choice of remedies, and the skills to choose between them.

THE REMEDIES

Homeopathic remedies are most commonly available as tablets made of sugar of cow's milk, or *Saccharum lactose*, commonly known as *sac lac*; this has been found to be an ideal medium for the potentized remedy. *Sac lac* comes in several forms: hard or soft tablets, globules or powders. Most homeopathic pharmacies will automatically make up remedies in the form of hard *sac lac* tablets unless they are specifically asked otherwise.

Listed below are the different forms a homeopathic remedy can take. In each case a few drops of the potentized homeopathic medicine in alcohol are used to medicate the base substance.

Soft tablets (*sac lac*) dissolve quickly and easily under the tongue. These are also easily administered to babies, by holding a tablet against the inner cheek until it dissolves, or crushing one between two spoons (see p. 36).

Hard tablets (*sac lac*) do not dissolve as easily as the soft tablets. They should be chewed and held in the mouth for a few seconds before being swallowed. They can also be crushed and given as a powder.

Globules (*sac lac*) are tiny round pills, like poppy seeds. A few grains should be dissolved on the tongue and not a lidful as is sometimes suggested.

Sucrose (*plain sugar*) is sometimes used, especially for pocket travel kits. A few grains should be dissolved on the tongue. They can (like the globules) be tipped onto the palm of the person taking the remedy, or straight on or under the tongue.

Liquid potencies. Homeopathic remedies can be made up in liquid form for children or adults known to be allergic to cow's milk. The remedy is added to an alcohol base, supplied in dropper bottles; the dose is either administered neat on the tongue or diluted in water for babies and children, in which case five drops should be added to a little water and if possible held in the mouth for a second or two before being swallowed.

Powders (*sac lac*). Most pharmacies will make up remedies in powder form. These are wrapped individually in small squares of paper and are convenient if you need only a few doses of an unusual remedy that you are unlikely to want again, or if you need to send small quantities by mail, especially abroad. They should be dissolved on or under the tongue like soft tablets or added to a small amount of water and held in the mouth for a few seconds before swallowing.

Wafers. Selected pharmacies can provide remedies as wafers, which, like powders, are wrapped individually. The wafers are made of rice paper, which are useful for people sensitive to milk *and* sugar.

Homeopathic remedies will keep their strength for years without deteriorating: remedies made over a hundred years ago still work well. They should be stored in a cool, dark, dry place with their container tops screwed on tightly, well away from strong-smelling substances: strong smells cause them to lose their potency. Don't keep them in the bathroom cabinet alongside perfumes and cough mixtures, or in a spare-room cupboard with mothballs. A sealed plastic container like an ice cream tub is good for storing loose bottles or you may choose to purchase one of the ready-made homeopathic kits available from many pharmacies, which can be adapted to your own specifications if you wish.

It is wise to keep all tablets out of the reach of children as a matter of course. If your child eats your entire first-aid kit in one glorious secret feast, don't panic. Your bank balance is the only thing that will suffer! A single dose at a time is a single dose, whether it is one tablet or one bottle of tablets. If your child eats a full bottle of, say, *Chamomilla 6* (or even *Chamomilla 30*) it will have roughly the same effect as taking one tablet.

HOW TO TAKE REMEDIES

Carefully tip a tablet into the lid of the bottle. If more than one falls out, tip the others back so that only one remains. Tip it on to the palm of the person taking the remedy and then replace the lid on the bottle. You can touch your own tablets, but if you are giving the remedy to someone else try to avoid touching it, although in practice this is difficult when giving remedies to babies, and tablets touched by their mothers or their homeopaths still work well!

Never put back tablets that have fallen out onto the floor or anywhere else, or that you have given out and are unused. In so doing you may contaminate your stock. Always throw them away.

It is preferable not to eat, drink (except water), smoke or brush your teeth for ten to twenty minutes before and after taking a remedy as this gives it the best possible chance of working, although in practice remedies given to toddlers who eat before and after still work well. The ten-minute gap makes sure that residues of food do not affect the action of the remedy.

Many homeopathic remedies available in the chemist or wholefood shop give dosage instructions on the bottle, suggesting different doses for adults (two tablets) and children (one tablet). This is questionable given the dilution process which means that the minute quantities make the size of the dose more or less irrelevant. I suggest that you take one tablet at a time, whatever your age!

Tablets for babies can be crushed between two spoons and the powder tipped dry on to the tongue. This avoids the danger of choking on a hard tablet and a powder is also hard to spit out, unlike a tablet. A little water can be added to the crushed powder on the spoon, or the tablet can be dissolved in a clean glass with a little water. Stir it vigorously and then give as needed, a teaspoonful at a time. Scour the glass and the spoon (with boiled water) after use so that the next person to use them doesn't get an inadvertent dose of the remedy.

THE POTENCY

Homeopathic remedies come in different potencies. The 6X, 6C, 12C and 30C are all safe for home prescribing. The 6X and the 6C are the most widely available and are the best potencies to use for minor complaints; 12C is slightly stronger than 6C, and 30C is stronger still, so fewer doses are needed. These higher potencies tend to work faster and are useful for more serious complaints, such as bad burns or head injuries with concussion. If you are ordering a remedy from a pharmacy I suggest you order it in the 6C or 12C potency to start with. As you gain experience in prescribing, you'll begin to know when one of the other potencies is more appropriate. At the end of the day, however, it is the remedy that counts more than the potency. The correct remedy will work in any potency.

HOW MANY DOSES AND HOW OFTEN

• **Prescribe according to the urgency of the case.**
Having selected the remedy, you will need to decide on the dose. This depends on the urgency of the case: frequent doses for acute stress that is recent and less frequent doses for on-going stress or past stress. The dosage chart (p. 44) will help you to decide how often to take your remedy.

- **Take the remedy less often (increase the gaps between doses) once it starts to work.**
Once you see that a remedy has started to work – when you notice a definite reaction or change or improvement – you can continue with the same remedy but take it less often, i.e. increase the gaps between the doses.

- **Stop on marked improvement.**
Once there is *marked* improvement – a strong positive reaction – it is essential to stop the remedy. This is the opposite of the instructions you receive when taking orthodox medicines (for example, anti-biotics), where it is necessary to finish the whole course of tablets. A homeopathic remedy acts as a trigger, a catalyst: it stimulates the body to begin to heal itself, and once that has happened the body's own healing process will take over. In some cases, taking another tablet after this reaction has occurred can stop the remedy working, and if too many are taken it is possible to start proving the remedy with your symptoms becoming more severe. You may even develop symptoms that you didn't have before. If this happens discontinue the remedy and your symptoms will clear up.
It's rather like a pebble which creates healing ripples when thrown into your pond. You need to get the pebble as close to the middle of the pond as possible, so that the ripples reach right out to every part of you. Remedies that don't fit can miss the pond altogether or just ripple out from the shallows, thereby helping with only some of your symptoms. If you feel much better *in yourself* you will, in most instances, get better even if your physical symptoms remain the same for a while or get slightly and temporarily worse.

- **Stop if you feel markedly worse. It may be part of a natural cleansing process.**
If symptoms have been suppressed (physical or emotional) then as the body heals itself with the aid of a homeopathic remedy, those feelings or physical symptoms can surface temporarily. Go with the flow – your body may need to have a good clear out, especially if you have been coping remarkably well with a lot of emotional or physical stress.

You may simply feel more tired than normal. This can happen as your body focuses all its energy on healing, especially if you need a good rest because you are over-tired. It is wise to sleep and rest as much as possible to work with this healing response and you should find your energy returning quite quickly.

If it is grief that has been the stress and tears that have been suppressed, and *Ignatia* the remedy that is indicated, then after taking it those tears may be closer to the surface and easier to express. It is important that these feelings aren't stuffed back inside again. There are many ways to express feelings without humiliating yourself in public – the general dos and don'ts for dealing with emotional stress as well as the specific ones will give you a few ideas to choose from if you get stuck.

Sometimes there is a more general cleaning out, or 'healing crisis' as it is often called, in the form of a cold or diarrhoea. Take it easy for a day or two; it should clear of its own accord and if it does it means that the remedy is working. If your symptoms are severe or if they persist then they may have nothing to do with the homeopathic remedy and you will need to seek expert advice.

Sometimes old physical symptoms recur that haven't been seen in a while. A well-selected remedy will occasionally push to the surface a complaint that has been suppressed in the past with, say, antibiotics. If you take a remedy for a particular stress and then feel worse initially, always ask yourself whether you have had this complaint before. This doesn't often happen with home prescribing but if it does the complaint will clear of its own accord, usually within a few days. Don't take another remedy at this point for the physical symptoms as this may suppress them again.

• **Repeat as needed, i.e. start again if the same symptoms return.** If your symptoms improve for a while and then relapse, a repeat dose of the same remedy may be necessary – but *only* on the return of the same symptoms. If your whole picture changes, then it is likely that you will need a different remedy. If your symptoms keep returning and only clear up while you are taking the remedy (and for a short time after) then it is simply alleviating your symptoms and you will need to find another remedy or seek the advice of a homeopath who can prescribe more accurately.

- **Repeat the remedy if you inadvertently antidote it.**
Any strong-smelling or strong-acting substance can affect the action of a homeopathic remedy. If you took a remedy that helped and then it stopped working, ask yourself if anything has counteracted (or antidoted) its effect. Some people have found that a spicy curry can have an adverse effect, as might a night of heavy drinking, but this is generally only true if the curry or the alcohol themselves had a stressful effect on your body, causing, for example, diarrhoea or a hangover.

Similarly, an unexpected emotional stress can cause a relapse. You may then have to decide whether to take a different remedy for the latest stress or repeat the last remedy which worked well for you. As a rule of thumb it is best to consider repeating a remedy that worked really well *unless* you have a new and clear picture to prescribe on that takes your current stress into account.

The following all counteract the effects of a homeopathic remedy to some extent. They are not necessarily 'bad', but as the action of remedy can last for as little as a few days or as long as a few months, they may be strong enough to stop it working and should be avoided while it is being taken and for several weeks afterwards. Be creative about finding alternatives; your local wholefood shop will help you with herbal cough syrup, fennel or Calendula toothpaste and mouthwash, grain coffees and so on.

Camphor: in 'tiger balm', deep-heat ointments and many lip salves.

Caffeine: in coffee, strong tea, cola's and to a lesser extent chocolate (if you feel 'wired-up' with any of the above then avoid them altogether whilst under stress).

Menthol/eucalyptus: in cough mixtures, Karvol capsules, 'tiger balm', Fisherman's Friend, Vick, Olbas Oil, etc.

Peppermint: in regular toothpaste, mouthwash and strong peppermint sweets. Natural, fresh mint in cooking and the odd cup of peppermint tea are fine.

- **Reassess your choice of remedy if you have taken six doses and have had no response, or if the symptom picture changes.**
If you have taken about six doses and there has been no change

whatsoever, then you may have taken the wrong remedy. Stop and reassess your choice of remedy and only take a further six doses if you are sure it's the right one. If you are under continued stress you may need to take your remedy for up to a week for it to help. If you aren't sure, it may be better to try out some of the practical advice given for your particular stress or consult a professional homeopath.

Did you have to choose between two remedies or might you have missed the *real* stress? You may need to delve relentlessly at times in order to uncover the original stress (see Sample Cases pages 47–71).

- **Consult your homeopath, if you are receiving homeopathic treatment.**
The long term treatment of chronic complaints is complex and if you are under the care of a professional homeopath you can inadvertently upset your course of treatment by self-prescribing. Get in touch with your practitioner if you are considering taking a remedy.

- **Seek the advice of a medical professional if you are suffering from long term chronic health problems, if you don't identify with the remedies in this book or if your self-prescribing doesn't help.**
You will need to seek professional help if you are suffering from long term, serious chronic health problems such as arthritis, asthma, hayfever, cancer, heart disease, AIDS, eczema, psoriasis, epilepsy, constipation, stomach ulcers, irritable bowel syndrome, etc. These complaints are always beyond the scope of the home prescriber, although if you do fall into one of these categories you can still prescribe on recent (acute) stress, be it physical or emotional. You might also consider seeking homeopathic advice if you are nervous about the possibility of inherited stresses (such as cancer, tuberculosis or heart disease, etc.) on either side of your immediate family (i.e. parents or grandparents). We can inherit both

physical strengths and weaknesses from our parents and homeo-paths have a comprehensive theory around the treatment of inher-ited weaknesses, which we call miasms. We can identify which one (or ones) have been passed on from the types of illness that you are vulnerable to – physical and emotional.

You will need to seek professional advice if you don't identify with any of the remedies listed under the stress section that applies to you. The remedies listed in this book are those which are com-monly needed for everyday stresses; a homeopath has many, many more to choose from.

Don't suffer in silence, soldiering on and coping if stress is af-fecting your health and self-prescribing hasn't helped. If you are in any doubt over what to do about your health and how to deal with the stresses in your life then it is better to play it safe and get some reassurance, expert advice and treatment than hope that it will sort itself out given time.

Always seek professional help from your homeopath or GP if your symptoms recur or do not improve.

CAUSE FOR CONCERN

The following symptoms may indicate serious illness and signal that you should seek immediate professional help. If you are worried about the general state of health of either yourself or members of your family, get appropriate help. If the picture is very clear or you know from past experience that you or your 'patient' is not seriously ill, you will be able to give the remedy and wait for improvement. But especially in the case of sick babies

DOSAGE CHART

Degree of seriousness	Potency	Dosage
Very serious stress/symptoms Symptoms need immediate attention and/or are accompanied by great pain, e.g. earache, head or back injury, second- or third-degree burns, cystitis after severe shock, etc.	6C, 12C or 30C	one dose every 5–30 minutes
Serious stress/symptoms Symptoms need help within about 24 hours and are not necessarily accompanied by pain, e.g. a cough after getting chilled, food poisoning from bad meat.	6C or 12C	one dose every 1–2 hours
Less serious Symptoms can wait a day or two to be treated, e.g. teething, flu after change of season.	6C or 12C	one dose every 4–8 hours
Not serious (i.e. tonic or longer term treatment) Symptoms are usually mild and need to be taken over a longer period of time, e.g. exhaustion after finals, anaemia and exhaustion after an acute illness or a growth spurt.	6X or 6C	one dose 3 times daily for up to 10 days

and children, if they do not show rapid signs of improvement you should always call for help.

Seek help if there is:
Bleeding: unexplained, from any part of the body, including the
     skin
Breathing: rapid – over 50 breaths per minute at rest in children
          under two
     shallow or laboured
     difficulties – with or without wheezing
Chest pain: severe
Convulsions
Crying or moaning, which is high-pitched or unusual
Delirium
Eyes: unusually sensitive to bright lights
     sunken or glazed over
Fever: above 104°F/40°C
     high, with a slow pulse (normal adult pulse is about 90
          beats a minute and 120 in a child)
     persistent, lasting for longer than twenty-four hours in a
          baby
     with thirstlessness
Listlessness, drowsiness, unusual, severe
Mental confusion, uncharacteristic
Neck stiff, especially if accompanied by severe headache
Pain that is severe, especially if accompanied by one or more of
     the other symptoms in this section.
Pallor, unusual which doesn't change – especially if it is all over
     the body
Stools, pale – grey or almost white
Urination profuse, accompanied by a great thirst
Urine: dark and scanty/bloody (certain foods can change the
          colour of the urine – beetroot for example, can turn it red
          – and this is nothing to worry about)
     scanty or absent
Vomiting: unexpected, repeated, severe, with or without diarrhoea
          which comes on some time after the onset of a viral
          infection

    green fluid
Weakness, extreme
Yellowing of the skin or whites of the eyes

If your child seems ill, even if he or she does not have any easily identifiable symptoms, always trust your instincts and get help. The same applies to yourself or anyone in your care.

Sample Cases

The following cases are all real cases from my practice or from patients who have self-prescribed. The names and some of the details have been changed to preserve confidentiality where necessary.

1. A SHOCKED NEWBORN

Jenny rang me to tell me that she'd had a baby boy (Ewan) at home, just as she had wanted, with her family gathered around her. The birth had gone well, although the labour had been unexpectedly fast and both she and Ewan were a bit shell-shocked. I made a house visit and on holding her new baby was struck by how shocked he *looked*, how much fear there was in his eyes and how much tension there was in his little body. Jenny was taking *Arnica* for her bruised soreness but was concerned to help her baby get over the shock of arriving on planet earth so suddenly. I told her to give him *Aconite 30*, one dose every two hours for a day.

She rang me four days later to report that he was very distressed a lot of the time, crying angrily in the day, waking screaming at night and having a difficult time going back to sleep again. Her doctor and the midwife had confirmed that there was nothing wrong with his physical health. She said, 'This may seem silly, but I think he's having nightmares, I think he's still working through the birth trauma. Is that possible? Is there anything you can do?' She told me that he wanted to be carried a lot of the time. I knew then that the stress of the birth had affected him deeply and prescribed *Stramonium 30*, once again every two hours, stopping if there was a reaction.

She rang the next morning euphoric. He'd slept a lot the previous day after only two doses of *Stramonium* and had slept more peacefully in the night, waking without the terrible screaming, feeding easily and going back to sleep without having to be walked and rocked.

If *Stramonium* hadn't worked, I'd have assumed that our diagnosis of birth trauma was wrong and would have started to think through what else was going on with this little baby. Babies can't talk and this makes it difficult to find out what is actually wrong.

Maybe his head was big enough to have got 'squashed' during the birth. Did he need a dose of *Natrum sulphuricum* or a visit to a cranial osteopath? Maybe Jenny's milk was slow in coming in, and he was screaming because he was hungry. Did she need a visit from her midwife? Maybe there was some tension at home that was affecting him. Did Jenny and her partner need to talk things through with someone? Maybe one of the post-natal interventions had distressed him. Maybe he was suffering from colic, or had something more serious (but not immediately obvious) that needed investigating by a paediatrician.

With stressed-out babies, you can only go a step at a time, using their symptoms *and* your gut instincts to guide you.

2. A TEETHING BABY

Carole's baby, Ben, weighed nearly ten pounds at birth and then went on to gain weight at an almost alarming rate on breast milk alone! He had a large head and a long body. He was hungry for what seemed like most of the time and from three months was very grateful to have some fruit and vegetables, moving quickly on to yoghurt, cottage cheese and eggs. He loved all food, especially eggs! At three months he started teething and seemed to find this particularly stressful. Having previously slept well, he started waking four to eight times a night and was generally difficult to please (having been a contented little soul). He had one bright red cheek and was sweaty at night especially on his head.

Carole asked me whether she should give him *Chamomilla*. It seemed to fit from reading the picture in her homeopathic first aid book – he had a bright red cheek – but because he wasn't particularly angry she wanted to check with me first. I suggested that *Calcarea carbonica* was, in fact, a better fit (see page 277). Ben was a big baby – not fat, just juicily plump! I asked her about his feet and she admitted reluctanty that they were clammy and well, yes, they did smell! She described him as a cheerful, happy baby with a large, stubborn streak that had come out rather strongly since he'd started teething. The feet and the sweaty head at night, the love of eggs, the cheerfulness, stubbornness *and* teething confirmed my choice of remedy.

He had a few doses of *Calcarea carbonica 30* that day and slept well for about a week, then started to 'play up' again. Carole needed to give him a weekly dose of *his* teething remedy for about a month and he finally managed to push through his bottom two teeth. A few months later he started teething with his top teeth and needed the same treatment to help him through the physical stress. He has maintained this pattern through his teething years.

It is as if all his energy is going into building his body and his big bones and there's none left over for his teeth! Some babies find teething very stressful and need a lot of help in order to maintain their equilibrium. I dread to think where he (and his mum) would be now if they hadn't had some homeopathic help through this time!

3. A BAD FALL ON THE HEAD

Robin's nine-month-old baby, Alice, climbed onto the sofa in her first serious climbing expedition, and fell backwards, hitting the back of her head on a pile of wooden bricks. She was in great distress but the skin wasn't broken and Robin knew it wasn't a serious enough fall to warrant a visit to casualty/ER. An egg developed at the back of her head quickly so Robin gave her a dose of *Arnica* for the physical stress, knowing that the swelling would go down quite quickly. Alice stopped crying within a minute of taking the remedy and fell asleep.

Over the next week Robin suspected that Alice was teething because she was more bad-tempered than usual and woke frequently at night, screaming. She asked to be picked up but soon started screaming again as if she was in pain. Nothing comforted her for long. Robin began to feel exasperated – her happy, contented baby had turned into a 'ratbag' and the nights are now very difficult. She gave Alice *Chamomilla 6* four times daily for her teething but it didn't help at all. She was convinced that Alice was teething and that *Chamomilla* was the right remedy and so she gave her a few days of *Chamomilla 30* in the hope that a higher potency would work. It didn't.

Luckily she kept good notes so she got them out and gave me a ring. I asked her when, exactly, Alice started to become irritable. And Robin said immediately 'Oh my goodness!' She was able to pinpoint that her crying had started on the day she had her fall. So much was happening with her other children that she hadn't connected the two events. She remembered giving Alice the *Arnica*, her going to sleep and then her waking up and being out of sorts ever since. I knew that Robin's baby was in pain and I knew that she didn't have earache or a sore throat because Alice had taken her to the GP the day before just in case. And because *Chamomilla* hadn't worked I knew that it probably wasn't teething either. I was almost certain then that little Alice was suffering from a headache (caused by her fall) – a surprisingly common but difficult-to-diagnose symptom in infants who can't talk.

I told Robin to give Alice a single dose of *Natrum sulphuricum 30* and as it dissolved in her mouth she smiled angelically again, and that night she slept well for the first time in a week.

4. WINTER COUGHS AND COLDS

Sonia's son David (age seven) seemed to have a constant cough and cold every winter from about the age of three. She had tried eliminating cow's milk and all dairy products from his diet, but this hadn't helped at all. As a baby he had been healthy except for a bout of whooping cough when he was two years old. She couldn't understand why he was so poorly so much of the winter. It couldn't be school as he was fine during the summer.

Her doctor had said there was nothing much he could do, that there was no point in giving him antibiotics, because they wouldn't be of any help for a viral infection.

The next summer she decided to watch him very carefully as winter approached and try to pinpoint the time when his health started to go downhill, to see if there was a particular stress in his life that she'd missed. There was. October came and with it his usual cough and cold. The only difference in his life that week had been the weather. After a glorious Indian summer the weather had turned cold and wet and his nose had started to run more or less immediately.

˜ So now Sonia knew that the stress in David's life that was causing his catarrh and cough was the weather, specifically cold, wet weather. She poured over her homeopathic first-aid books to see if she could find a remedy that matched his symptoms – she had noticed that his glands were usually swollen when he had a cough, that he was generally sensitive to the cold and had always needed wrapping-up well, even as a baby. Several remedies were indicated for people who are stressed by cold, wet weather. She read through the pictures and immediately identified her own son when she got to *Silica*: generally, with the embarrassingly smelly, sweaty feet; emotionally, with being shy and sensitive, as well as physically with the lingering winter coughs and colds (see page 338).

She decided to give him a low potency (*Silica 6*) three times daily for up to a week, knowing that she could repeat it if she needed to. By day four his cough and runny nose had cleared.

Sonia rang me to ask whether she could keep *Silica* to hand in the winter and give it at the first sign of a cold rather than waiting for it to become chronic. I agreed that it would be a good idea, as long as it worked, as long as David only needed to take it occasionally. We talked about her seeking the advice of a professional homeopath who could prescribe on the underlying, inherited weaknesses if David needed more than the occasional course of this remedy.

5. SICK FROM A REPRIMAND

Nine-year-old Tamsin came home from school very upset one day. She burst into tears as she told her mother, Anne, how her teacher had shouted at her in front of the whole class. Something she'd never done before. Tamsin felt dreadful at having been told off, worse that the whole class had witnessed this indignity and worse still that some of the children had teased her afterwards, adding insult to injury. She didn't know whether to scream or cry and said she hated them all and never wanted to go back. Her mother tried to talk it through with her but Tamsin just stormed off saying that no one understood her.

She didn't want much supper, saying that she had a stomach ache and when Anne went in to check on her at 11 p.m. she found her still awake chewing over the whole experience and planning what she would have said and wishing she hadn't just stood there and pretended that she didn't care.

The next morning she woke with a raging sore throat. Anne knew why. She also suspected that antibiotics wouldn't help, would only supress what was an acute reaction to emotional stress and so she looked up Tamsin's symptoms in her homeopathic handbook. It was very clear that she needed an urgent dose of *Staphysagria*. Unfortunately her local wholefood shop didn't stock this particular remedy so she had to ask a homeopathic pharmacy to send her some which meant waiting for twenty-four hours.

Anne suggested that Tamsin write a letter to her teaching telling her how she felt, as well as what she thought of her. This she did willingly, writing three long, very angry pages. Anne had Tamsin gargle with salt water and drink lots of hot lemon and honey to soothe her throat but it was still very sore the next morning when the remedy arrived. She gave her one tablet every two hours and by the evening it was much better. Tamsin slept well and woke up more cheerful, and said that she wanted to go to school. She decided not to give her teacher the letter but did want her mother to write a note explaining about her absence. Anne suggested that it would be better to talk to her face to face and said that she would make an appointment to go and talk to her as soon as possible.

6. POST EXAM EXHAUSTION

Jake, aged 18, had a tough time in his final year at school. He'd decided to take four at once and had found it really hard work. During the year his dad had given him the odd course of *Kali phosphoricum 6* to help with tiredness when he'd been particularly low (see page 301) but that was nothing to how he felt now. He was absolutely shattered.

He gave himself a week to rest and eat well and thought he'd pick up quite quickly, but he didn't. He didn't even have the energy to go out and enjoy himself and after a week of feeling dreadful he asked his dad, Tony, if he had any magic pills that could maybe help. Tony sat him down and asked Jake to tell him what his symptoms were.

Jake said that the worst one was that he was suffering from twitchy legs which would start up any time he sat down, which made it impossible to relax. They were worse in bed at night, starting to twitch and jerk when he was dropping off to sleep, which would wake him up again and meant he wasn't getting the sleep he needed. He said he'd lost the ability to relax. He also had a bursting headache most of the time, as if his brain cells were worn out with the stress of studying, although this was better in the fresh air, and his eyes felt strained – sore and gritty.

Tony had noticed that Jake had been moodier than usual and had been particularly uncommunicative, worse than anything he'd pulled out of the adolescent hat so far.

He remembered reading about a homeopathic remedy for restless, twitchy legs in people who have been under a lot of mental strain and rifled through his books until he found it – *Zincum metallicum* (see page 352). Luckily he lived near a homeopathic pharmacy and nipped out for a bottle in the 30th potency. He told Jake to take one every two hours for the rest of the day and then twice daily for a day or two at the most.

The next day Jake felt much worse – he was more tired than he'd felt before – but his headache had gone and now he came to think about it, yes, his twitchy legs had finally relaxed. Tony realized that, in relaxing, Jake's body was feeling the build-up of tiredness from the previous months and all he needed now were a few long, uninterrupted sleeps. Within a couple of days Jake felt his energy – and his good moods – return.

7. A DIFFICULT ADOLESCENCE

Fourteen-year-old Gemma was having a hard time at school and at home. Her parents had separated when she was twelve and her father had moved away so she didn't see him as often as she would have liked to. Her mother (Maureen) had been preoccupied with her own sadness about her relationship ending and had been working harder than usual to pay the bills. As an only child, Gemma had felt increasingly lonely over these past two years. She came home to an empty house each day and would flop in front of the TV for an hour or two before tackling her homework.

At school she had been the brunt of some unkind teasing because her puberty was slow in coming – her breasts hadn't developed and her periods hadn't started. She still looked in many ways like a 'little girl'. The teasing made her want to cry and as she often couldn't hold her tears in, the other kids had even more ammunition with which to get at her. They called her 'cry baby' and ostracized her.

Because she didn't want to bother her mother with even more worries she didn't tell her what was going on at school, but one day Maureen came home unexpectedly early and found Gemma in floods of tears and so it all came out. Gemma was adamant that she didn't want her mother interfering at school so they talked about how Gemma was going to deal with the situation.

Maureen looked up the various stresses that Gemma was stockpiling – the grief, delayed puberty and the teasing – and found *Pulsatilla* listed under each one. A few doses helped to heal some of the raw emotional wounds and gave her some inner strength to fight her tormentors at school.

8. DRIVING TEST NERVES

Deborah, who was twenty-four, asked me if there was anything she could take for her sinusitis. She'd used a nasal decongestant which had worked whilst she was taking it, but since stopping it her sinuses were beginning to block up again. She also had some back pain. And a vaginal discharge. She'd looked up her physical symptoms in a homeopathic first aid book and couldn't find a remedy that matched them.

I asked whether she had had any particular stresses recently. She told me that she had a driving test coming up in one week's time, that it was interesting that I'd asked because she *was* incredibly anxious about passing and had been having anxiety nightmares for two weeks. I asked whether she suffered from exam nerves at school and she laughed and said she was frightful, always getting herself into an absolute lather of anxiety, suffering from acute lack of self-confidence, knowing she was going to fail and mostly doing rather well. She realized that her worries were irrational, that she was capable of passing, but couldn't help herself and was frightened that her nerves would cause her to make a silly mistake. Deborah confirmed that her physical symptoms had started once she'd started to get anxious about her driving test.

On looking up anticipatory anxiety and lack of self-confidence in the index, we found *Lycopodium* under each symptom (see page 305). She read through the remedy picture and grinned in self-recognition, confirming that she did indeed identify with the emotional state described.

I suggested she take *Lycopodium 6*, one tablet three times daily, leading up to her test, stopping if she felt better and then starting again if the anxiety came back. Her nightmares ceased immediately and she had more energy. Physically she felt better, and emotionally she was more confident and philosophical about the outcome of the driving test. On the day of her test she calmly and confidently passed.

N.B. A homeopathic medicine can't perform miracles. Deborah could only have passed her test if she had been fully prepared for it. The greatest difficulty with anticipatory anxiety is that it can prevent people from doing their best in certain situations like public speaking and exams. It is then that homeopathy is wonderful – in dealing with the emotional stress that can hamper their performance, it enables people to do their best.

9. A SUMMER COUGH

Peter rang to say that he'd had a bad summer cough and cold and wasn't managing to shake off the cough – in fact it seemed to be getting steadily worse. He hadn't taken anything homeopathic, thinking that it would just sort itself out given time. He had been taking it easy, although he hadn't actually taken any time off work.

The cold had been a pretty standard one – lots of sneezing and a runny nose. The cough was now worrying him because he felt he couldn't get enough air into his chest, especially when he was outside. He described it as 'a sort of choking'. He would cough up a bit of watery phlegm.

He lived on a main road, in a part of town that was very flat and built-up, and usually cycled into work. Since he'd had his cough he hadn't felt like cycling because he'd noticed that it often made the cough worse.

I asked Peter about the stresses in his life, and he said that there was nothing special going on. Work and home life were both fine, and he actually felt pretty good in himself. It seemed as if this cough and cold had come out of the blue. Then I remembered that the weather had been hot and close for at least a month, with no rain and very little wind, and that the newspapers had been full of warnings to asthmatics and people with chest problems to stay inside because the air pollution (from car exhausts) was consistently exceeding WHO safety levels. I mentioned this to him and he jumped on it immediately, saying that he had started with a little cough the first week of the hot weather. He admitted to not wearing a protective mask when cycling because he felt so silly.

I prescribed *Acid sulphurosum* 12 three times daily for up to two days and then to stop and start it as needed, i.e. to carry on taking it if it helped but only if and when the cough was bad. He rang back a week later to say that it had helped more or less immediately, that he'd only needed to take the first day's tablets and then one or two a day over the next few days.

I suggested that he think very seriously about cycling at all when the air was bad and that he wear his mask at all times when cycling around town, that it was better to look silly and be healthy – the stress of looking silly wasn't going to make him sick!

10. A NEAR DEATH EXPERIENCE

Frances never dreamed that her journey to work that fateful morning would change her life so drastically. She sat on the train in the rush hour, along with hundreds of other passengers, crammed into the carriages like so many sardines, reading her book and wishing she didn't live so far away from her work place so that she could just stroll around the corner to work and not waste two hours every day commuting.

Suddenly, there was a noise that she hopes she will never hear again. A terrible screeching and shrieking; the sound of metal smashing and tearing; then people screaming, louder and louder till the noise was right on top of her. Her carriage felt like it was thrown up in the air. Everyone rolled around like pieces of driftwood on a crashing wave. As the reality of the situation hit her, she realized that the train had de-railed and was colliding on the tracks and that she might be facing the end of her life. She thought of her family, her husband and her children in a rising tide of panic and at this point she simply blacked out.

When she came round there was an eerie silence, punctuated by the moans and cries of the injured. A terrible sight met her eyes: people were strewn in various stages of batteredness, some with limbs askew, obviously broken, with blood pouring from head injuries and clothing torn. The carriages were scattered up and down the train tracks. People soaked in blood were climbing out of them. Frances found that by some miracle she was relatively uninjured, just bruised and grazed. She clambered out of the carriage in a sort of daze and walked the length of the train to where firemen and police had already gathered and were attending to the wounded. Once it was established that she wasn't hurt she was taken to the nearest station and actually continued her journey to work, still in a daze. Her boss sent her home having called her husband first to pick her up.

By the time Frances got home she was in a frightful state. She cried uncontrollably on and off all evening and her husband called me to see if there was anything homeopathy had to offer. I asked him to tell me what had happened and what she was saying and doing. She kept repeating the words 'I could have died, it was so terrible.' And he said that every time she talked about the accident her eyes would fill with terror and she would start trembling and pace the room.

I told him to give her *Aconite* every ten minutes (luckily he had some in the 30th potency in the house) and to call me back in an hour (see page 255). He said that after the third dose she suddenly relaxed, stopped trembling and asked to go to bed. She slept well that night and needed to repeat the remedy on a daily basis for a week. In the case of terrible shock, when symptoms suggest what is now called post traumatic stress disorder, a homeopathic remedy can be repeated until the symptoms subside. Frances needed counselling to help her to deal with the feelings that surfaced after the shock abated, including a sense of guilt that she had been spared while others had died. At each stage that she wasn't able to heal and move on she used a homeopathic medicine to help her.

11. SICK OF THE DENTIST!

Martin rang me in a dreadful state. He had what sounded like a serious chest infection, had been in bed for three days with what felt like flu (aching and a high temperature), had a painful cough with green phlegm and was feeling acutely depressed and totally exhausted. He hadn't seen me for about six months because he had felt generally well. At the start of this 'flu' he'd taken several remedies, none of which had worked. He had no idea why he was ill. Although he'd been working incredibly hard he hadn't felt stressed by it, in fact, quite the reverse – work was exciting and stimulating and he couldn't wait to get back to the office!

I asked him to get his diary and go through everything he'd done in the week leading up to his falling ill. Actually it had been Christmas week and he'd had a really nice time with his family and a lovely rest. He'd been careful not to overeat or drink too much and was genuinely mystified as to why he was ill. And then he said 'Oh my goodness! I'd forgotten about that. I visited the dentist the Tuesday after Christmas to get it over with before I went back to work and he did a huge filling replacement.' Martin hadn't ever had a filling replaced that he could remember and apparently his dentist hadn't protected his mouth from the amalgam with a rubber dam (sheet). He said he remembered looking at the new filling afterwards in the mirror and being surprised at how black his tongue was but he hadn't scraped it clean.

So then I knew that he was suffering from mercury poisoning from the amalgam dust that he'd absorbed and checked his physical symptoms. Yes, he had a coated tongue which was indented around the edges with the imprints of his teeth, he was much thirstier than normal, sweaty with his fever and had smelly breath. I told him to take *Mercurius solubilis* 30 every two hours and to ring me the next morning. He said he could feel his vitality returning within an hour of taking the first dose, that the pain in his chest eased after a couple of hours, his fever came down by the evening and he'd slept really well for the first time in a week. His depression had lifted and he felt that all he needed to do was build his strength up with some good food and a little gentle exercise and he'd be fine within a day or two. I told him not to take any more *Mercurius* unless he needed to, i.e. unless the cough started to return or he started to feel weak and woolly.

I also suggested that he make sure his dentist protect his mouth for future fillings (whether they were replacement fillings or not), and that he have the *Mercurius* standing by just in case he needed it.

He rang me two weeks later to say that he'd been to the dentist for another filling and even though his mouth had been protected he felt awful afterwards. He'd taken *Mercurius* and it hadn't helped. This time he had a sore throat and he said, rather angrily, that he wished he hadn't gone to the dentist for a yearly check-up, that he was really beginning to resent the effect it was having on his life and health. On further questioning he told me that *this* time he'd had to have a really deep filling and the local anaesthetic hadn't worked fully. It had been very painful and in order to get it over and done with quickly, the dentist had worked 'hard and fast', which had meant that Martin had a lot of pain in his tooth and jaw afterwards. He said his whole mouth felt traumatized and his tooth was still sensitive, especially to cold drinks.

He talked about the dentist as 'that torturer' and said that he had been having angry conversations in his head with him, partly because he had a final appointment booked for the following week. He said those close to him were finding him difficult – touchy and irritable.

It is interesting that two separate visits to the dentist had produced such different results. One had been physically stressful with the mercury poisoning causing mainly physical symptoms, and the other had been more emotionally stressful with the effects more noticeable on the emotional body (rather than the physical). I suggested he take *Staphysagria 30* every 2–4 hours over the course of a day for the recent physical and emotional trauma (see page 341), and that he give dental treatment a rest for at least three months, unless he had something really urgent that needed attention. That he'd become vulnerable to 'dental' stress and needed to build up his reserves before he went back. He readily agreed!

12. AN OVERWHELMED MOTHER

I called on Susan to find her looking pretty exhausted. She was cooking her three older kids their evening meal with the three-month-old baby on her hip and said she hadn't sat down all day, except to breastfeed. Either the baby wanted carrying or she'd been running around after the other children and then she'd had to shop and cook and hoover/vacuum and attend to the fire *and* the nights had been terrible because it seemed as if the baby was teething already. Her husband was on shift work which had been a strain for the whole family. She had decided to start work six weeks ago which meant that she was spending her evenings at the computer once the children were in bed. It was suddenly all too much. 'But this is what I wanted so I have to put up with it. I mustn't complain.'

She coughed as she 'whizzed' around the kitchen. Her face was pale with deep, dark circles under her eyes. She snapped at the kids when they asked her for anything. She said her back hurt all the time with having to carry the baby (large at birth, he had carried on as he'd started out and put on masses of weight), and she also had a touch of cystitis.

I asked her whether she was getting enough rest. She snapped that she couldn't, she had too much to do, and anyway she was all right when she was rushing around, as long as she didn't stop.

I could see she badly needed a dose of *Sepia* (see page 334) and a good rest, otherwise she was going to suffer from more than a little cough and a touch of cystitis, so I simply offered her a remedy for her physical symptoms. She said she didn't want one and that she was fine.

A few days later she rang asking for help because she felt herself to be going down with 'flu, she was aching all over and feeling miserable. I gave her *Sepia 30* to take every two hours and by the next day she was feeling much better. Once she was feeling better she was able to talk about how she had barely done anything for herself since the baby had been born, about how all the different demands of babies and children and partner and house and work were beginning to get to her. She resolved to remedy that pretty quickly, as well as have some early nights to balance out the stress of broken sleep.

It's not uncommon for women with large families (more than one child!) to feel overwhelmed with the work-load, especially if they have to go back to work fairly soon after the birth and even more especially if they are single parenting. Susan needed the odd dose of *Sepia* while she was breast-feeding to help her through this emotionally and physically stressful time in her life.

13. A TERRIBLE SIGHT

Margaret decided to make a career change at the age of thirty-seven, a year after the death of her mother. She had spent the best part of her adult life working behind a desk and decided she wanted to go into the helping professions. She wished to be more useful, to do something that gave her a sense of purpose. She had cared for her mother until her death from cancer and, while she had found the final years tough, she had enjoyed the nursing part of caring for her, so she found it an obvious decision to train as a nurse.

She loved going back to college, liked studying again and quickly learnt the practical nursing skills. She enjoyed her new life with her fellow students, and made easy and welcome contact with patients who quickly learnt to appreciate her gentle ways. She passed her exams effortlessly and began her working life in the Casualty Department/ER.

Her first day was more than an education. The firemen brought in a family whose house had gone up in flames as they slept . . . a mother, father, two children and a baby. All, except for the baby, were very badly burned. The smell was terrible and the sight of their charred and disfigured bodies was more than Margaret could bear. Both the children died that night and Margaret went home feeling utterly devastated by what she had seen. She just could not get the images of those poor children out of her mind. She felt numb emotionally and knew from her training that she was suffering from shock. The firemen had all been upset as well, and had called several times for a progress report. She wondered how they managed to cope with such a terrible job.

Margaret couldn't sleep that morning and by the evening felt like she was treading in treacle. She felt completely spaced-out, nothing seemed real, and she was totally exhausted. She called one of her nursing friends who was taking a homeopathy course and asked whether there was anything that might help her. Her friend picked up the confusion and apathy in her voice and rushed around with some *Opium 30* (see page 321). She held Margaret's hand while she gave a dose every five minutes until some life came back into her eyes.

Margaret then called in sick for that evening's shift and went to bed for a long, healing sleep. It took her quite a while to get over the shock altogether, and her Staff Nurse referred her to the hospital counsellor to help her do so. But it was the homeopathic remedy that helped with the acute phase of the shock and which helped her return to work without feeling utterly discouraged about going on.

14. A TOUGH MENOPAUSE

Barbara had been incredibly healthy all her life, having the odd cold but rarely anything else. So it was with great surprise and distress that she started to feel ill in her mid-fifties, for what seemed like most of the time. Initially she didn't bother going to her GP because she kept thinking 'it' would go away. But it didn't and eventually she started putting two and two together and wondering whether she was sick. She had seen her doctor who had confirmed that she was menopausal. She rang to ask me what to do.

Her symptoms were quite severe and she was really desperate. She was suffering from hot flushes with sweating, both day and night, pain in her joints and general lethargy. She said she felt like an 'old crock', could barely get out of bed in the morning and was hobbling around in pain. Her libido had completely disappeared. She felt very low and depressed and just wanted to shut herself away, to be on her own. She said she didn't want to talk about what was going on because she didn't feel comfortable talking about her feelings and was finding her husband's attempts to be sympathetic really irritating.

I asked her about her menstrual cycle and she confirmed that it was all over the place and that her periods were heavier than normal. Her doctor had offered her HRT. All her friends were extolling the virtues of HRT, but since she had never taken medicines for anything, instinctively she felt that she didn't want to start now – if there was an alternative. I suggested that if she didn't want to go on HRT she should give homeopathy a chance, but that she needed to sign on with a local homeopath who would take her whole case history. She went to a colleague the following week who prescribed *Natrum muriaticum* and within a couple of weeks all of her symptoms had abated and within a month she felt back to her old (not so old!), healthy self. Over the following years Barbara needed to take *Natrum muriaticum* from time to time to help her hormones adjust to the stress of her menopause and is relieved that she didn't relent to the pressure to medicate herself needlessly with HRT.

15. A SAD ENDING

Andrew rang in distress. His wife had died a week previously after a prolonged and difficult illness. He was devastated by her death, even though he had been fully prepared for it, and was finding it hard to adjust to life without her. Was there anything I could do, homeopathically, to help him over the emotional stress?

I asked him to talk through what was happening in his life and he told me that his sons were staying with him for a couple of weeks and that they were all trying to put a brave face on it together, but that he wasn't managing terribly well. The funeral had been and gone and that had been very stressful, but mostly what he felt right now was terribly lonely and unbearably sad. He said he couldn't bear to go through his wife's things, even though he knew he had to.

Physically he was fine, eating well and sleeping at night, and so I made a few practical suggestions.

I validated his feelings and said that this was going to be a tough time and that he was doing really well. I asked whether his sons were struggling with *their* grief, and whether he was holding his back in order to protect them. He said that was exactly what was happening. So I told him to 'go for it' and 'let it all hang out'. That this was *his* time, and his feelings were more important now and that he needed to attend to them without worrying about how others could or couldn't cope.

I suggested that he make a time each day to go through his wife's effects and allow himself to really, really grieve as he did so. To allow memories to surface, to talk about them and to cry if that is what he felt like doing. And that when he had finished he could sit down and write her a letter. He cried as I made this last suggestion and I said that however painful it would be, it would open up a place for healing to come into his life and enable him to begin that process of letting go of the past in order to be able to move forward without carrying a great, big suitcase full of grief. He sighed a big, huge sigh and said that he knew he had to do this and would try. I said that I thought it would be better to wait for a few days to see if he really needed a remedy rather than prescribe now and risk suppressing what was really a healthy emotional response to a painful situation.

He rang a week later with relief and calm and a new strength in his voice. He said it had been hard, harder than nursing his wife in those last days, but he'd completed his tasks in his own way. He had sorted through her clothes and papers in one big, ten-hour session, rather than eking it out over days and laughed as he told me he'd used up an entire box of tissues in the process.

He said that the letter had been excruciating and he had put it off day after day but had finally sat down and written it, and was astounded by what poured out. He laughed and said it was the most cathartic thing he had ever done. He wrote sixteen pages – a love letter to his true love – and used up another box of tissues. He had made all sorts of important connections and been able to 'say' things that he hadn't done when she had been alive.

Although he still felt sad most of the time, he said he didn't feel consumed by grief now. His sons had watched him go through his emotional cleansing with a mixture of horror and envy and one of them had finally allowed himself to let some of his own grief out – encouraged by his father's example.

We both agreed that he didn't need a homeopathic remedy, that he was doing fine and that he would ring me if he got stuck. It is really important to acknowledge healthy grief, however painful it may seem, and to step in only if appropriate and absolutely necessary. If I had prescribed *Ignatia* when Andrew had first called, he may have felt soothed emotionally, but it may have been a suppressive prescription in that he might not have been motivated to go through *his* grieving process (see page 298). The problem then is that the grief goes in deeper and becomes more difficult to deal with and to heal – and, of course, more painful when it finally surfaces.

I do not believe people should suffer, especially if they are suffering needlessly, but there are times when we have to enter a dark place and deal with our most painful feelings, in order to come out into the light again.

16. BROKEN NIGHTS

Jan had to give up her job as a nursery school teacher (which she loved) five years ago in order to look after her elderly mother who had a stroke and was increasingly dependent, although looking like she might live for quite a few years to come. Jan was finding it difficult to sleep at night, was suffering from headaches and indigestion, felt tense and exhausted for what seemed like most of the time and completely lost her get up and go. She knew she was run down.

Jan's mother was a difficult patient, demanding and irritable and resentful that she had lost her independence, that she has to ask someone else for help with almost everything. Jan found herself seething with anger when her mother ordered her about, and had trouble keeping her own temper under control at times.

Her mother had been calling out in the night for help for weeks now, at least twice a night, wanting a drink or thinking it was morning and wanting her breakfast at 3 a.m. Jan looked up resentment and broken sleep in her homeopathy book and found *Nitric acid* (see page 314) under both stresses, but it didn't really fit.

She thumbed through the other emotional stresses, stopping at anger and then at bullying, and realized that it was the constant, imperative demands that were making her feel abused. She looked up bullying and loss of sleep and found *Nux vomica* under both, and when she read the picture, smiled with relief (see page 317). She knew she might need an awful lot to get her through the years ahead of her, so she started with the 6th potency.

17. A BLACK CLOUD

Nick was happily self-employed for about twenty years, running a café. He turned over enough money to pay his bills and support his family – and have a good holiday once a year. And then the recession hit and business started dropping off. The three factories near his café closed down, which meant he lost a lot of regular business. He advertised and tried to diversify but after two years of struggling, his accountant advised him to close down before he was forced to do so.

Over those years he'd found himself increasingly anxious and had slept badly – lying awake at night problem-solving and wondering what on earth he was going to do, how he was going to survive, feeling despondent and hopeless about becoming unemployed. His marriage suffered with lots of petty arguments, and he completely lost all interest in sex. Luckily his children had left home and were doing well.

The day he closed his café down was the worst day of his life. He felt a black cloud descend and walked home with a heavy heart. He'd never been able to understand why people would want to take their own lives, but he did now – he thought about suicide often. He had been to church that Sunday for the first time since getting married but it hadn't helped much. His future looked utterly bleak. He was fifty-three, had no saleable skills and no job. In a bad recession.

His wife brought home a book on homeopathy from the library with a glint in her eye, and excitedly showed him the chapter on failure and made him read through *Aurum metallicum* (see page 269). They both recognized him immediately. Nick didn't want to go to the doctor because he knew that he would probably be offered antidepressants and he knew they would only be an emotional sticky plaster/band aid at best. He wondered whether the same applied to homeopathic medicine. He sat down and read the introductory chapters and decided to give it a go.

He took *Aurum metallicum 30* twice daily for three days and, whilst they didn't solve his financial problems, they did help him emotionally and physically (with sleeping) and gave him the inner strength to deal with his stresses without them wrecking his health. He realized that by putting all his energy into his work he'd neglected other areas of his life, so he and his wife began to make plans for their future that took these into account.

18. RETIREMENT SLUMP

Stephen was worried about his seventy-six-year-old father, James, who retired, reluctantly, six years ago and seemed to have been going downhill ever since. He completely lost his get up and go, not bothering to get shaved most mornings and often padding around in his slippers and dressing gown until midday. Stephen's mother died fifteen years ago of cancer and once his father had recovered from his grief, he had thrown himself into his work. He had a small import/export business which he had built up over thirty years and had finally decided to retire when he reached seventy so his partner bought him out.

Initially James had been euphoric, had thrown himself into travelling and reading books he'd always wanted to read. But after a couple of years he seemed to lose interest in these pastimes and this also coincided with his best friend (and his golfing partner) dying and his only daughter getting married and moving away.

It was then, about two or three years ago, that he had started to slow down. He had retreated into a shell, happy to potter about on his own, but not doing very much apart from listening to the radio, watching the TV, heating tinned soups and doing a little shopping. Stephen noticed that the last time he had visited him his father had seemed particularly spaced-out and seemed to be regressing back to what he had heard others call a second childhood. James made a joke about how he was losing his marbles, that he would spend ages in front of the tinned soup shelves in the supermarket, unable to choose between them. His health was beginning to suffer with one cold after another, especially in the winter months, and he complained of feeling tired.

Stephen wondered whether there might be a homeopathic remedy that could help him and was delighted to find 'boredom' listed as an emotional stress and even more pleased to recognize his father described under *Baryta carbonica* (see page 271). He took over a bottle of the 6th potency and told his dad to take one tablet three times daily for his cold. He also talked to him about eating a better diet so that his body could get its full complement of vitamins and minerals and suggested that he stock up on fresh fruit and vegetables. His father laughed at him and said that he didn't get where he was by eating fresh foods.

Whilst Stephen recognized that his dad needed some practical help with sorting out a reasonable diet, he felt this wasn't the moment to give him a hard time about it. He resolved to wait until the homeopathic remedy had helped a bit, and if it didn't, to take him to his GP or the local professional homeopath. He also resolved to give some time each week to his dad, to take him out, maybe to get him playing golf again.

Baryta carbonica did perk him up and clear his catarrh and then he was able to admit that he had become bored. 'I don't like growing old, I don't want to make an effort and I can't be bothered,' he said petulantly. But he was physically very fit and certainly didn't deserve to put himself on the dust heap. So Stephen sat down and had a brainstorming session with him, about his life – just as his father had done with him when Stephen first went to work as a young man and was finding it hard to adjust to. Out of that session his father decided to offer to do some fund-raising for a local charity – he'd seen a plea in the local paper, and it was something he rather relished having a go at. He also planned to sign on for an art class at the Adult Education College – it was something he'd always wanted to learn. So now, as an added bonus, he'd be getting out of the house and meeting other people. He agreed that he needed to eat properly and sorted himself out a meal plan that was easy *and* included fresh fruit and vegetables – every day.

19. TOO MANY LOSSES

Jane rang to ask whether I could help her seventy-nine year old mother, Mary, who was in a sorry state. She was at an age where her friends were dying one after another with three of her close friends dying in the past few months. I asked her to describe how her mother was dealing with all this emotional stress in her life and whether it had affected her physically or emotionally or both.

Mary was plainly depressed, although she was putting a brave face on it, partly because she believed that it wasn't right to bother others with her feelings, but also because she had never liked others to see her crying. Jane remembered her mum shutting herself away to cry when her gran (Mary's mother) died. What worried Jane was that her mum seemed harder and more bitter, resentful that she was left behind – although not particularly wanting to die herself. Physically she was tired and pale, sleeping badly and suffering from constipation. She had also been plagued by cold sores, something she had always suffered from occasionally, but which were particularly severe at the moment. It had been these that had given Jane an excuse to offer to ring me. Mary had said that if there was anything homeopathic that could help she'd be very happy to give it a try. I asked how Mary reacted to Jane's sympathy and she laughed and said she'd learnt a long time ago to keep a bit of a distance when her mother was upset because she hated people 'fussing' around her and said it only made her worse.

I asked a few questions about her general symptoms and found out that she was a warm-blooded person, had been over-fond of salt in the past and had been persuaded to cut down. I suggested Jane give Mary *Natrum muriaticum* 6 three times daily for up to a week (see page 310). But I also said that it *was* a first-aid prescription and that if it didn't help I would have to take her full case history in order to work out something more specific for her.

Jane rang back ten days later to say her mother was much better, both in her spirits and her body. That 'cold sore remedy' had really worked and she was sleeping better, too. Mary asked if she could have a big bottle of them! I told Jane to tell her how she could repeat them but to be very careful to take them only occasionally, as and when she really needed them.

20. A BROKEN HIP

Seventy-six year old Sandy fell and broke her hip two weeks ago. She was taken into hospital where she needed surgery and was violently ill from the anaesthetic, with repeated vomiting. What with the shock of the accident, the fracture itself, the operation and the reaction to the anaesthetic, she found it very hard to mend and went down with a chest infection for which she needed a course of antibiotics – on top of painkillers and sleeping tablets. What with these and ten days of standard hospital fare (lots of strong tea and over-cooked, prepared meals) by the time she arrived home, although she was on the mend, she was badly in need of building up.

Her daughter-in-law, Amy, came to stay, to look after her for a couple of weeks but after three days felt worried about how low she was. Sandy had lost a lot of weight in hospital. She looked very thin and pale and Amy thought she was probably anaemic. She had no appetite and was very, very tired – she complained of feeling very heavy, she said that even her arms felt heavy, too heavy to hold a book. And talking of complaining, she seemed to do nothing else! She was very miserable, nothing was right, and despondent about ever getting well again. She said all her joints ached.

Amy had used homeopathic medicines for her children when they were little and found it particularly helpful after her youngest one had broken his arm falling out of a tree. She could see that Sandy had had a series of stresses and definitely needed some help to recover.

She got hold of her homeopathic handbook to see if there was a remedy that matched her collection of symptoms. *Calcarea phosphorica* had Sandy's specific stresses in its picture – the broken bones that are slow to mend, the stress of recovering from illness as well as the shock (emotional stress – see page 281).

She was pleased to note that there were a few other confirming symptoms, Sandy had been feeling the cold acutely since coming home and would snap at Amy if she left the door open – she could feel a draft from twenty yards away!

Sandy was still taking painkillers and sleeping tablets but after only three days of *Calcarea phosphorica* 6 (four times daily) could do without the sleeping tablets and was beginning to eat better. After a week she had reduced her painkillers and had some colour in her cheeks. It took her a long time to recover fully and she actually needed to take *Calcarea phosphorica* for three weeks before she decided to give it a rest for a week and see what happened. Her improvement continued and she only needed to take it once more, this time for a week only, after she began to get out and about and the pains started to return again.

In addition to the homeopathic remedy she also agreed to cut out tea until she had fully recovered and to let Amy feed her little, nutritious meals every 2–3 hours to build up her strength – also to follow the exercises the physiotherapist gave her, without grumbling!

EMOTIONAL
STRESSES

INTRODUCTION

Our feelings inform every aspect of who we are, and their healthy expression is an important component of every strong immune system. We need to exercise and rest them in a similar way to our bodies for our emotional well-being, strength and flexibility.

We need to address our emotional house-keeping, and dust and clean out our emotional cupboards on a regular basis so that rubbish does not pile up in our psyches. Far too many people are suffering from emotional repetitive stress injury with, for example, on-going unpleasant or difficult situations at work or at home, or repeated problems that have been swept under the carpet.

Emotional stresses can range from mild all the way through to severe. Their effects will vary depending on your inner strengths and weaknesses. They can pile up, one stress on top of another, creating a load that is hard to carry, a burden that affects your health and vitality. Physical complaints that come our way as a result of emotional stress are debilitating and unpleasant – dismissing them as psychosomatic can add insult to injury.

The problem is that feelings can't be seen. A physical injury will usually get a lot of attention – the worse the injury, the more the attention. If you suffer an emotional injury, however, there is no blood, nothing to actually see. If you have learnt to hide your feelings then that injury can fester internally, unable to heal and making you vulnerable to similar injuries, which will be felt all the more strongly.

Our mental processes need attention, too – the brain can be compared to a muscle that needs exercise, that needs to be stimulated and stretched to develop; to be able to concentrate well and easily; to be able to remember (both in the short and long term); to be able to think things through and make decisions and judgements; to be creative with concepts and ideas. Is your mind fit, is it getting the exercise it needs? Has it become a bit flabby from under-use? Or has it been over-stretched and become tired and slow? Develop an on-going awareness of how your mind responds to the stresses in your life so that you can attend to its needs.

Ask yourself whether (and how) your emotional stress is limiting you, and from what. Sometimes answering this question alone gives people the motivation they need to do something about it. You may find it useful to read more than one section of the emotional stresses themselves in order to identify what remedy you think you may need, as well as what action may be helpful.

Homeopaths have a deep respect for the inter-connectedness of the physical and emotional and mental bodies and take emotional injury as, if not more, seriously than physical injury. Use the guidelines/advice below to problem solve with your emotional stresses, those from your past, those around you right now, as well as to plan for your future – to develop healthier ways of handling emotional stress in your life. Use them to encourage your children to be aware of their feelings too.

Your feelings count
Develop an understanding of how people and events affect you emotionally. If this is hard for you, because of your personality make-up or because you were brought up to hide your feelings, then consider learning about them through a self-help group, through psychotherapy or counselling or communications skills training.

Your feelings need listening to and taking seriously, whatever the situation, and however strong or apparently 'inappropriate' they may seem. It is your awareness of them that will enable you to heal them. Be honest with yourself about the depth of your feelings and try to get to the root of their cause.

If you are having difficulty knowing what you are feeling then take some quiet time to be with yourself and to let the emotions surface. So often, our busy lives keep our deeper feelings hidden whilst we attend to the daily grind. Allow yourself to daydream – to let pictures, thoughts or sensations come into your mind, without censoring them. These can help you to understand what you are going through.

When you know that you are under emotional stress, don't pretend that nothing is happening, or ignore or swallow feelings (or signals from your body), or hope they will go away. After a while they might seem to disappear but they will simply sink into your unconscious where they will lie in wait for the next time!

Be kind and considerate towards yourself, in your thoughts and feelings, and compassionate if the emotional stress has been particularly painful, as you would be towards a good friend who is hurting. Being hard on yourself will only add insult to injury and make healing more difficult. It isn't helpful to compare yourself to others in a similar situation who have 'sailed through'.

Many people make efforts to 'snap out of it', repeating harsh words that may have been used when they were children. Ask yourself whether you would speak these words to others or whether you are only nasty to yourself! You may find it useful to question the messages you grew up with regarding the expression of feelings: girls should be good, should listen to others, shouldn't get angry or be noisy; boys shouldn't cry, be soft or weak, should be assertive, brave and strong. Many children are brought up to squash themselves into a mould created by others, and then they continue to play the same game as adults – conforming to expected 'norms' rather than developing their own emotional maturity. The critical messages that we carry from our childhood are often at the root of many difficulties in dealing with emotional stress and can also be at the root of many relationship misunderstandings and conflicts. They often have the words 'ought', 'should', 'must' attached to them.

Your feelings give you feedback about how events and people are affecting you. They will help you understand whether you are stressed and how that stress is showing itself. Accepting your own feelings will help you to accept other people's. And stop wanting to change them. It is unnecessarily stressful to want to change circumstances that are outside of your control – and other people's behaviour fits into that category. You can only change your own behaviour – and when you do you'll be surprised at how others close to you will change in response.

How we handle emotional stress and, in particular, emotional trauma, is more significant in terms of its effect on our health than the trauma itself. Many people have learnt to cover up their true feelings to protect others (and themselves) from pain. This suppression has profound effects, trapping people in an endless cycle of hurt and isolation that can be hard to break.

Pressure cooker
Suppressed emotions can back up, creating a blocked drain or a pressure cooker situation. It is important that we cleanse ourselves emotionally as well as physically in order to stay healthy. We have very few rituals that encourage the healthy expression of strong emotions, and little encouragement to learn about them, especially when we are under emotional stress.

Take some time to 'indulge' in the feelings that have come your way – anger, sadness, resentment, shock, etc. Work through them so that you don't end up carrying them around . . . and around and around. Be creative about this. For example, express anger in the privacy (and safety) of your own home – kick or punch a cushion or bean bag and have a good scream, take a bat or tennis racket to the bed or sofa. (Warn neighbours if necessary, so that they don't misinterpret the noises and ring the police!) Have a good scream in the car (with the windows wound up) on a quiet road. If you feel sad, cry as much as you need to: on your own or with others, whichever works for you. Use a stimulus if you are finding it difficult to cry, like music or a sad film.

Sometimes we need to really sink down into our feelings and wallow around in them to fully understand their place in our lives. We need to choose the right time and place to do this as other people (especially those who habitually suppress their own feelings) can find it hard to take and may try and talk you out of it or, worse, be critical of you.

Don't forget that holding in so-called 'positive' emotions (like love) is stressful too. As an encouragement to yourself, make a list of the people who matter to you and ask yourself whether you would regret not having told them how you feel about them if they were to die suddenly. This isn't a callous thing to do. It does happen.

Talking it through
Talking about emotional stress with a tried and trusted friend, a counsellor or psychotherapist will help you to understand and accept what you are going through, and release some of the pressure.

You may need to 'de-brief' after a painful experience, to tell your story over and over. You may need reassurance – for example, after a painful loss you may want to be told (over and over again) that your baby's death was not your fault, that there was nothing you could have done to prevent it. You may need to be told that your elderly mother's heart attack wasn't because you both had a blazing row the day before she died, or that your dog didn't die of a broken heart in kennels whilst you were on holiday. Or you may need the emotional support of someone who has suffered a similar experience, someone who can sympathize with what you are going through.

Be careful to talk to people who are going to support you in a caring way. Some people inadvertently encourage others to squash their feelings because they find it hard to see their friends in pain. Don't be put off by friends' or relatives' embarrassment or judgemental responses. Your feelings may be different to theirs. This doesn't make either of you right – or wrong!

Some people find it difficult to ask for help – out of pride or a fear of exposing themselves to more hurt. If this is the case with you, pick your listening ears carefully and remind yourself how honoured *you* felt the last time someone in need came to you. It is easy to forget that it is a sign of strength, not weakness, to ask for help.

Some people don't want to talk about their feelings, are quite content with the methods they have for dealing with emotional stress. It is important to respect this: some people are very private and have their own personal ways of being true to themselves and their feelings.

Get some outside help
When the going gets tough, remember you are not alone, even though it may feel like it. Use support networks in times of need. Help lines, support groups or classes as well as experts can all be useful in providing information, advice and/or reassurance. Don't suffer in silence.

Ring a help line if you need to talk and don't have anyone close to you or simply want some outside advice. Help lines like the Samaritans have a twenty-four-hour service for those who are seriously depressed or suicidal. Some organizations help by listening, giving practical advice if appropriate. Some will put you in touch with others who are in a similar situation.

Get some professional help, from a counsellor or psychotherapist trained in what you are going through, i.e. one who is skilled in working with, for example, bereavement, marriage guidance or sexual abuse. A counsellor can help if:

- You are having difficulty with a particular emotional stress.
- You are finding life a struggle.
- You cannot let go of the past.
- You find yourself repeatedly involved in stressful situations, and want to learn new ways of dealing with them.
- You suspect or know that your problem is linked to low self-esteem – if you measure yourself against others through what you do for them. Some people do far more than is asked of them, hoping for acknowledgment and appreciation, and then when they don't get it they feel resentful and may then (perversely) redouble their efforts to 'please'. This is an unhealthy self-perpetuating cycle. Other symptoms of low self-esteem include: lack of self-confidence; feeling responsible and guilty when things go wrong (that aren't your fault); thinking others are better than you; feeling worthless. Sometimes people cover these feelings up with a show of arrogance or bravado but they simmer away underneath, undermining everything they do.
- You become stuck in blaming others for what is happening 'to you' because of 'them'. You make yourself vulnerable to sinking into negativity and may find yourself repeating the experience in a similar form at a later date, thereby creating a world full of people who are out to get you.
- You become stuck in self-blame, feeling like a victim of what life throws at you, unable to break the cycle. You can only deal effectively with what has happened once you stop blaming yourself.
- You are suffering from an emotional wound that isn't healing.
- You are suffering from depression (especially if it is accompanied by an altered sense of reality), phobias, sexual difficulties, inexplicable physical sensations or complaints that are not diagnosable. Don't struggle on your own if you feel yourself

sinking deeper and deeper into, for example, depression. It really is easier to heal if you get help earlier rather than later.

- You are experiencing difficulties in your intimate relationships, say, a repeating pattern of abuse in your relationships (at home and/or at work).
- You find yourself stuck in a tornado of strong emotions (that may be related to a particular event) and talking about them with friends or writing about them hasn't helped.

Ask your doctor or homeopath to refer you to someone whose work they know, rather than picking a name out of the *Yellow Pages*. Don't put up with patronizing or dismissive treatment from professionals (especially if you are seeking help with depression). You and your feelings deserve to be taken seriously and to be dealt with kindly and courteously.

Check out local groups, including self-help groups, that will meet your particular needs. Just knowing that you aren't alone will help. Find out if there are any assertiveness training courses – they have a good track record in helping people to feel more in control of their lives and to develop effective communications skills.

Keep reaching out, however many dead ends you find yourself up against, until you get the help you need.

Write about your feelings

The expression of emotional trauma gives a boost to the whole body, including the immune system. And this effect can be achieved through writing. Writing is a private, personal form of confession. It is a way to acknowledge our deeper feelings to ourselves, to confide our inner truths to ourselves, to engage in our own healing. Whilst this method doesn't work for everybody, putting upsetting experiences (past or present) into words has profound psychological and physical benefits for many people and is worth trying because it is something you can do any time, anywhere.

The key to doing it successfully is to 'let it all hang out', to allow the feelings to come to the surface without inhibiting them. Many people avoid doing this because they think they will feel bad or even worse than they already do. They usually will. But it is only temporary. The feelings of peace and resolution that follow will make it worth while.

Some people keep a diary or journal in which they record the daily trivia of their lives, what they did, who they saw, etc. Whilst this can be interesting it won't provide a medium for self-healing. Using a journal for understanding and coming to terms with an emotional trauma needs a different approach and is helpful when there is a specific difficulty or problem that needs dealing with. Use the following guidelines to help you to do this:

- Make space for yourself – a quiet room where you won't be interrupted.
- Write for half an hour (or more if you want to) for at least four days in a row.
- Don't worry about your handwriting, grammar, spelling or sentence structure.
- Write about your deepest feelings, those you've kept to yourself. Just let them flow out of you without censoring them.

You will find that as you write your feelings will surface and it is important that you just let them. The benefits of doing this exercise are that you will come to terms with difficult experiences; you will make all sorts of connections between, say, old feelings and current problems; you will gain insights into yourself and others; your immune system and nervous system will relax; you will eventually be able to forgive yourself and/or others for hurtful behaviour; through dealing with old or unfinished business you will be able to put these problems into a broader, more balanced perspective. The greatest benefit is the physical and emotional sense of resolution, the peace that comes with the ending of inner conflict, with the healing of old (or new) hurts.

This, then, is more like a personal confession with the added bonus that you give absolution to yourself on your own terms. Confession is structured into the way other institutions work from the Catholic Church to Alcoholics Anonymous but your experience will be based on your own chosen values.

Include the small details – who said what, what you thought and felt, what you wish you had said and done, and so on. As you write you will be surprised at what surfaces once you get the superficial details out of the way. You may make important connections to other events in your life, or experience unexpected feelings – for example, you find there is a sense of loss and sadness under the anger and self-righteousness after a friend betrayed you. This exercise will allow you to access your feelings and understand better how an experience has affected you, and will help you to decide what to do about it.

Or you can make this a more specific exercise by writing a letter to the person (or each person) involved in a stressful situation. One that you are *not* going to send. Put these writings in a safe place, where they cannot become 'accidentally' mixed up with your correspondence, and sent out by mistake! As with the exercise above, don't censor your thoughts or feelings – let your language be fully expressive, however unpleasant it is. No one is going to see this letter. It will help you to resolve your feelings so that you don't carry them around inside you – where they can fester and cause you harm. Afterwards, you may decide to write a letter you do send, one which covers the issues in a way which will not generate ill will.

Keep a journal, and write something on a daily basis. Use it to record experiences, feelings and dreams. You will notice repeating patterns in your life and it will help you to keep in contact with your emotions. Your dreams provide a rich source of information from your unconscious, from the deeper, emotional parts of yourself. You'll need to keep pen and paper next to your bed and make a strong mental note to remember your dream *and* write it down before you do anything else after you wake up, because they can evaporate so quickly.

Repeating patterns in dreams or repetitive dreams are nearly always trying to tell you something about yourself. See if you can unravel the cryptic puzzles that your unconscious feeds you. It can be fun as well as personally rewarding. Some people even ask their dreams for help in times of emotional (or physical) stress.

Your needs count
Respect yourself and your needs. Many people who take care of the needs of others, neglecting themselves and their own needs in the process, become martyrs or resent those around them who have been taking them for granted. Put yourself first so that you can care better for those close to you.

Reassess your responsibilities and your duties. Have you taken on too much? How many times do you say to yourself and others 'I have to—' or 'I've got to—' or 'I should/ought to—'? You may have a behaviour pattern that needs challenging and changing.

Treat yourself as you treat others, as you want others to treat you. People often put themselves at the bottom of a very long list and then are surprised and hurt when others treat them the same way, as if they weren't important.

Protecting yourself (be prepared!)

Think ahead and prepare yourself for situations where you know you are vulnerable to emotional stress and plan your strategies carefully.

There are times when we need to 'pretend' to feel something we don't or choose to act as if we felt something we don't. It's Monday morning (again) and you feel tired and irritable – try putting a smile on your face and breathing out your tension and exhaustion.

There are times when it isn't necessarily appropriate to express our feelings, times when we would expose ourselves by expressing them. Simply putting a smile on our face when we are feeling sad or angry can help to alleviate the pain – like putting a plaster on a blister. You'll need to deal with the cause of the blister sooner or later but it will enable you to walk without pain for a while.

You may need to hide your feelings in certain situations to protect yourself from the unkind (however unintentional) or inappropriate responses of others. Consciously putting our feelings to one side, in order to deal with them later when it may be safer, can be a smart and sensible thing to do.

Be willing to take a stand if people behave badly towards you or those close to you. Sometimes we allow others to attack us, to be unkind or rude or nasty, because we worry about *their* feelings, or because we are concerned about how others see us, or because we haven't learnt how to stand up for ourselves.

Letting others know

Sometimes we need to talk directly with someone who has hurt us. It is important that we are able to do that without hurting their feelings in return, otherwise there is a danger that the emotional stress will escalate (see Conflict, p. 98).

You may want to find a way to express difficult feelings directly to the person who has hurt you, to let a friend or colleague know how their behaviour or their words have affected you and to tell them what you need. This isn't always easy or appropriate, in which case you may find writing is more helpful (see p. 100).

Sometimes people behave badly because they are having a bad day and it has nothing to do with you directly. You just happened to be there. It can be a relief to find this out, and a good opportunity to let that other person know that they don't live in a vacuum! We can remind a friend or colleague, unconsciously, of someone else in their lives and they can behave towards us as if we were that person. This is known as projection. It can be useful to clear up this sort of misunderstanding quickly.

It can be stressful to listen to others who tell you what to do based on their own experience. You may need advice but we each need to find a solution that suits our particular situation, one that takes our needs and wishes into account.

The healing power of laughter
Learning about yourself and accepting who you are will make it easier to see the funny side of things. Taking yourself or others too seriously or hanging on to unrealistic expectations is always stressful. Learning to laugh at yourself (and others) can relieve an awful lot of tension and encourage you to be realistic in your relationships, to put them in perspective. Laughter can transform an impossibly difficult situation into a challenge where you end up feeling better, especially about yourself.

But if laughter is your way of avoiding your deeper feelings then beware. Don't grin and bear it, or be coerced into 'cheering up' when you feel upset.

Strengths and weaknesses
Be honest with yourself about your own strengths and weaknesses. Admitting your limitations will help you to avoid unnecessary, unhealthy emotional stress. Be realistic about your capabilities and get help if you need it (see p. 000). Or reconsider whether there is a stress in your life that you could choose to avoid – for the moment. You might need to remind yourself from time to time that you don't have to win every game, come top of the class every time, get top grades in your exams – and so on.

Appreciate your strengths. Accept compliments from others (as you would a nice present) and allow warm, good feelings to settle throughout your body. This is one of the ways we recharge our emotional batteries.

Congratulate yourself on your achievements, on your successes. Don't think this is tempting fate, or worse, encouraging arrogance. Taking credit for your successes is healthy and life-enhancing, and helps to put the difficult times into perspective.

Don't pile it on
At times of high emotional stress it makes sense to cut down on additional unnecessary strains, both physical and emotional. This will give you the best chance of getting over what you are going through and ensuring that it doesn't affect your health.

Don't numb emotional pain with alcohol, drugs, cigarettes, caffeine, junk food and/or work. Don't neglect yourself, especially if you feel like doing so. It is especially important to look after yourself through trying times – to eat and sleep well, to take some sort of regular exercise, and to make sure you have a daily routine that keeps you in touch with the outside world – even if it is only to go shopping.

Learning from experience
You may want to reflect on your current relationships and consider what it is you want to say or do in order to bring them 'up to date'. It is often love and affection that people wish they had expressed to those who have passed away, for example. Remember – it is never too late to tell someone close to you that you love them. Don't be hard on yourself if you have lost someone and you regret not having said or done certain things with or for them.

Each knock, each blow, each struggle can be used to help us learn about ourselves, to come to terms and make peace with our strengths and weaknesses, and with our differences. We can use the information that we gather about ourselves – and others – to plan ahead and to become wiser and healthier.

Homeopathic treatment
I have included some common 'first-aid' remedies for emotional stresses at the end of each of the following chapters. You can refer to

the table (on pages 88–91) for an at-a-glance guide. It is important to choose a remedy based on your whole picture (use the prescribing guidelines on pages 33–46 to help you). You will need to seek professional advice if your emotional stresses are either severe or long-standing.

Emotional Stresses Chart	Aconitum napellus	Ambra grisea	Anacardium orientale	Apis mellifica	Argentum nitricum	Arnica montana	Arsenicum album	Aurum metallicum	Baryta carbonica	Belladonna	Borax venata
Betrayal								•			
Boredom									•		
Bullying									•		
Conflict											
Criticism											
Depression							•				
Disappointment											
Embarrassment		•							•		
Excitement											
Failure					•		•				
Fear	•				•		•				•
Guilt							•	•			
Homesickness											
Humiliation											
Jealousy				•							
Loneliness								•			
Loss								•			
Mental strain					•						
Reprimand											
Resentment						•					
Shame								•			
Shock	•					•				•	•
Transitions			•				•		•		•
Uncertainty					•		•				
Worry	•	•	•		•		•				

Emotional Stresses Chart	Calcarea carbonica	Calcarea phosphorica	Capsicum	Carbo vegetabilis	Causticum	Chamomilla	Cocculus indicus	Coffea cruda	Colocynthis	Conium maculatum	Gelsemium
Betrayal											
Boredom											
Bullying											
Conflict					•	•		•			
Criticism											
Depression											
Disappointment		•									
Embarrassment											
Excitement							•				
Failure											
Fear											•
Guilt											
Homesickness			•								
Humiliation								•			
Jealousy											
Loneliness											
Loss					•						•
Mental strain		•					•	•		•	
Reprimand											
Resentment											
Shame											
Shock		•		•							•
Transitions		•									
Uncertainty	•				•						•
Worry	•										•

Emotional Stresses Chart	Ignatia amara	Kali phosphoricum	Lachesis	Lycopodium	Natrum carbonicum	Natrum muriaticum	Nitric acid	Nux vomica	Opium	Phoshoric acid	Phosphorus
Betrayal					•				•		
Boredom								•			
Bullying			•								
Conflict							•	•			•
Criticism	•							•			
Depression		•	•			•					
Disappointment	•					•				•	
Embarrassment											
Excitement		•							•		
Failure								•			
Fear			•								•
Guilt	•										
Homesickness	•									•	
Humiliation	•			•		•		•			
Jealousy			•								
Loneliness	•										
Loss	•					•					
Mental strain		•			•			•		•	
Reprimand	•								•		
Resentment						•	•				
Shame	•							•	•		
Shock	•							•			
Transitions				•		•					
Uncertainty										•	
Worry		•		•		•		•			

Emotional Stresses Chart	Picric acid	Pulsatilla	Sepia	Silica	Staphysagria	Stramonium	Sulphur	Tarentula	Veratrum album	Zincum metallicum
Betrayal		•			•					
Boredom				•			•			
Bullying				•	•					
Conflict		•			•					
Criticism				•	•					
Depression		•	•							
Disappointment					•					
Embarrassment		•					•			
Excitement										
Failure				•					•	
Fear						•	•			
Guilt										
Homesickness										
Humiliation		•			•					
Jealousy		•								
Loneliness		•								
Loss		•			•			•		
Mental strain	•			•						•
Reprimand					•		•			
Resentment					•					
Shame					•					
Shock						•				
Transitions		•	•				•			
Uncertainty										
Worry				•						

BETRAYAL

Betrayal is hard to live with – so many feelings come up when we have been 'conned', when we find out that someone has betrayed our trust, whether that someone is a teenager who's stolen the housekeeping and spent it on drugs; or a business partner who's been involved in fraudulent activities; or a partner who has had an affair. Betrayal can come into ordinary everyday friendships and working relationships, when, for example, someone breaks a confidence, or 'goes over your head' without talking to you first.

Feelings that surface when you find out someone has lied to you can range from shock and anger or even rage, to humiliation and disappointment. A betrayal is always stressful, whether it is a close friend or a work colleague who breaks your trust because it can involve the loss of a relationship – even if it is the loss of a relationship as it was, with a rebuilding based on a new understanding.

The most painful thing for many people is having to readjust their 'vision' and see others as they are rather than who they would like them to be (based on expectations of how *they* would behave in their place). We all tend to repeat our patterns of behaviour, including the deceptions. It can be very hard to come to terms with the fact that someone who has deceived you once is capable of doing it again. It is important to be realistic about the future, based on what has happened, without expecting either the worst or the best.

Sometimes a betrayal hurts so much that it makes us ill. The guidelines below are to help you protect yourself from future deceptions.

Do:
- Remember that someone who has deceived you once is capable of doing it again. So think carefully before confronting someone who has lied to you more than once. They are capable of lying again, or making false promises to change.

- Look at your own part in what has happened, without blaming yourself. Did you suspect that things were not as they seemed and did you turn a blind eye to the clues, or ignore your gut feelings? Does this situation mimic a similar situation from your past which you had buried, which has caused a blind spot of your own and made you vulnerable?
- Consider, without blaming yourself, whether you might have set yourself up so that others are more likely to lie to you, rather than negotiate with you or be honest with you.
- Alter your expectations of others based on their behaviour and who they are rather than who you wish they would be.
- Consider renegotiating the boundaries with those who have betrayed you but with whom you have to carry on living or working. For example, your partner had an affair and says that it wasn't a big deal and anyway the two of you had never talked about whether that was okay or not. But you'd always assumed it wasn't, and your partner hadn't – apparently. It may be time to make the assumptions explicit.
- Get a third person to referee if you feel anxious about renegotiating on your own – a counsellor or psychotherapist, a colleague or business consultant.

Don't:
- Put your head in the sand and hope this one will go away.

Homeopathic treatment
The following remedies are to help with the emotional effects of an unexpected betrayal.
- *Aurum metallicum (Aur.)* See also p. 269.
  Deception and betrayal – especially at work, possibly with a financial loss.
- *Natrum muriaticum (Nat-m.)* See also p. 310.
  Betrayal with a sense of loss and deep hurt. Cannot express the sadness.
- *Phosphoric acid (Pho-ac.)* See also p. 323.
  Betrayal (especially of friendship) with disappointment and shock – feels defeated and humiliated.
- *Pulsatilla nigricans (Puls.)* See also p. 330.

Betrayal with disappointment and sense of loss. Feels let down, lonely and sad. Can't stop crying.
- *Staphysagria* (*Staph.*) See also p. 341.
  Betrayal with humiliation. Feels furious – may pretend nothing is wrong. Angry thoughts make it difficult to sleep at night.

BOREDOM

Boredom can be seen as a healthy stress: it lets us know that change is needed. It can act as an impetus when we become stale, leading to a change in career or attitude, or the development of new skills.

It can be stressful if we become apathetic about what's happening in our lives: if we become stuck in a job that isn't challenging; if we get bored at home with the relentless tedium of babies and/or small children; if children are understimulated at school; if we lose a sense of purpose after retirement. A lack of structure to our days – especially if we are out of work – can be a huge stress.

If the initial signs and symptoms of boredom aren't listened to and dealt with it is easy to sink into apathy and find it difficult to get motivated. Sufferers can lose their self-confidence, become indecisive and finally lazy and indifferent to what is going on around them – and even to those closest to them. There may be a feeling of resentment, a feeling that no one is doing anything to help.

First, ask yourself what is causing the boredom. Is it a consequence of another stress that hasn't been resolved, such as anger at having lost your job? If this is so, the shock or shame of redundancy, i.e. the feelings which lie behind the apathy, need to be dealt with first.

You will then need to make a special effort to get that creative energy, that spark going again.

Do:
- Be prepared to do anything to get yourself out of a rut.
- Be creative – use daydreaming, your imagination, to come up with ideas.
- Write a list of your skills and strengths and pin them on your wall. Remind yourself what it is you have to offer so that when times are hard you have created a mental lifebelt for yourself.

- Seek the advice of a careers or business counseller to help you focus on what you are going to do.
- Take up a new hobby/interest – or an old one. Join a local club or sign on with an adult education class.
- Offer to do some local voluntary work.
- Plan for your future, however grim or difficult it may seem. Keep exploring and building in things to work towards – sooner or later something will come up for you.
- Consider a complete career change if you are out of work – including starting from scratch, doing something you'd never, ever have considered before.
- Consider going back to 'school'. Take a course in something you've always been interested in but never had the time to pursue before – whether it is art, photography or car mechanics. Enjoying yourself will give your morale a much-needed boost and this will ripple out into every area of your life.
- Keep a domestic routine going, keep fit and physically active and eat at regular times.
- Build *some* structure into your life – something to do every day, something to get up for.
- Get out of the house every day – to walk or shop, to visit a friend, etc.

Don't:
- Sink into despondency and give up! If one thing doesn't work try something else. Some people need to work inordinately hard to get themselves going again once they've been out of work for a while or have become bored through looking after, say, small children for many years.
- Isolate yourself. Reach out into your community and let people know you are there.
- Get addicted to television – limit the number of hours you watch a day, otherwise you may sink into passivity, and develop couch potato-itis, which is very hard to cure.

Homeopathic treatment
The following remedies are to help those who have become temporarily stuck in a boredom rut.

- **Baryta carbonica** (*Bar-c.*) See also p. 271.
  Bored and indecisive. Lacks self confidence. People of any age regress emotionally. Can't decide what to do and doesn't feel capable of doing anything.
- **Nux vomica** (*Nux-v.*) See also p. 317.
  Bored and irritable. Becomes sedentary and loses former drive. Takes to alcohol and/or drugs and fritters time away.
- **Silica** (*Sil.*) See also p. 338.
  Bored and floppy. Lacks grit. Can't seem to get going – keeps putting off things until the next day, but it never comes! Completely unmotivated.
- **Sulphur** (*Sul.*) See also p. 345.
  Bored and lazy to the point of idleness. Won't do what they say they are going to do. Make plans but lack initiative. Lose interest in looking after themselves.

BULLYING

In the power struggles that go on between people in all walks of life, and of all ages, bullying is a special type of persecution. People can feel threatened by others at work, at home, at school or in a public place. Unkind criticism, unpleasant rudeness and nastiness can all be upsetting for those on the receiving end. Sarcasm, irony, humour and silence are more subtle ways in which one person can bully another. Discrimination of any kind can involve bullying, whether over race, sex, religion, age, class, size, height (small men can suffer as horribly as tall women) or looks. Those who are sick can be unintentionally bullied by well-meaning but harassed health care professionals. The elderly and those with a mental or physical disability can be bullied by those caring for them, including the social services. Children in groups can be especially cruel, behaving like pack animals, hunting out those who do not fit in and picking on them mercilessly.

Common emotional reactions to bullying include humiliation, fear, anxiety and shame. Those who have been bullied experience a loss of self-confidence in themselves and a loss of trust in others. Children who are bullied at school may refuse to go, may regress emotionally, and can become aggressive themselves. Some people are more sensitive to being bullied than others, either because of their character or because they have been bullied before – especially if it was traumatic and/or repeated.

Common physical complaints include stomach aches, headaches, insomnia and tiredness, especially in children. Adults may suffer from rashes and backache or more serious complaints like irritable bowel syndrome and migraines.

In order to learn how to deal with bullies, we need to be familier with what we will and won't put up with, as well as our limits when handling people who try to transgress those personal boundaries. It may mean saying 'no', something that many of us are not taught to do. If people aren't responding to your requests, aren't respecting you or are actually ignoring you when you try to stop them from bullying you, then you will find it beneficial to learn some basic assertiveness skills. Start by practising 'no'. You may want to do this with a friend: get them to goad you and have you say or shout 'no' until they really feel you are not to be messed with. Then do the same exercise with 'yes' – we need to be able to say yes and mean it, for our 'no's to be heard.

If you are harassed in a public place, especially at night, then you need to be especially cautious. Walk tall even if your confidence is a pretence. Breathe deeply and evenly, loosen your shoulders, look resolutely ahead – or get a friend to meet you, or take a cab if you feel seriously unsafe.

Some of the advice that follows is to help you to look at strategies for dealing with bullying so as to minimize its stressful effects. Pick those that are relevant to you and you particular situation.

Do:
- Check out your civil rights regarding, for example, noisy or offensive neighbours.
- Consider reporting harassment or bullying to an appropriate authority, i.e. head teachers or school governors if your child is being bullied at school by a child or a teacher; your union if you are being harassed at work.
- Keep notes (including dates) of unpleasant incidents in case you need to follow through with an official complaint.

• Learn skills for dealing with bullies. Teach them to your children
  or learn together if you can. There are many possible strategies
  for dealing with a difficult situation where you are feeling
  harassed: have one or more up your sleeve and practise them
  when an opportunity presents itself:
  — Respond in your own time (if there is time to play with).
  Carefully plan your strategy for dealing with a bullying boss or a
  threatening neighbour. Silence can make bullies feel uncomfortable and let them know that you aren't going to react without
  thinking.
  — Get out if you can. It is sometimes possible to walk away from
  trouble, to get out of a situation where you are feeling under
  attack. There are times when you don't have to stay and take it,
  and many creative options for removing yourself, like suddenly
  having to go to the toilet or to make an urgent phone call.
  — Ignore them. Consider ignoring those who are getting at you,
  pretending they have not spoken, acting as if they don't exist.
  You can even do this politely!
  — Use distraction. This is a powerful technique that can be
  extremely effective, especially if the persecutor is someone close
  to you. Change the subject, do something unexpected like
  jumping up to answer a doorbell (which hasn't necessarily
  rung), or if you are desperate you can spill your cup of tea (not
  on anyone!)
  — Smile. Smiling or even laughing at bullies as if they are
  ridiculous (which they often are) is a great tension release and
  gives the message that you are not taking them seriously.
  However, this can make them really angry, and needs using
  very carefully.
  — Decide it isn't your problem. Tell yourself that this person has
  a problem, that they are stupid or ignorant or both, that their
  behaviour isn't personal and make a determined effort not to get
  drawn into their foolish game. Even if you are pretending. When
  we act as if we are confident the feeling can follow.
  — Confront the bully. Some people need to be told directly that
  their behaviour is unacceptable. This is a challenge for those who
  hate making a fuss, who want peace at any price. For it to be
  effective, it needs to be done in a way that does not add fuel to

the fire: the anger that you may feel can come across non-verbally so try to be aware of your body language. You may appear aggressive even though you are trying hard not to be! Taking a surprisingly sudden firm and loud enough position can disarm a cowardly bully. Take another person along as a support, someone who can referee if things get heated. If you decide to confront your persecutor in writing, ask someone else to read the letter before you send it, to make sure you haven't left any inflammatory barbs in.

— Freak out! A well-chosen volcanic eruption (if you have it in you) can bring an awful lot of people to their senses. A very loud 'for goodness sake, stop it' may be all that is needed – the element of surprise is all-important. It can also attract some anger which will be directed at you, so beware.

- Teach children to understand the difference between teasing and bullying. Check that the teasing hasn't deteriorated into something spiteful or even become a verbal, emotional bullying. Encourage them to turn teasing back on the teaser, to put it back where it belongs!

Don't:
- Allow yourself to be pushed into an attacking position without thinking it through. Look at your options for dealing with a situation where you are feeling bullied, frightened and/or undermined – especially if you don't have to stay and take it.

Homeopathic treatment
The following remedies are to help those who are being or have been bullied or harassed to regain their self-confidence.
- *Baryta carbonica (Bar-c.)* See also p. 271.
  For children or adults, who regress as a result of bullying, who become emotionally withdrawn and mentally 'stuck'.
- *Lycopodium (Lyc.)* See also p. 305.
  For the intellectual type who gets bullied, at work or at school, who feels humiliated and suffers from low self-confidence and anxiety.
- *Silica (Sil.)* See also p. 338.
  For those who are painfully shy, who unwittingly attract the

unwelcome attention of bullies because they find it hard to stand
up for themselves (although they will stand up for others).
- *Staphysagria (Staph.)* See also p. 341.
Feels humiliated and indignant and very angry. May hide it behind
a nice smile, but seethes inside and replays the incident at night in
bed, saying all the things they wish they had said at the time.

CONFLICT

Conflict occurs when two or more people disagree with each other.
It may be a minor argument which is easily resolved, or a more
serious one leading to ill-feeling and resentment.

Potential for conflict exists in every area of our lives: at home, in
the workplace, at school, in shops, on public transport. We all
struggle with inner conflict too, when we have to reconcile what we
want to do with what we have to do.

All conflict needs to be talked through with people we trust, so
that we can understand, resolve and integrate it into our lives, rather
than allowing it to grate on our nerves and make us ill.

Conflict isn't all bad: it may add spice to a relationship. It
challenges us emotionally and alerts us to look at those sides of our
character that we'd rather hide from ourselves, and others. Relationships without conflict (at home or at work) are often static, surviving
only while no one rocks the boat.

Any confrontation that stresses you needs dealing with so that it
doesn't make you ill. Common emotional responses to conflict are
anger, humiliation, anxiety or fear if there is a danger of one person
hurting another. Allow yourself to be aware of how conflict affects
you – both positively and negatively. Some people almost enjoy
conflict because they have a fighting side to their character, others
are 'allergic' to conflict after growing up with adults who were
always arguing. For many people anger is a difficult emotion: it may
be suppressed, so that it festers as resentment, or expressed in
uncontrolled and uncontrollable eruptions. It is a powerful force in
all our lives, part of that rich spectrum of emotions that makes us
who we are. It can be empowering rather than destructive, when
used appropriately and consciously. A raised 'don't-mess-with-me'

voice to gain the attention of squabbling children, or when you have tried everything else (reason, sympathy, repeated requests, negotiating, etc.) with an unreasonable teenager; an enraged yelling to distract an attacker. It is good to know how to access and use it in certain situations to protect yourself.

But it isn't healthy to be feeling angry a lot of the time. If you know yourself to be an 'angry' person then seek the advice of a homeopath (and possibly a counsellor) to understand what lies behind the aggressive position you have taken up.

Anger which is suppressed is the most dangerous of all. Inside, a pressure cooker situation can develop with anger bursting out at unpredictable times, and depression simmering away alongside it. Or worse, the anger can't get out and people direct their anger against themselves through self-destructive behaviour such as anorexia or taking drugs.

Do:
- Become familiar with your own patterns for dealing with conflict and expressing anger.
- Encourage your children to understand the place anger and conflict has in their lives.
- Learn techniques for dealing directly with conflict. Assertiveness training is a good start and will help you with the practicalities of facing anger (in yourself and others) effectively (see p. 14).
- Communicate openly with those involved about how indirect conflict is affecting you, for example work colleagues or siblings who are always arguing. Suggest that they find some way to resolve their situation.
- Absent yourself from situations where there is unacceptable conflict. You don't have to endure more than you can reasonably bear.
- Get help – don't try and deal with potentially explosive situations on your own, especially if there's a chance you'll get physically hurt if you do.
- Try and understand what happened from your own perspective as well as the other person's, not to excuse anyone's behaviour but to explain it and put it in context. This will help you in the end to forgive everyone concerned – including yourself.

- See the funny side of what's happening – sometimes well-placed laughter can diffuse tension in a conflict that has run out of steam but carries on because no one knows how to stop it.
- Consider resolving the conflict – in person or in writing. Use the following guidelines to help bring about a satisfactory/peaceful resolution:

    — Start by expressing any genuine appreciations (general or specific) that you have for the other person. This will put your complaint in a context where it will be more likely to be heard.

    — Be specific about your complaint without apportioning blame. Stick to what happened from your perspective and be brief but clear about the effects of the other person's behaviour on you (or, for example, your child or anyone else you are speaking for).

    — Make a clear and specific demand or recommendation. This could, for example, be for an apology, a guarantee that it won't happen again, some sort of compensation, an explanation, etc.

    — Get a clear agreement on the above or negotiate if necessary, but make sure that any compromises are acceptable to you as well. Say what action you will take should this agreement be broken.

    — End on a positive note, with an appreciation if possible for the other person and/or something they have done. Even a small, genuine thank you goes a long way towards building good will back into a relationship which may have soured.

Don't:
- Assume that because you are in conflict with someone close to you it's the end of the relationship – it may herald a productive and rewarding transformation.

Homeopathic treatment
We all find ourselves in situations where we get angry, whether it is justified or not, from time to time. Those one-off situations can be stressful in themselves, more so if they are unusual. They can leave us feeling depleted and shaken – and so stressed on occasions that physical symptoms develop. This is where you might consider taking a homeopathic remedy.

- *Causticum (Caust.)* See also p. 286.
Incredibly sensitive to conflict because of a strong sense of justice and anxiety about others. Tends not to get involved if the conflict involves people they are close to. Puts energy into fighting bigger battles for others.
- *Chamomilla (Cham.)* See also p. 289.
General bad temper. Angry, irritable and snappy (touchy). After an outburst develops colic or diarrhoea.
- *Colocynthis (Coloc.)* See also p. 294.
Anger with indignation. Becomes ill after an outburst of anger – with cramps or shooting pains (anywhere).
- *Nitricum acidum (Nit-ac.)* See also p. 314.
Gets stuck in, will erupt in all sorts of situations. Finds it almost impossible to forgive, hangs on to grudges and old conflicts.
- *Nux vomica (Nux-v.)* See also p. 317.
Goes into 'fight' mode in a conflict situation. Uncontrollable outbursts of anger. Impatient and stressed out – has so much to do, explodes over little things that go wrong. Furious at the time rather than afterwards.
- *Phosphorus (Phos.)* See also p. 325.
Sensitive to conflict *and* will intervene to make peace in any situation – from parents who are arguing to a fight in the street.
- *Pulsatilla nigricans (Puls.)* See also p. 330.
Sensitive to conflict, wants peace and wants others to think well of them. Cries easily in conflict situations, although may struggle to suffer in silence.
- *Staphysagria (Staph.)* See also p. 341.
Anger with indignation. Anger is kept under control (suppresses it) but eventually snaps and ends up trembling and feeling bad afterwards. Replays the situation endlessly in their mind.

CRITICISM

Constructive criticism, tactfully and thoughtfully presented, can help us to grow by making us aware of the effect we have on others, or by encouraging us to examine our behaviour and to make necessary changes. Incessant, harsh or negative criticism, however, can erode a person's self-esteem, leaving the recipient feeling blamed or attacked, and can even cause physical symptoms to develop.

Some people use fault-finding to control others, in the mistaken belief that they can change another person. Children can be particularly vulnerable to criticism because the seeds of our self-esteem are sown in childhood, and unreasonable, harsh or repeated criticism can erode away at a child's sense of self – making them feel that they don't count for much.

Some people are resilient to criticism because of their own high self-esteem, or perhaps because of arrogance. Others take it personally, either because they are generally sensitive to it or because they have been criticized a lot in the past. They find it difficult to know when the criticism is unfair, and may take it too much to heart, focusing on what seem to be their bad points and not realizing how much they are appreciated.

Any criticism, whether well-meant or unkind, may trigger distress, making us feel small, hurt, angry, weepy and trembly, defiant or sulky.

Do:
- Learn your own response to criticism, so that you can take constructive criticism in the spirit in which it is offered.
- Develop strategies for dealing with it so that it doesn't make you ill. Talking to someone close to you is a good start so that you don't let your feelings build up inside you. Talk to people who aren't bothered by criticism and find out how they deal with it. Seek the advice of a counsellor or psychotherapist if you can't develop strategies that work for you.
- Protect yourself from unkind criticism by:
  — checking out what is being said rather than taking it at face value.
  — responding to your gut feelings if you know that this criticism is unreasonable.
- Remind yourself that you deserve to be treated with respect, that however fair this criticism is, it should be delivered in a way that isn't damaging to you.
- Remember you can always ask for some positive feedback if the criticism comes undiluted and you have the (wrong) impression

that you aren't valued. Some people simply forget (or have never learnt) that they need to make sure people feel appreciated first, not to soften the blow but to put the criticism in a context where it will be more easily accepted.

Don't:
• Come away from a situation where you've been criticized feeling it's all your fault, even if you were in the wrong. Everyone makes mistakes – we all have a right to learn from them rather than be hauled unceremoniously over the coals.

Homeopathic treatment
An incident of harsh criticism can have a similar effect to shock and this is where homeopathic treatment can help.
• *Ignatia amara (Ign.)* See also p. 298.
  Swallows criticism – gets a lump in the throat or a sore throat, from all that they didn't say.
• *Nux vomica (Nux-v.)* See also p. 317.
  Furious after criticism. Intolerant of contradiction, although extremely critical themselves. Gets angry in response to criticism although can cry, which makes them more angry.
• *Silica (Sil.)* See also p. 338.
  Vulnerable to criticism because they find it difficult to fight back. May invite more criticism than they deserve.
• *Staphysagria (Staph.)* See also p. 341.
  Chews over what they wish they'd said, feels a strong sense of personal injustice, seethes with resentment and gets all sorts of physical complaints.

DEPRESSION

Strictly speaking, depression isn't a stress, it's a *result* of stress, but I have included it here because it is so commonly experienced and often triggers the realization that we have been under unacceptable stress. It can affect anyone, at any age.

Depression may result from suppressed anger, from grief, loss, loneliness, mental strain or disappointment. People sink into a sad place inside of themselves which, at its worst, is a black hole, frighteningly dark, empty and hopeless, from where the future looks bleak. They can become self-absorbed, losing interest in things that formerly gave them pleasure and finding it difficult to engage with others (especially if those people are happy) without feeling worse.

Depressed people can project their feelings on to their environment and the world in general, seeing misery everywhere. A serious depression is terrible, a sort of half life, where people put what little energy they have into going through the motions, feeling deep down that there is little point.

The following common symptoms of depression are experienced in a variety of combinations (those in italics more often accompany a severe depression and should be taken seriously):

- Exhaustion, which isn't helped by sleep.
- Insomnia: an inability to get to sleep, restless or light sleep or waking in the early morning and being unable to sleep again.
- Loss of interest in appearance.
- Loss of appetite.
- Excess smoking, drinking, drugs, or even work to dull the pain.
- Loss of libido.
- Lack of motivation, feels helpless and hopeless.
- Inability to cope with extra demands, difficulty making decisions.
- Everything seems to take a long time, even small tasks.
- Thinking, remembering and concentrating are all difficult.
- Lack of joy.
- Sadness, unhappiness.
- Crying, sometimes for no apparent reason.
- Loneliness – in spite of (or sometimes because of) having friends or family around.
- A feeling that no one can help.
- Self-pity, absorbed in sad thoughts about self.
- Low self-confidence, low self-esteem, low self-worth, a sense of inferiority.
- Guilt, anxiety, either blaming others or oneself.
- Negative, pessimistic thoughts that churn around and around.
- Gloom, a feeling of flatness.

- Indifference to family, close friends and/or loved ones.
- A feeling of pointlessness.
- Increased irritability.
- Mood swings.
- *Feeling numb, apathetic, dazed. May just sit and stare.*
- *Feeling imprisoned, separate – as if nothing is real.*
- *Despair – as if a cloud hangs overhead.*
- *Suicidal thoughts, life is bleak.*

If our lives become unbalanced with too much or too little work, relationship difficulties, work problems, any major physical change and of course, any serious emotional stress, then depression can result.

Economic and social factors are at the forefront of much depression: poverty, bad relationships, inadequate housing, financial problems, unemployment and so on.

People with close friendships and/or a spiritual dimension to their life are less likely to suffer from depression. People who are brought up to value appearances, to conform to external goals may struggle with their own self-identity, their sense of themselves dependent on meeting others' needs and on others' approval. The media (especially television) has an important effect on how people see themselves and the goals they set. We are constantly assailed with unreal role models – women with careers, families and 'perfect' figures who cope without a struggle; men as strong leaders who are active and competitive.

Adults who were neglected as children (with a lack of love, affection, acceptance and/or approval) carry that neglected and needy child into adulthood, hidden in a grown-up body. They may find it difficult to relate to other adults because of their feeling of worthlessness, and difficulties in their grown-up relationships can reawaken the childhood emotions which can then act as a trigger for depression. These patterns need to be understood and acknowledged for healing to take place.

Depression can often be overlooked by those who haven't experienced it, or haven't acknowledged it in themselves, either suppressing it or coping on their own without any help. Mild depression can go unnoticed if people are able to hide their deeper feelings as they go about their daily life – they might seem quieter than usual, but that's all. As depression deepens other more noticeable symptoms develop, and these can worsen until finally, if ignored, people can suffer a complete nervous breakdown. It is always easier to deal with depression if help is sought earlier rather than waiting for a crisis situation to arise.

Depression never surfaces in a vacuum. There may be an inherited weakness and those who have low self-esteem are often more vulnerable to it. Some people are more optimistic and positive than others, and therefore less likely to become depressed than those who are naturally negative.

It is a mistake to assume that depression is caused only by emotional stress: depression can be set off by a physical stress. Alcohol can cause it in some, especially those with a weak liver. A serious head injury or prolonged lack of sleep or a deficient diet can all cause depression.

'Depression', like stress, is a word that people use without knowing what it means for *them.* Sometimes exhaustion is mistaken for depression and vice versa. Many people's depression goes undiagnosed because their overworked GPs don't have time to look beneath the superficial complaints that patients present. When the diagnosis is made they may be given a prescription for a drug they know nothing about, including its possible side effects, and which does not take the cause of their symptoms into account.

Depression can be scary and unfamiliar, making it hard to deal with, especially for those close to someone who is depressed. Sometimes families close ranks when one member becomes withdrawn and they organize themselves around the depressed person and carry on as if nothing unusual is happening, hoping maybe that time will sort it out, not wanting to face up to the reality of the situation. This can make the depressed person feel more alienated. Those close to someone who is seriously depressed may also need support – as well as information and advice.

You will need to seek professional help (from a homeopath *and* a counsellor or psychotherapist) if you have been suffering with a long term depression or if your symptoms of depression are severe – that is, if you feel suicidal, that you've lost touch with reality, or that you are separate from everybody and everything, or if it seems as if your feet aren't solidly on the ground when you are standing or walking.

If you are close to someone who has passively lost the will to live or who is talking about suicide, get them appropriate, competent, professional help if they won't do so for themselves. Sometimes those who are suicidally depressed drop clues rather than speak directly about how they feel: 'There's no point in doing anything' or 'I wish it were all over.' It isn't interfering to get help for them. It may save their life. If you are close to them you have a duty at least to try.

Do:
- Try and work out the cause of your depression. It *may* be emotional stress, but if it is a physical stress this will need dealing with instead of, or as well as emotional stress.
- Check that any medication you are taking is not causing or contributing to your depression. Antibiotics, steroids and the contraceptive pill, as well as many other ordinary everyday medications, are capable of causing depression as a side effect. Ask your doctor to reassure you about this, or you can look up your medication in one of the many books available that list common drugs and their side effects, and discuss the alternatives with your GP – especially if you are on long term medication. It may be possible to take a break from the drug or change the prescription.
- Remind yourself that *this too will pass*. Put your depression into perspective (or get some help with this) and remind yourself that it won't last forever, even if it *feels* like it will.
- Take one day at a time and spend some time every evening going back over the day and list the ways in which you *have* coped. List each achievement, however apparently insignificant, from getting up in the morning to eating lunch, visiting a friend and brushing your teeth. *All* these things count when you are depressed.
- Make an effort to do something enjoyable and pleasant every day: a walk, a bath, listening to music, playing with your dog or cat; or, once a week, go on an outing to the theatre or cinema.
- Re-appraise your life/lifestyle. Go back over the previous year or two and list all your stresses; then remember the time before

you became depressed and ask yourself whether your daily routine had become relentlessly hard work, with no time to yourself, and no time for fun. Start thinking about how (and whether you are willing) to make some serious (and not-so-serious) changes.

- Find a way to express the pain that lies under your depression *in your own way*, with or without the support and guidance of a counsellor or psychotherapist.

- Spend some time on your thought processes – they have tremendous power in our lives, in sickness and in health. Harness this power to enhance your health rather than reinforce your depression. Depressed people spend a *lot* of time thinking unhappy thoughts and unfortunately, it isn't possible to change your thoughts simply by wanting to. The following steps may be helpful – be creative with them, skipping those that don't work for you, or get some professional help if you can't do it on your own, if it simply makes you feel worse:

  — Get curious. Without being critical or judgemental work out what happens to your thought processes, especially when you are feeling low. Do you have any repetitive thoughts? What are they?

  — Write down your most depressing thought, the one that repeats itself over and over, the one that represents the core of your depression.

  — Expand this message by looking behind it. For example: 'No one can help me . . . because they don't care about me . . . because I don't need anything . . . because I am worthless.' Where did this message or thought come from?

  — Be honest with yourself about the reality of your message. How true is it?

  — Ask yourself what the positive 'payoff' of this message is. How does it help you and what does it protect you from? And how is it working against you now? For example: 'No one can help me . . . because no one did when I was a child and I learnt to be independent and not ask for anything. That protected me from hurt [positive payoff] but now I feel imprisoned by it, trapped.' Turn it around, i.e. 'If someone could help me what would they have to do?' and then 'If someone could help me what would I have to do?'

— Ask yourself if you are willing to let go of this thought, this message. You need an unequivocal 'yes' to be able to go to the next step. Choose the words that best describe how you feel able to begin to change this message. For example, 'Although I sometimes *feel* alone I recognize that I am not actually alone. I want some support right now. Maybe it's OK to ask for it.' You may be able to move away from your entrenched position towards one where 'maybe' you could ask for help.

— Say the new message out loud, taking a deep breath as you do so. Say it into the mirror. Say it without thinking about the words, without caring particularly whether it actually happens, without willing it to happen – turn it into a mantra or prayer.

- Ask someone close to you, someone you care about and trust, to tell you they care about you and/or love you or to write it down. If you are depressed to the point where you feel you can't do this, then dig out some old cards or letters from people who care about you and try and take in their warmth.

- Consider some radical action, an unscheduled break such as a weekend retreat or a few days away. The break you have been promising yourself for five years but have never taken! A visit to family or a friend who has moved to another part of the country, someone you miss who you know will make you feel better, who will be able to give you some of what you need. You may find yourself saying that you can't take time off, that you can't afford to. In this case ask yourself what would happen if you became ill with, say, a bad flu.

- Make practical changes if your depression is the result of a difficult relationship or lousy work situation. It's *never* as difficult as it seems when you're apparently stuck in it. Get some marriage guidance counselling if your relationship is on rocky ground and making you depressed. Consider a job change or even a departmental move if your current work situation is untenable.

- Search deeply and honestly in order to try and find out what it is you need. Ask yourself 'What do I really want? Right now?'

- Find something that makes you laugh (or smile) and do it on a daily basis. Even when depressed, most people can find it in themselves to laugh at their favourite comic, comedy show or funny book.

Don't:

- Blame yourself for your depression. This will only make it more difficult for you to heal yourself. It isn't your *fault*, and neither is it anyone else's. It will be a combination of circumstances: your inheritance, your history, your character and your situation. You do have some say in how you will deal with it so don't let self-blame stop you.
- Don't measure yourself up to others at a time like this, it will only add insult to injury. Your depression is unique to you, just as all your other feelings are. Snapping out of it is the emotional equivalent of ignoring a badly sprained ankle and carrying on as if nothing had happened. That ankle will take longer to heal and be vulnerable to re-injury. Ignoring your feelings is as damaging to your health as ignoring hurt in any part of your body, physical *or* emotional.
- 'Suppress' your symptoms with orthodox medication and carry on with your life, except as a short term measure. The drugs will help ease the pain but the underlying cause or causes will remain undealt with. There are risks of side effects *and* dependency, drugs dull people's reactions, making them emotionally numb, and they can take away the motivation to make necessary changes. N.B. Serious, long term depressions *always* need professional medical attention.
- Neglect yourself – even though you may feel like doing so.

Homeopathic treatment
The homeopathic remedies listed in this section are to help with acute depression, where you can easily identify its cause. Don't self-prescribe on a deep-seated depression. Do remember to write down what you have taken, why you took it and what the results were so that if you need to seek the advice of a homeopath you can give him or her this information.

- *Aurum metallicum (Aur.)* See also p. 269.
  Despairing depression, commonly caused by a business loss or a personal failure of some sort. Everything seems black. Feels ˙ worthless.
- *Kali phosphoricum (Kali-p.)* See also p. 301.
  Depression from over-excitement. With simple exhaustion.

- *Lachesis (Lach.)* See also p. 302.
  Depression from suppression (physical or emotional). Depressed and suspicous. Feels much worse on waking in the morning.
- *Natrum muriaticum (Nat-m.)* See also p. 310.
  Quietly and deeply depressed. Sad and resentful. Comes on after a loss or a disappointment. Hides feelings: may not realize the depth of their emotions and especially doesn't want anyone else to see them.
- *Pulsatilla nigricans (Puls.)* See also p. 330.
  Depressed and weepy. May have suffered a loss. Feels lonely, wants sympathy, and feels better for it, and also feels better after crying.
- *Sepia (Sep.)* See also p. 334.
  Worn out, depressed and irritable. Feels better for crying but wants to be alone and doesn't want to be comforted. Indifferent to close friends and relatives (including their children).

DISAPPOINTMENT

A disappointment is usually associated with loss of some sort. It may be a dream or expectation, or it may be more concrete – a failed exam, a job that didn't materialize, a relationship that didn't work out.

Identify whether you are experiencing the shock of bad news, or perhaps a sense of humiliation or failure, before you consider straightforward disappointment. The words you use to describe what has happened as well as your feelings will guide you: 'I've had some dreadful news, I feel really confused'; 'It was a terrible shock – I don't feel anything, well, sort of numb'; 'I feel so disappointed – like all the stuffing has been knocked out of me' or 'No, I don't feel a failure, I just feel despondent about it all.'

The positive side of disappointment is that it can spur us on to make a re-evaluation of our goals, aspirations and dreams, whether these relate to a job, a relationship or a study project. Sometimes when we don't get what we thought we wanted, we find out what we do want and are able to act upon it.

Some disappointments can be a huge blow, can be hard to get over and can cause a terrible despondency.

Do:

- Step back and get a sense of perspective: the job you were turned down for is not the only one. Even if you have applied for 300 jobs, the one that has your name on may still be around the corner.
- Use every disappointment as an opportunity to become a stronger person. What can you learn from this experience? Did you leave studying for your exams until the last minute, thinking you were bright enough to cruise through them? Did you make certain assumptions about this relationship without checking them out first?
- Get philosophical: maybe this job wasn't meant to be. It probably isn't helpful to read these words right now, but it can be useful to have some sort of broader framework within which you can accept the blows that fate seems to deal out from time to time.

Don't:

- Keep banging your head against the same brick wall. Change your tactics if what you are doing isn't working – get some help with this if you can't see any other way forward.

Homeopathic treatment

If you find yourself lacking in motivation after a disappointment then consider one of the homeopathic remedies below. They will help you to heal the emotional wound and get you going again. If you sink into depression after a disappointment see pages 105–113 for some additional help.

- *Calcarea phosphorica* (*Calc-p.*) See also p. 281.
  Disappointment with exhaustion. Becomes discontented and dissatisfied and full of negative thoughts.
- *Ignatia amara* (*Ign.*) See also p. 298.
  Acute disappointment with shock – especially after a disappointment in love.
- *Natrum muriaticum* (*Nat-m.*) See also p. 310.
  For those who have suffered many disappointments, who have suffered inwardly and on their own, who have sunk down into grief, but who may be putting on a brave face in spite of it all.

- *Phosphoric acid (Phos-ac.)* See also p. 323.
Disappointment with apathy. Becomes exhausted, physically *and* mentally. After a relationship disappointment grieves silently.
- *Staphysagria (Staph.)* See also p. 341.
Disappointment with resentment and indignation. 'How could this happen to *me*?'

EMBARRASSMENT

Most people dislike feeling exposed, especially if it involves having done something stupid or silly in public. Embarrassing incidents can make us blush and break out in a sweat every time we think of them – *and* they can be hilarious, if only we can see the funny side.

Some people are naturally shy and bashful. They can't bear to be embarrassed and hate the idea that others may be laughing at them. They find social situations difficult and are nervous at parties, where they feel awkward. Teasing, however 'good-natured', upsets many people as it usually seeks to ridicule the object.

Do:
- Remember, no one actually dies from embarrassment! However close they get to wishing they could.
- Avoid people who are unkind or nasty, who go out of their way to embarrass you in social situations. You don't have to put up with being deliberately embarrassed.
- Confront people who make your life difficult, who find it amusing to embarrass you because you rise so easily to the bait. Tell them how their behaviour affects you and ask them to stop.
- Recount the embarrassing episode to a good friend who will laugh over it *with* you (not at you) and by so doing help you to feel better about it.

Don't:
- Brood on an embarrassing incident. Remind yourself that everyone else involved has probably forgotten it already.

Homeopathic treatment
- *Ambra grisea (Ambr.)* See also p. 257.
  Naturally shy and anxious and easily embarrassed in social situations. Blushes furiously. Feels awful afterwards.
- *Baryta carbonica (Bar-c.)* See also p. 271.
  Shy, serious and sensitive. Hates to be teased and because of that tends to attract it.
- *Pulsatilla nigricans (Puls.)* See also p. 330.
  Shy, sensitive and easily embarrassed. Blushes easily. Feels victimized.
- *Sulphur (Sul.)* See also p. 345.
  Tends not to think of others and therefore can put both feet in it and feels bad afterwards about what they have said or done.

EXCITEMENT

Wonderful, exciting things can be stressful too! Christmas, parties, falling in love, celebrations, getting married, new babies, winning a large amount of money: the full force of unbridled joy or excitement can be overwhelming, especially if it is unexpected. Joy is a powerful emotion and needs to be expressed.

Excitement can lead to over-excitement: some people go up and can't get down again. This is most clearly seen in children who can become wild with excitement. People may cry as well as laugh with happiness, may want to scream with excitement. If these feelings aren't expressed, contained or calmed, it may be difficult to sleep. They may feel as if they are going to burst with excitement, then get headaches, can't eat and become exhausted, even mildly depressed.

Excitement has a similar physical response to fear, and because of this some people mistake the signals their bodies give them – feeling fearful or anxious in situations instead of interpreting the signs as excitement.

Excitement and joy are energizing, motivating emotions: they light up the dark corners of our lives and make us feel good. If we express them they can be contagious, lighting up other people's lives as well.

Unfortunately many people are brought up *not* to get excited because of the fear that it will get out of control. Some people grow up with the belief that they mustn't make too much noise about the good things they have because someone will take them away, or they will have to share them. They are brought up not to boast about their happiness or successes, and they damp down their enthusiasm in an attempt not to arouse envy in others. This is a big mistake: the suppression of happiness is as stressful as the suppression of any other emotion.

Do:
- Express your feelings fully without harming yourself! Do a dance, a jig, a whirl, give yourself a good shake, sing your favourite song at the top of your voice, hug someone close to you.
- Ground yourself by doing something physical like cooking or gardening or having a bath, or go for a run or a fast walk.
- Share your excitement with others – without censoring it, without damping it down. You *won't* be tempting fate – happiness shared simply doubles it and spreads it to others, like any other feeling. There is plenty of room in the world for *lots* more joy, happiness and excitement.
- Try 'redefining' your fear or anxiety just in case there's some excitement lurking unacknowledged. For example: it's your wedding day and you are overwrought with nerves. Everybody has told you, repeatedly, that it's normal to be nervous. Try saying to yourself, silently or out loud: 'I'm incredibly happy. I feel really excited.' Breath deeply. If you fill up with warmth and feel relieved, then go on saying it and ditch the 'nervous' message. If it doesn't 'fit' then try and find out what is making you nervous and deal with it if you can.
- Question thoroughly that belief that says 'It'll all end in tears' for yourself or your children. Sometimes it does, but usually only when you openly expect it to.

Don't:
- Suppress your happiness to make other people feel okay.

Homeopathic treatment
- *Coffea cruda (Coff.)* See also p. 293.
  A pleasant surprise causes over-excitement and then cannot unwind, especially to sleep.
- *Kali phosphoricum (Kali-p.)* See also p. 301.
  Nervous exhaustion from over-excitement.
- *Opium (Op.)* See also p. 321.
  Sudden, unexpected surprise or sudden joy. Feels dazed, out of touch with reality, as if it's all a dream. Finds it hard to express the excitement.

FAILURE

Failure is always stressful, the more so if it has been preceded by a period of hopefulness, of anxiety and hard work. We are more susceptible to feeling a failure if our external goals are the guiding light in our lives. Having put all our eggs in one basket, if we fail, our whole world crumbles, and this can be devastating.

In a business, the stress of losing one's livelihood is all-encompassing. It may include the loss of a home, of position, money and possessions, and relationships may also crumble under the strain. When this happens we have to face starting again from scratch, self-confidence and self-esteem in tatters. Flunking an important exam can cause a sense of failure, especially if expectations were high, and especially if the individual concerned has based their life plan on passing. Losing a court case is stressful, more so if a lot is tied up in winning, either emotionally or financially or both. People can feel they have failed when a relationship doesn't work out.

Common emotional reactions to failure are shock and then the need to blame somebody for what has happened: some blame other people – their husband or wife, the government, a business partner, even God. They may feel humiliated, betrayed, angry. A pervasive sense of impotence and a loss of self-confidence are common, as well as despair and a desire to give up. It is then that depression may set in.

Do:
- Use each failure to re-examine your goals, dreams and aspirations.
- Find some inner strength/peace via meditation, prayer, silent reflection or writing in a journal. You need this now more than ever.

Don't:
- Forget that behind every successful person are many 'failures'. It is our ability to bounce back and to try again that makes us strong and enables us to succeed.

Homeopathic treatment
The following remedies can take the edge off recent feelings of failure, but if you have been suffering for some time it is important that you seek the advice of homeopath and/or counsellor.
- *Argentum nitricum (Arg-n.)* See also p. 262.
  Failure with constant state of anxiety. Frightened of taking on a new project in case they fail again. Energy becomes scattered and can't persevere at anything for long.
- *Aurum metallicum (Aur.)* See also p. 269.
  Failure with black despair. Usually a business failure although it can be any failure, often where a loss of money is involved.
- *Nux vomica (Nux-v.)* See also p. 317.
  Failure with humiliation. Turns to drink and tries to keep on going. Becomes irritable and eventually burns out and loses all ambition.
- *Silica (Sil.)* See also p. 338.
  Failure (business or examination) with sense of inadequacy. Can't get going again, frightened of taking anything new on in case they fail.
- *Veratrum album (Verat.)* See also p. 351.
  Failure with loss of money and/or position. Feels angry and humiliated at losing their position and all that came/went with it.

FEAR

Fears can be rational – as a child you were bitten badly by a dog and have been frightened of dogs ever since. Or they can be irrational – you don't know where the fear comes from but it is always there, a part of who you are, or, perhaps, you are frightened of something that logically you know cannot hurt you.

We all fear different things, and you may never be able to answer satisfactorily why you are afraid of thunder or the dark. It is probably more useful to ask yourself how your fears affect you, and whether they limit you in the course of your life. For instance, a strong fear of crowds may stop you travelling, or going shopping or to the cinema. Other feelings may underpin a fear. For example, a fear of heights or of flying can be linked with a deeper fear of losing control in someone who likes to be in charge, a fear of being alone can be caused by emotional trauma. Fear may be a symptom of a longer term emotional stress such as anxiety or even anger that hasn't been dealt with and has been displaced on to something more ordinary.

When frightened, people experience scary, repetitive thoughts and catastrophic fantasies. The mind can seize up, making it difficult to know what to do next. Physical symptoms are similar to anxiety, only more so – a fast pulse, sweating, pallor (colour draining from the face), palpitations and trembling are all common.

Remember that in many circumstances fear keeps us safe. Its positive function is to alert us to danger. It is when irrational fears disable us in ordinary, everyday situations that we need to get help. If a fear becomes a phobia, consider consulting a psychotherapist skilled in working with phobias.

Do:
- Avoid situations that bring out your worst fears (like watching *Raiders of the Lost Ark* if you are terrified of snakes or going on a cruise if you are scared of water). You do not have to put yourself through unnecessary stress. If you find yourself sweating and anxious on a cliff top walk then find another path further inland – far enough away for you to feel at ease and be able to breathe normally again.

- Seek out alternatives: travel by bus if you are frightened of the tube, take B roads at a slower pace if motorways terrify you. It may take longer but it will be worth it.
- Use commonsense measures to make your life easier: leave a night light or a landing light on if you are frightened of the dark. The same applies for children – your job as a parent is to make the world a safe place for your child and if they are frightened of the dark (for whatever reason) it is unnecessarily cruel to try and train them out of it.
- Ask for help in difficult situations: ring up a friend or neighbour and ask them to come over and be with you if you are freaking out in a violent thunderstorm. Don't make light of your fears – if you are terrified then say so. People are usually honoured to be asked to help out in an emergency.
- Talk yourself through a difficult but unavoidable situation that you can't easily get out of, for example if you're caught up in a crowd and can feel fear and panic rising:
  — Use reassuring words and phrases and keep repeating them. 'I've been through this before – I can get through it again.'
  — Remind yourself that this is (just) an endurance test. It won't go on forever. All you have to do is get through it.
  — Ask for some inner strength/help: find a quiet, calm place inside of yourself (close your eyes if necessary to do so). Some people find prayer helpful.
  — Take slow breaths: start with taking one slow breath. Don't bother about it being deep or long. In fear we tense up and breathe shallowly and this deprives us of much needed oxygen. Breathing will help you deal with a frightening situation better. Once you've started, take another breath and then another. And then keep going.
  — If you can't breathe because you've become rigid with tension then scrunch up all the muscles of your arms (including making your hands into fists) and shoulders and jaw as tight as you can. Then let them go as floppy as you can and as you do so take that first slow breath. Keep repeating this until you can breathe more easily. Feel your feet on the ground, whether you are standing up or sitting down.
  — Imagine you are heavy – if you are lying down especially. Feel

your body sink 'through' the bed (it can't but it will help you *not* to hold yourself hovering above the bed with tension and fear).

— Concentrate if you are actually in danger, i.e. if you are in a situation where your worst fears are realized. For instance, you are on a motorway overtaking a coach and one of your tires blows out. It's vital that you don't go out of control along with your car.

— Watch out for hyperventilating: if you breathe rapidly and shallowly, taking in too much oxygen, you will increase your sense of panic and become faint and dizzy. Breathe into a *paper* bag or your cupped hands in order to increase your intake of carbon dioxide and you will quickly feel better. (See also p. 163.)

Don't:
• Be pressured into joining a group activity if you know that you will be terrified: like climbing the Eiffel Tower if you have a fear of heights. Send your friends up with a camera and ask them to take photos for you.
• Push on if you find that you're panicking half way through or up: you can usually turn back and however awkward or humiliating it is, it will be less stressful for you and much better for your health.
• Get angry with yourself over apparently irrational fears; it may be that a childhood trauma that has been buried in your unconscious has surfaced as a fear.

Homeopathic treatment
Homeopathic treatment can help with acute or recent fear and several remedies are listed below, as are some common constitutional remedies where fears are part of a bigger picture. If your fears are chronic or on-going then you will need the expertise of a professional homeopath and/or a counsellor to help you overcome them.
• *Aconitum napellus (Aco.)* See also p. 225.
  Fear (can border on terror) with anxiety. Fear of death, i.e. before an operation, a plane flight or during labour. Frightened in a crowd or a busy street, or in the underground.

- *Argentum nitricum (Arg-n.)* See also p. 262.
  Fear of heights with an irrational, frightening impulse to jump. Looking up at tall buildings evokes a fear of heights. Looking down at rivers whilst walking across a bridge causes panic. Fear of losing control in any situation: fear of flying, of being late, on motorways overtaking lorries in the fast lane, of exams. Claustrophobic: fear in tunnels.
- *Arsenicum album (Ars.)* See also p. 266.
  Fear of death. Fear of losing control especially when flying. Insecure: fears are worse when alone. Fearful when seeing or hearing of accidents because 'it might happen to them'. Fear of robbers: looks under the bed at night. Fear of becoming ill, especially of cancer, especially if a close friend or relative has it.
- *Borax venata (Bor.)* See also p. 276.
  Fear: of downward motion, of going down in lifts, of flying – but only of landing; of sudden noises.
- *Calcarea carbonica (Calc-c.)* See also p. 277.
  Fear of heights with vertigo. Generally anxious and frightened about lots of things: feeling crazy, dogs, insects, catching diseases or infections (especially in an epidemic) but also of cancer.
- *Gelsemium sempervirens (Gels.)* See also p. 297.
  General agoraphobia. Fear of losing control: becomes paralysed with fear. Anticipatory fears, before any ordeal: when flying, before an exam or interview or giving a public talk.
- *Lycopodium (Lyc.)* See also p. 305.
  Anticipatory fears: before an exam, interview or performance. Fears getting lost (even in familiar territory). Claustrophobic.
- *Phosphorus (Phos.)* See also p. 325.
  Fear of the dark; of being alone; of illness. Fear of thunderstorms: of both the thunder and the lightning. Nervous and highly strung, but easily reassured.
- *Stramonium (Stram.)* See also p. 344.
  Fear of the dark which borders on terror, impossible to reassure. Fear of ghosts. Fear of small spaces (claustrophobic). Fear of water: even looking at it may cause panic, although generally it is a fear of getting in water especially the head being covered by water.
- *Sulphur (Sul.)* See also p. 345.
  Fear of heights with vertigo. Fear for others: if loved ones are late

home, will fantasize that they've had an accident and wait up until they return, then not say anything. Claustrophobic.

GUILT

Guilt, regret and blame are part of a package that people often loosely describe as feeling 'bad'. It accompanies an expectation of how we 'should' or 'ought' to have behaved, but failed. Perhaps you decided to place your elderly mother in a residential home because she can no longer look after herself, and because you cannot take her into yours. She is not happy about this. You cannot change your decision, but you feel increasingly guilty, regretting that you can't change your plans, vacillating between blaming yourself for being a bad daughter and your mother for making you feel so bad.

Guilt and blaming act as a brake on our emotional health and can eat away at us inside, contaminating our interactions and relationships. If these feelings are not resolved then ill health can ensue.

Guilt usually relates to something that happened that we can't change. The most positive effect is that it provides us with a moral code by which we decide what we can and can't do in our lives and our relationships, and it stops us from breaking the law. And the very presence of guilt can alert us to the need to sort out an emotionally stressful situation.

Sometimes the values we grow up with are overly strict, are punishing in themselves: some children are taught a distorted sense of what is right and wrong, and too many rules by which to run their lives. Some religions, for example, encourage their followers to look on themselves as 'miserable sinners' who must strive against impossible odds to escape the fires of hell.

People can feel remorse for feelings they 'shouldn't' have and for uncharitable thoughts. Anger, resentment, revenge, hatred, rage and passion have all been labelled 'bad', and for some it is a taboo to express or even feel them.

Guilty feelings may prompt you to reassess messages or beliefs you have been carrying from your childhood, which are causing you unnecessary stress in certain situations. Often these messages aren't conscious – we do things 'because we have always done them that way' or 'because we were brought up to do them that way'. But they form a part of the picture of who we are. They may prevent us from feeling good about ourselves.

Do:
- Use guilt as an incentive to explore and perhaps change your beliefs. The more you reproach yourself, however much you think you deserve it, the more likely you will be to get stuck. It takes a conscious effort of will to make a change, to discard outmoded beliefs that you have carried from your childhood. Try starting with something easy and fun: eat soup for breakfast; leave the washing up until the morning; send a bunch of flowers to a good friend just because you feel like doing it and not because it is their birthday.
- Make a list of the 'shoulds' and 'oughts' in your life: the more there are the easier it is to feel guilty every time you do not live up to these standards.
- Question your own expectations that dictate how you (and others) should think, feel, behave in different situations. Start noticing when and how you feel guilty.
- Find a way to get the reassurance and information you need if you are blaming yourself for something outside your control, for example, for your doctor to tell you (as often as you need it) that it wasn't your fault your baby miscarried.
- Make amends in any way that feels right to you, if your guilt is tied up with an incident in which you know you have hurt someone else.
- Examine your own moral code on a regular basis: your integrity depends on it.

Don't:
- Blame yourself for something you have done wrong – we all make mistakes, and deserve to be able to learn from them. If you castigate yourself for your mistakes you will add to your stress load.
- Allow others to persuade you to feel guilty because you chose to say 'no' in order to look after your own needs first or because you have behaved in an uncharacteristically assertive manner.

Homeopathic treatment
Homeopathic treatment can help with guilt in its everyday, acute manifestations, but if you have suffered it for a lifetime – perhaps starting with a manipulative parent or a hell-fire religious upbringing, which has led to many unsatisfactory relationships – it is essential that you seek professional help to undo the past damage and write yourself a new 'life script'.

- *Arsenicum album (Ars.)* See also p. 266.
  Guilty and anxious. Great desire for perfection in all they do for themselves and in all others do for them as well. If they think they have done something wrong, tends to blame others rather than themselves.
- *Aurum metallicum (Aur.)* See also p. 269.
  Guilty and depressed. Feels full of remorse, that they have neglected their duty at home or at work. Blames themselves for mistakes.
- *Ignatia amara (Ign.)* See also p. 298.
  Guilt and loss. Feels bad *and* sad, that they have done something wrong, almost as if they have committed a crime.

HOMESICKNESS

For many people homesickness is just an occasional twinge when the familiar sights and smells of home are a long way away. For some, however, 'home' is where the heart is, a sort of bedrock in an unstable world: going away from home can be an almost unbearable stress, making even short trips unthinkable. Some children suffer from homesickness so badly an overnight stay with a friend is torture. Children who have been unwillingly sent away, to boarding school for example, can suffer horribly from being separated from their home and family – as can young adults during their first days at university – or those who need hospital treatment. Unfortunately, many children suffer in silence, having been made aware of the sacrifices their parents have made to give them this 'special' education or holiday trip, or because they know rationally that their medical treatment is unavoidable and necessary.

People who travel for a living are vulnerable to feeling homesick at times, especially if they are missing a special occasion at home, a birthday or a wedding, for example.

Common reactions to homesickness in adults or children are quiet depression, a change in character, distracting behaviour, and/or weeping. Physical symptoms vary from insomnia, headaches and exhaustion, to sore throats, colds and even cystitis.

Do:

- Take some sights and smells from home with you when you travel: photos, a picture, a special pot pourri that you use in your bedroom, a favourite cushion for your bed. It'll be worth it – you can make yourself at home away from home.
- Choose your holiday venue carefully if you know that you (or a member of your family) gets badly homesick.
- Let each child move away from you and from home in their own time: some children are happily packing overnight cases before they reach the age of two and others struggle, not wanting to go, way into adolescence.
- Encourage children to tell you how they feel about going away from home, to be open and honest about staying, for example, with an elderly relative.
- Seek help for a child who has become worryingly home-bound.
- Remember that some people become homesick when moving and leaving a much-loved house that has years of happy memories. Don't leave hoping that the sad feelings will just go away in their own time. Say your goodbyes by spending a little time in each room in turn. Let yourself remember the good times and then say goodbye, moving on when you are ready. It's fine to cry if you feel sad and encourage children to do likewise. Children are open to doing this, especially if they are very attached to their home and don't want to go.
- Be thoughtful with an elderly relative who has had to go into a nursing or residential home, especially if they have had to leave a much-loved pet behind. They will need as many mementoes and comforts from home as their new place will allow. This is worth asking about before you make final arrangements about where they will stay.

Don't:

- Put yourself under unreasonable stress by travelling away from home for longer than feels comfortable to *you*.
- Send your child away to boarding school without a lot of careful thought, especially if your child is sensitive, young (under the age of nine) and you know they will find it hard to adapt to life away from home.

Homeopathic treatment

The following remedies are for acute homesickness.

- *Capsicum (Caps.)* See also p. 283.
  Homesick and melancholic in stubborn, sensitive, excitable types. Nostalgic for home. Sleeps badly away from home.
- *Ignatia amara (Ign.)* See also p. 298.
  Desperately homesick – yearns for home. Weeps on own into pillow at night. Tries to put a brave face on but looks unhappy.
- *Phosphoric acid (Pho-ac.)* See also p. 323.
  Homesick and apathetic. Becomes mentally and physically sluggish and dull.

HUMILIATION

Humiliation is a more serious stress than embarrassment and accompanies something we did or something done to us that made us wish the earth would open and swallow us. It involves feeling unpleasantly exposed with a deep sense of mortification and/or embarrassment that is hard to erase. Many different situations may lead to humiliation, from forgetting our lines in the school play with all the parents watching and then bursting into tears, to being jilted by a much-loved partner.

Humiliation, like so many strong emotions, is often experienced alongside other feelings: the shame of bungling a public appearance can be tied up with a sense of failure; the humiliation of being jilted in favour of a more 'attractive' person can come with a sense of loss or jealousy or betrayal.

Humiliation can be a strong emotional reaction to abuse, especially sexual abuse, which may leave you feeling blemished in a way that is hard to put right. You may blame yourself for what happened and feel that there is something wrong with you. Or you can end up feeling resentful and angry, blaming others for what happened to you.

The positive side of feeling humiliated is realizing because of it that something needs addressing – in ourselves and/or our relationships.

Do:
- Separate the wood from the trees. What actually happened? How did it affect you? How were you responsible? How were others responsible?
- Ask yourself whether this experience reminds you of other such incidents in your life that you swept under the carpet, that are riding on the back of this new experience and making you feel doubly (or trebly) bad.
- Find a way to come to terms with what happened, to stop blaming yourself or others. You can't wipe out what happened but eventually you *will* be able to think about it without cringing or feeling ill.
- Find some way to put what happened in perspective. This can feel like an impossible task, but while it may be very difficult to do, it will help a lot.
- Take appropriate steps to protect yourself from this happening again.

Homeopathic treatment
It is important that you take the whole picture into account when choosing a remedy, one that addresses the cause as well as the effect.
- *Colocynthis* (*Coloc.*) See also p. 294.
  Humiliation with anger. Feel furious and gets cramps as a result.
- *Ignatia amara* (*Ign.*) See also p. 298.
  Humiliation with shock and numbness. Feel that they have done wrong and blame themselves in an attempt to rationalize the experience.
- *Lycopodium* (*Lyc.*) See also p. 305.
  Feel easily humiliated because they are easily offended and suffer from low self-confidence and anxiety.

- *Natrum muriaticum (Nat-m.)* See also p. 310.
  Humiliated and deeply hurt. Feel got-at by someone they trusted and suffers inside because of that.
- *Nux vomica (Nux-v.)* See also p. 317.
  Feel humiliated and angry, especially if they feel scorned or reproached by others. Take an aggressive position (although may not express it).
- *Pulsatilla nigricans (Puls.)* See also p. 330.
  Feel humiliated and exposed. Blame themselves for what happened.
- *Staphysagria (Staph.)* See also p. 341.
  Humiliation with indignation, especially if 'told off', or have the sense they have been reprimanded. Blame others for their hurt pride but may not show it.

JEALOUSY

Fear of the loss of someone (or something) close to us – in other words feelings of possessiveness – can cause jealousy. It is an emotion rooted in a complex mixture of reactions from anger and hurt to rage and fear of abandonment, whether it is a child who feels jealous at the arrival of a new baby or an adult whose partner has left them for someone else, or who has been passed over for promotion at work.

Envy is where we covet something already belonging to someone else, whereas jealousy runs much deeper, leaving people feeling needy, afraid that there won't be enough for them too, that they will lose something important to them.

Emotions that accompany jealousy range from feeling slighted and tearful to angry and plain murderous. Jealousy can sometimes seem irrational, with no apparent cause, and can be a particularly destructive force in any relationship. However, it may be a sign that something is not being dealt with, or worse, that some deceit has been 'sniffed out' by a sensitive partner.

Some people experience jealousy more strongly than others. Those who don't feel it may be scathing about the seemingly extreme reactions of a jealous person, who may entertain violent thoughts – and occasionally acts on them.

Sometimes people suppress jealousy, professing to feel all right after a traumatic emotional upheaval. These feelings may then surface as anger, fear or anxiety: children with new baby sisters or brothers can have more tantrums or be scared 'their' baby will die. People who become easily jealous may have been brought up in an environment in which affection or attention was scarce. Or they may have lost something or someone they were close to – to someone else – leaving them with a feeling of loss accompanied by jealousy.

Jealousy can spur us on to deal with difficulties in a relationship, and help us adjust to a new situation or confront behaviour which is unacceptable to us. Or it can help us to face parts of ourselves that have been neglected – to uncover aspects of our personality or our past that we haven't faced before.

Do:

- Be honest with yourself about the depth of your feelings – the passion involved in full-blooded jealousy can be scary. Try and get to the root of where they came from.
- Use feelings of jealousy to renegotiate the terms of an intimate relationship. You will need to talk things through if, for example, you have agreed to an 'open' relationship but find that your feelings are unexpectedly painful; or if you start seething at the amount of time your partner spends with her parents.
- Help jealous children to understand their feelings. Children (of any age) who find it difficult to verbalize their feeling may be helped through drawing or painting, or through playing with dolls. Dolls' house dolls are particularly useful – they can be given actual names or just labelled 'mother', 'child', 'baby', etc. All sorts of interesting situations can be played out, and it is fun to have a dustbin you can dump various individuals in from time to time! Don't judge what your child does with various members of the family – just acknowledge the action and the feelings that go with it. You don't need to comment beyond accepting and empathizing by saying something like 'That's how I feel at times'.

Don't:

- Judge yourself harshly for feeling jealous – you are not a bad person, you just have strong emotions that need dealing with.

- Be critical of your children or others around you for feelings of jealousy, however irrational they may seem. Feelings aren't rational – by definition. They give us information not just about what is going on in the present, but also about how our past is impinging on our current lives. We need to try and understand them, put them in context and then respond to them, hopefully appropriately.

Homeopathic treatment
Homeopathy can help those who are out of balance as a result of jealous feelings. Only use the following remedies if they fit the whole picture well.
- *Apis mellifica (Apis.)* See also p. 261.
  Jealous and aggressive. Becomes sensitive and restless – to the point of hyperactivity in children.
- *Lachesis (Lach.)* See also p. 302.
  Jealous and possessive. Becomes 'wild' with jealousy, angry, spiteful and malicious.
- *Pulsatilla nigricans (Puls.)* See also p. 330.
  Jealous, clingy and insecure. Feels hard done by – may even say 'It's not fair'.

LONELINESS

Loneliness is a sort of emotional desert. There's no colour in our life, but mirages of what we want plague us from the inside as longings come in the form of dreams and fantasies – longings that seem unattainable. It's a hard stress to endure – the feeling that you are all alone, that no one would care if you dropped off the face of the earth tomorrow.

Everyone feels lonely at times – adolescence can be miserable, as can old age, especially after a partner dies. Those who are disabled may have to endure unbearable loneliness, mothers at home with small children can feel surprisingly lonely. And then we can feel lonely in some quite unlikely places – on holiday, for example, in a place where you don't speak the language, the food is unfamiliar and you are surrounded by strangers.

Permanently lonely people often feel that they don't count, that they don't have a place, that people don't like them, that nobody values them. They long for a feeling of connection – with anybody – but their neediness may push others away. Perhaps anger and a sense of rejection keep them isolated – it's hard sometimes to break through that shell.

Children may feel neglected at home because their parents are busy working, looking after younger children or are unable to show affection.

In an adult, loneliness can be a pit into which we fall and which can be hard to climb out of. It may lead to depression, or be a symptom of depression. Don't try to deal with it on your own: seek professional help if you find yourself swamped with loneliness.

The positive side to loneliness is that we can reach parts of ourselves that we would ordinarily miss when distracted by work, friends, family and things to do. Time spent alone gives us the opportunity to just be with ourselves, our thoughts and feelings. To take stock. Sometimes loneliness provides a spur for dealing with something difficult that we have been avoiding.

Do:
- Explore your inner loneliness. Find out where it comes from – a miserable childhood, a bereavement or loss or incident of abuse is often at the root. An event like moving house or becoming a parent for the first time can also be incredibly lonely, especially if you don't have a network of friends or relatives to help you adjust. Write in your journal and see what comes out.
- Acknowledge the lonely times – allow yourself to wallow in self-pity, to really feel your loneliness, without blaming yourself or being self-critical. For a time.
- Try to navigate yourself out of your desert. It won't necessarily be easy. Even if you limp from oasis to oasis, you'll get out eventually – or you'll find a happier, more nomadic existence.
- Do something, every day, that will get you out and about in contact with others.
- Have a conversation with somebody every day – by phone if necessary, or by letter if you aren't able to get out or phone someone.

- Identify what you are missing in your life and be creative about possible solutions.
- Join a local group – it doesn't matter what it is. You may feel lonely initially (it is possible to feel more lonely *with* people than when you are on your own) but you'll feel better for having tried and you might make a friend.
- Get a pet – a dog or a cat if you are at home all day. They can be marvellous company. (Remember, though, that pets cost money in food/vets/insurance fees, etc., and dogs need training to be really lovable.) Or put a notice in your local newsagent's window offering to walk dogs – that way you can get the enjoyment without the responsibility. There are far too many pets on their own all day every day, and far too many lonely people on their own every day. It's about time they got together!
- Be aware of children who are going through lonely times and be supportive. It always helps if, when we are lonely, we feel there is someone out there who values us, who loves us, who sees what we are going through.

Don't:
- Hide away – make sure somebody knows you are there.

Homeopathic treatment
Use the following remedies only if the whole picture fits really well. If your feelings of loneliness are deep and dark then you will find it helpful to talk about them to a homeopath and/or a counsellor.
- *Aurum metallicum* (*Aur.*) See also p. 269.
  Lonely and despairing – usually after a loss or series of losses.
- *Ignatia amara* (*Ign.*) See also p. 298.
  Feels lonely and neglected – because they are. For children or adults who have been starved of affection.
- *Pulsatilla nigricans* (*Puls.*) See also p. 330.
  Lonely and needy. Weepy at the slightest hint of a sympathetic ear (and shoulder). Feels better for company and for crying.

LOSS

Loss may be experienced through any separation, not just death. It can be felt in a divorce, by both sets of parents and any children involved; a move, especially if it is to a different area; irreconcilable conflicts at work or with friends/family; by children going to school; through the normal passages of life (children may feel the loss of childhood as they move into young adulthood or the elderly the loss of youth). It can include the loss of a precious possession through, say, a robbery; the loss of independence through disability, ill health, poverty or old age; and, of course, the loss of ambitions and/or dreams at any age, but especially for those who face a mid-life crisis.

The loss of a loved one is one of the hardest of stresses and can be almost unbearably painful. Suddenly there is an empty hole in one's life, and the feelings that accompany it include shock (numbness, denial and disbelief), which can be especially intense after an unexpected death; grief (expressed or kept inside); anger (from irritation to rage); resentment and a desire to blame someone or something for what happened; guilt especially if there is 'unfinished business' or regrets about harsh words spoken or love not expressed; hopelessness; depression with despair about the future – and so on.

Death through murder or a natural catastrophe is a tragedy that is always accompanied by a difficult package of feelings that includes grief, anger, shock and the need to apportion blame – to hold someone to account for what happened, to find meaning in what may seem a senseless act. Sudden death, through an accident or war, or for some unexplained reason such as a cot death is always devastating.

Death is always confrontative – we face our own death and/or our own fear of death when someone close to us dies. Some people deal with this by pretending it isn't happening, others become distressed, frightened and anxious.

Relief sometimes accompanies the death of someone who has been ill or suffering for some time. Those close to them may have grieved before the death so that afterwards they feel joy that the sufferer is free at last. Some people feel free unexpectedly at the loss of a domineering parent – the sense of liberation can be energizing, especially if there is no guilt. The loss of a child, however, can be unendurable – whether that child dies through miscarriage, abortion, at birth, in infancy, or in adulthood. Couples who face infertility struggle with the loss of the children they never had but desperately wanted, often after many years of trying.

Sometimes the depth of our emotions can feel intolerable or even ridiculous as the pain of an old, ungrieved-for loss rides on the back of a new loss and threatens to overwhelm us. These feelings can pile up inside creating a pressure cooker situation, and it is this which causes health problems.

Everyone has their own way of grieving – there is no right or wrong way. For some it takes weeks, months or even years for feelings to surface and then they all come rushing out at once. Others grieve slowly and steadily, on their own or with friends. Some are confused as anger or even rage surfaces. Feelings can sometimes pass and then return unexpectedly.

Special dates become painful: birthdays, anniversaries and of course, the day of the death itself. If the loss happened at a special time such as Christmas then that period, when everyone else is celebrating, acts as a stark and painful reminder as feelings and memories come flooding back.

Death is still largely a taboo subject. We have relatively few rituals to help people through this time except for the cremation or burial, after which the bereaved are often expected to get on with their lives, especially if they have children to care for. People often don't know what to say to someone who has suffered a loss, especially a death – especially where they judge that loss to be easy to get over, i.e. an abortion or a miscarriage.

Many people are taught that to show feelings is a sign of weakness, that you literally 'grin and bear it' – even when 'it' is a death. People who are by their nature very emotional, who grow up in families where expressions of emotion are discouraged, can feel like the cuckoo in the nest, and suppressing their feelings can be terribly stressful. Other families encourage the expression of emotions – so that those who are naturally introverted can feel a pressure to be something other than they are.

The loss of a pet can be a sadder event for some people than the death of a person. For some a pet is all they have in the world – they feel more loved by their pets than by any of the humans they know. That loss can take place not just through death – elderly people going into a home are rarely allowed to take their pets. That separation can feel like a huge bereavement.

People can feel a strong sense of bereavement when they lose a physical part of themselves – after the amputation of a leg, for example – which can affect all areas of their lives. To a woman, the loss of the uterus or a breast, bound up as they are with her sexuality, can damage her sense of self. Those who have been sterilized or had a vasectomy can suffer similar feelings, as they come to terms with losing their fertility.

The life-changing diagnosis of crippling disease such as multiple sclerosis, AIDS or cancer can be devastating as people come to terms with the loss of their health and their future as they had seen it.

Some losses are unexpected: perhaps you retire and fulfil a lifetime's dream to live by the sea, but you find that you miss your old house, your friends and neighbours and the local shopkeepers. Or your children grow up and leave home and the peace and freedom that you longed for (especially throughout their adolescence) are overshadowed by feelings of emptiness and even jealousy if your child has married. Some situations are almost comical, but need taking seriously nonetheless: when Mrs. Thatcher was voted in again some people were grief-struck as their hopes for the future were dashed.

Some of the following advice applies specifically to bereavement, some is more general. Pick and choose those that feel appropriate to you and your circumstances.

Do:
- Acknowledge the loss whatever it may be: a friendship, your independence, your home, someone close to you.
- Write a letter to the person (p. 81) you have lost. This will provide you with a focus for your emotion in a way that nothing else can and help you to come to terms with it. Express your appreciation of all that you have shared together, for what that person has meant to you; reminisce about the good times and the bad; list

any regrets, especially if you have hung on to grudges or resentments; talk about how this loss is affecting you and finish by writing your hopes and wishes – for both of you.

You can even write to a lost object, to a house that was taken away from you after your business went bankrupt, or to the treasured piece of jewellery that was stolen or, of course, to a beloved pet. We sometimes project profound and meaningful emotions onto the things in our life and the loss of them can be as painful as the loss of a person.

- Remember that your feelings won't come out all at once. Go easy on yourself and take it a step at a time.
- Go with the flow – express what feels right and true to you in your own way and your own time. Remember, this is your loss and your feelings will be different to those of other people who have been through a similar experience.
- Remember that you *will* learn to live with this loss, *and* you may never get over it, especially if it is the death of a child – however much people (kindly but misguidedly) tell you that you will.
- Seek the support of a bereavement counsellor if your emotions are hard to come to terms with and/or if you are feeling alienated from those close to you. The apparently irrational feelings that can surface, especially after the death of a child, can drive parents apart if they aren't dealt with or if they become acrimonious or blame each other.

Don't:
- Spend time with people who find your feelings difficult until you are ready and able to cope again.
- Let others tell you what to do or how to behave. If others suggest that the time to grieve is over, find a way to tell them that your grieving will be over in your time, not theirs.
- Feel pressured to grieve as quickly as possible. Unresolved grief always returns, on the back of another loss, and can then be overwhelmingly difficult to cope with
- Hide your feelings from your children or those close to you in a misguided attempt not to worry them. They will pick up the more subtle (usually non-verbal) signs of your distress and worry more than if you had been straight with them in the first place.

You can't protect others, especially children, from your feelings – neither should you. Your children are learning how to be adults from your behaviour (not from what you tell them to do or say!) Try not to overwhelm them, however, and use language appropriate to their age and maturity.

- Ignore or dismiss the feelings of loss that accompany a situation that doesn't rationally seem to deserve them – for example, you put all your expectations into having a natural birth and you ended up with a Caesarean; or you dreamed that your wedding day would be the best day of your life – and it wasn't.
- Worry if you become unbearably nostalgic for a while or temporarily introspective and want to be on your own more than usual. These are a healthy part of coming to terms with loss.
- Shut yourself away to lick your wounds in solitude if you find yourself sinking into a deep depression – this is a sign that you need some help.
- Give up if your hopes or dreams are dashed. Update or rewrite them, setting yourself an easy goal so that you can begin to rebuild your self-confidence – and your hopefulness.

Homeopathic treatment
I have included several remedies for the acute shock, grief and depression that accompanies loss but it is essential to seek the advice of a homeopath if your health suffers and home prescribing doesn't quickly help.

- *Aurum metallicum (Aur.)* See also p. 269.
  Grief with deep, black despair. Everything seems dark, as if there is a black cloud over everything.
- *Causticum (Caust.)* See also p. 286.
  Grief, especially after the death of a friend or a parent. Cries easily. Becomes negative and gloomy and full of anxious forebodings.
- *Gelsemium sempervirens (Gels.)* See also p. 297.
  Paralysed with grief – maybe after the death of a child. Finds it hard to cry. Becomes dull and sluggish.
- *Ignatia amara (Ign.)* See also p. 298.
  Recent grief with shock after the loss of a child, a parent, a friend or a pet. Fights the tears, swallows the feelings and gets a lump in the throat.

- *Natrum muriaticum* (*Nat-m.*) See also p. 310.
  Grief – usually not so recent. Or a new grief awakes the sadness (unexpressed) from other losses that haven't been dealt with.
- *Pulsatilla nigricans* (*Puls.*) See also p. 330.
  Grief-struck and weepy. Cries easily, especially when talking about what has happened, and feels better for it.
- *Staphysagria* (*Staph.*) See also p. 341.
  Resentment after loss. Feels angry and abused. Thoughts of blame go round and round, especially when trying to sleep at night.
- *Veratrum album* (*Verat.*) See also p. 351.
  Loss of social position (after a move or a bankruptcy for example) is intolerable. Feels angry and blaming and becomes busy (hyperactive) to compensate for feelings that are whirling around inside.

MENTAL STRAIN

The brain can be compared to a muscle which needs to be well exercised in order to remain fit! And it is possible to overstrain it, through working it too hard for too long without adequate rest. Typical mental stresses include having to study hard for an exam; a heavy period at work with long hours; preparing to teach or lecture; writing to meet deadlines; unusual responsibility with, say, having to make too many decisions; having to learn a lot of new information too quickly – and so on. Some people say, after a period of overwork, 'My brain feels tired/worn out' or 'I can't think any more, I can't make another decision.' Thinking, remembering, decision-making, reading and talking become harder. We have the feeling that we want (and need) to rest, to simply stare at a blank wall until our brain recovers!

Our mental processes do not exist in a vacuum: they have a relationship with our emotions which differs from person to person. Some people are ruled more by their hearts, reacting strongly with their feelings in many situations, whilst others are ruled more by their heads, reacting rationally in those same situations. Rational types tend to be able to tolerate more mental strain than those who are more emotional, and for this reason can become, in the long run, more out of balance (without realizing it) because their feelings aren't letting them know when they are mentally stressed.

Do:

- Take your mental stress load seriously – a combination of a build-up of mental *and* emotional stresses can lead to ill health and ultimately to burning out.
- Start balancing out the mental stresses in your life to recharge your mental batteries: go home on time, don't take work home with you for a week (or longer if necessary), get some extra sleep, do something fun to make you laugh or take some exercise. And then do it again – until you feel your mental energy has returned.
- Pace yourself. This is a learnt skill, we all have different 'speeds', some people are naturally slower than others. Working at your own speed, however slow it is, will be healthier for you than trying to work fast to match someone else's pace – and you'll make fewer mistakes.
- Learn to 'space out' on a daily basis. Give your mind, your thinking brain a rest – sit and gaze vacantly out of the window or at your garden or at a flower, without actively thinking. Let your mind wander – let thoughts come and go without directing them.
- Take a mental holiday. Shut your eyes and imagine that all you can see is black velvet. You can do this sitting at a desk or table with your head resting in your hands (elbows on the table) and your palms cupped over your eyes. Let your body relax and breathe deeply. Let your thoughts pass through your mind until there are none left, just look at them without reacting to them and sit there on your own little island of peace. You'll be surprised at how refreshed you feel (mentally) afterwards.
- Be realistic about what you can, and can't do. Working within our limits keeps our stress at an acceptable level.
- Consider carefully before taking anything else on if you are stretched to the maximum: now may not be the time to agree to fund raise for your local charity. The more you give the more people will ask you to do. *You* are the only person who really knows what your limits are. It's not up to others to work that out.
- Delegate – it may be more hassle in the short term, but it will be worth the investment.

- Set yourself manageable goals, especially if you are studying for an exam or have a seemingly impossible task to perform like moving house. Do it in manageable chunks and congratulate yourself on each completed task, at each step of the way. Reward yourself with breaks that balance out the mental stress and help you to come back to your task refreshed and enthusiastic.

Don't:

- Think you are superhuman because you know you can cope with impossibly large work loads – you too have your limit and once you've gone over it you will find it harder to build yourself back up again.

Homeopathic treatment

The most common reaction to mental stress and strain is exhaustion. Homeopathic treatment can give your poor worn-out system a much-needed boost of energy, a kick start, and help restore some of your former vitality. The homeopathic remedies are all for mental strain from overwork or a lot of studying, which has been stressful to the point of exhaustion or insomnia, etc. If self-prescribing doesn't help quite quickly then do seek professional advice – there are many more remedies a professional homeopath can choose from.

- *Argentum nitricum (Arg-n.)* See also p. 262.
  Brain gives out after a period of anxiety leading up to an exam or a speech. Becomes dull, confused and forgetful. Excitable and nervous.
- *Calcarea phosphorica (Calc-p.)* See also p. 281.
  Mental strain with exhaustion and headaches – especially in those who have over-studied.
- *Cocculus indicus (Cocc.)* See also p. 291.
  Mental strain with trembling, exhaustion and dizziness. Becomes dazed and confused and forgetful.
- *Coffea cruda (Coff.)* See also p. 293.
  Mental strain with overexcitement. Becomes oversensitive and restless.
- *Conium maculatum (Con.)* See also p. 295.
  Mental strain with dizziness. Exhaustion with whirling vertigo.

Brain seizes up – can't even read. Depressed in a melancholy sort of way.

● *Kali phosphoricum (Kali-p.)* See also p. 301.

Mental strain with nervous exhaustion. Sensitive (to light and noise especially), jumpy, mildly depressed and mentally sluggish.

● *Natrum carbonicum (Nat-c.)* See also p. 308.

Mental strain with exhaustion and depression. Gloomy and melancholic. Worse for any exertion – mental or physical. Can't think.

● *Nux vomica (Nux-v.)* See also p. 317.

Mental strain in workaholics. Feels burnt-out from overdoing everything.

● *Phosphoric acid (Pho-ac.)* See also p. 323.

Mental strain with apathy. Can't concentrate, doesn't want to talk or think. Headaches from overwork or overstudy.

● *Picric acid (Pic-ac.)* See also p. 329.

Mental strain with complete exhaustion. Heavy, tired feeling in body and mind.

● *Silica (Sil.)* See also p. 338.

Becomes ill or collapses only after the job (exam, research project, setting up a business) has been done. Irritable and resents offers of help.

● *Zincum metallicum (Zinc.)* See also p. 352.

Exhausted and twitchy. Restless legs. Can't relax, especially at night – legs jerk and wake people up just as they fall asleep.

REPRIMAND

A reprimand or telling off can be a minor, justified one-off affair or something much more serious. Sensitive people may find even a gentle reprimand stressful and will fall ill – with a stomach ache, headache or cough.

There are plenty of opportunities for people to feel told off in their everyday lives: a policeman giving you a ticket for parking incorrectly; a nasty letter threatening legal action because of non-payment of a debt; being hauled over the coals by your boss.

The stress of a reprimand doubles if it doesn't feel deserved or justified, and is worse if it is delivered in front of others, so that there comes with it humiliation, shame and/or hurt. If there is no possibility of redress, of being able to answer to the charge, then the sense of injustice may fester inside, increasing your stress load.

Some people are naturally sensitive to being told off. Others become sensitive, perhaps because they were repeatedly reprimanded as children, unjustly or seemingly unjustly; or as adults by parents who didn't temper their criticism with praise or approval.

A well-placed reprimand, however, will make us aware of behaviour that has been unacceptable, hurtful or worse. At times we benefit from the shock of someone close to us being angry so that we can be aware of our behaviour. Reasoning, negotiating and talking things through don't always work . . . as every parent knows!

Do:
- Ask yourself why it is that you (or your child) are sensitive to reprimands. If it is because of past experiences then it may be useful to try to heal the old wounds.
- Ask yourself whether the reprimand was a bad one or whether you have overreacted because you are sensitive – either generally, or with regard to this particular person and/or this particular situation.
- Check out fully why it is you are being reprimanded.
- Teach your children to be respectful of authority figures but not frightened – or rude and nasty. They will learn this mainly by example – your example!
- Take notes – there are some situations where you might want to ask for names and numbers, and to write down information which you can then check up on when you feel calmer. So often we get caught up in our feelings and then lose our heads, forgetting what was actually said afterwards.
- Ask for an apology after an unjustified reprimand.
- Think very carefully about what it was that you have done to attract this reprimand and make amends if necessary. You may have overstepped the boundaries of acceptable behaviour.

Don't:
- Freak out, adding insult to injury. If you can't rely on your temper then it may be better to say nothing rather than to overreact.
- Answer back if someone is being seriously unreasonable and you know that they are spoiling for a fight. Deal with them in *your* time, with support if necessary.
- Fight injustice on your own.
- Answer back if someone is being reasonable – there are times when we all need to eat humble pie and make an apology for a wrong-doing, however inadvertent it was.

Homeopathic treatment
Homeopathic self-prescribing can help in a situation where you or your child has received a telling-off and become ill as a result.
- *Ignatia amara (Ign.)* See also p. 298.
  Sensitive type – feels hurt and humiliated after a reprimand. Wants to cry but doesn't want anyone to see them doing so.
- *Opium (Op.)* See also p. 321.
  Shock from a reprimand. Becomes spaced out and can't think.
- *Staphysagria (Staph.)* See also p. 341.
  Reprimand with a strong sense of humiliation and indignation. May appear to take it well but feels hurt and seethes inside.
- *Tarentula hispania (Tarent.)* See also p. 350.
  Reprimand with an hysterical reaction in highly strung types. Becomes freaked out. Children become hyperactive and destructive – turning their anger on to 'things'.

RESENTMENT

Resentment may grow or fester in any situation where we cannot express grudges, complaints, hurts, irritation or anger; where we feel taken for granted; where we have to withstand someone else's unreasonable behaviour; where we and/or our feelings are ignored.

Resentment can build up where people are caring for dependents who are sick, disabled, elderly or, even, growing children. It may feel as if the attention they need is too much even though it has to be given, sometimes with little respite.

Some people control by giving so that they are always 'in credit' in a relationship. They may dislike asking for anything, thereby creating a neat little prison for themselves and a trap for everyone else! It is easy for resentment to build up under these circumstances. Many people are brought up to be 'unselfish', not to ask for anything and not to expect thanks. Some, however, struggle to suppress 'ungenerous' feelings, growing increasingly resentful and becoming martyrs in the process. Resentment may build up when others don't offer help when needed: it is easy to feel used. 'After all I have done for them, this is what I get in return.'

In order to be able to give with an open heart we need to make sure our own cup is full. Too many people continue to give at the expense of their own valid and important needs. This is like drawing endless supplies of water from a limited source – the well may run dry.

The first symptoms of resentment can be hard to spot. You may simply find yourself avoiding someone for apparently rational reasons. But if the 'unequal' relationship between you continues, other signs will surface, such as irritation, coldness and withdrawal, as resentment builds. You may chew over certain situations in your mind, talk to others about them, and be surprised at the strength of your feelings. People who have been trained to be kind and giving often find it difficult to come to terms with resentment. As it builds and festers, and if it isn't dealt with, it can develop into a more serious hostility – with vindictive thoughts and fantasies.

Yet, resentment does have a useful function. It lets you know that your feelings of being taken for granted need attention. You may need to redress the balance in a particular relationship, or get some help if you aren't able to do so by yourself.

Do:
- Assess your own personal philosophy with regard to giving and receiving. If resentment is ever-present in many of your interactions then you will need to examine your own attitudes and beliefs in order to avoid this particular stress.
  — Is it all right to ask for help or to give without being thanked or to work without being appreciated?
  — What are your expectations from the people you work with,

and are they different with people you are close to – at home, in your friendships?

— Are you inviting others to take you for granted because of the way you treat yourself? Are you kind and thoughtful to yourself and your own needs or do you give 'selflessly' without a thought to yourself?

— What are your models for giving and receiving? How did the adults in your childhood behave? Do you need to reject the messages they gave you?

• Express your resentments early in your relationships rather than letting them build up, when you run the risk of dumping them uncontrollably and causing a lot of unintentional hurt in the process. Deal with the situation – with sensitivity so that you don't inadvertently create more bad feelings. Be clear about what sort of outcome you want. If you are particularly bad at expressing resentments then practise with a friend who's good at it. If you just want a fight then it doesn't matter what you say or how you say it. If you want the relationship to continue and get stronger then you need to express yourself clearly, without apportioning blame (see page 102). The following guidelines may be helpful:

— Use 'I' statements rather than attacking the other person by telling them what they did wrong.

— Stick to your own experience, your own feelings.

— Describe how the other person's behaviour has affected you rather than attacking them.

— Make a simple request rather than wild threats.

• Write a letter to each person who has hurt or angered you. Letters that you are not going to send. You'll be amazed at what comes out – other resentments you didn't know you were harbouring, similar situations you had forgotten about.

Don't:

• Suppress your feelings with righteous indignation. There are always three sides to every story: your side, their side – and the truth! Expressing your side will give the other person an opportunity to state their own. This will help you both to understand each other better.

Homeopathic treatment
Homeopathic self-treatment can help you through the acute phase of feeling resentful, but it is important that you address the practical and emotional issues in your life that led to it building up in the first place – and deal with them so that, in learning from the experience, you can prevent the same thing happening again.

- *Arsenicum album* (*Ars.*) See also p. 266.
  Resentment with selfishness. Gives but keeps a mental score. Expects a return. Becomes cold and picky when unappreciated.
- *Natrum muriaticum* (*Nat-m.*) See also p. 310.
  Resentful and hurt. Has really given a lot, tends not to show how much and may even brush it off, then becomes hurt when unappreciated. Will not show that either.
- *Nitricum acid* (*Nit-ac.*) See also p. 314.
  Seething resentment. Angry at how they have been treated. Vindictive. Cuts off friendships. Finds it hard to forgive.
- *Staphysagria* (*Staph.*) See also p. 341.
  Resentment with suppressed anger. May be sweetness and light with those concerned, but explodes with anger when it finally comes out.

SHAME

Shame is a response to an event that leaves a person feeling under attack and blaming themselves. There is a sense of disgrace, of something dishonourable having been done. We can feel ashamed of ourselves or of others, depending on the circumstances. We can bring it on ourselves – through behaving badly, by doing something that is against the law of the land, or our own moral code; or we can experience it as a result of a traumatic event, like sexual abuse; or through someone close to us (someone we may have trusted) behaving shamefully.

It is an emotion that is hard to heal because it comes in a package with so many other feelings: disappointment, hurt, guilt, rage, etc., and because we have to face a side of ourselves (or others) that may previously have been hidden. But we can use it to confront an unpleasant facet of ourselves or others, and become wiser in the process.

Some adults (teachers and even parents) use shame as a punishment, and in sensitive children this can be devastating, leaving them with shattered self-esteem and a deep sense of badness that is hard to put right, leaving a kind of emotional toxic waste.

Shame is a common consequence of abuse, including sexual harassment; mugging; domestic violence or any situation where a person's safety or sense of self is violated. People blame themselves, in a misguided attempt to make sense of a difficult experience, or they blame others as a way to express anger. They can become withdrawn, suffer from a loss of confidence and trust in themselves and others, and have their self-esteem eroded.

Anxiety, nervousness and depression are all common in those who have been abused, with feelings of self-disgust in those who have been sexually abused. Children may regress, bed-wetting and suffering from a delay in their development (mental or emotional). They may become more overtly sexual if sexually abused, or aggressive. If the aggression is not seen as a plea for help then a more serious disease can develop such as anorexia, night terrors or obsessive behaviour. Abuse may perpetuate abuse: adults who batter their babies or those with a history of violence were often . abused themselves as children.

Shame can be a consequence of something we did that was, indeed, wrong. Something we regret, a mistake, an oversight or even a misunderstanding. Rather than hide away, facing up to the consequences of our behaviour and making amends can be a useful learning experience. Healthy shame provides an important check in our lives, letting us know when we have done something that goes against our own moral code, and it can give us the impetus to reassess and update our values – as well as our self-esteem.

Do:
- Find a way to sort out the wood from the trees. Do your feelings of shame stem from something you have done, or something someone else has done to you, or something someone else has done which has affected you indirectly?
- Find a way to make amends if you feel ashamed of something

you have done so that you can learn from it and preserve your own integrity.

- Make a commitment to dealing with your own shame so that you can forgive yourself and move on. Blaming yourself will keep you feeling bad about yourself and contaminate all your relationships.

- Look at how and whether you need or want to forgive others who have shamed you. Understanding other people's behaviour and motives can be helpful in our healing – and it can be very difficult to forgive, for example, a relative who sexually abused you when you were a child. You might want to remind yourself that you don't *have* to forgive this person (or persons); rather, that you may forgive them in your own time . . . as and when you are ready and able to. There are many steps to take on the path to forgiveness, one of which is to face the feelings and thoughts you have been carrying as a result of a particular experience. This is work that generally needs to be done with a counsellor or a therapist trained in working with people who have been abused, because it can be hard to come to terms with feelings of violent rage or hatred for example, and move through these feelings to a more accepting state of mind.

- Seek help if you have suffered abuse which has left an emotional wound that isn't healing: if you are experiencing nightmares, depression (especially if it is accompanied by an altered sense of reality), sexual difficulties, difficulties within your intimate relationships, inexplicable physical sensations or a repeating pattern of abuse in your relationships (at home and/or at work) where you feel powerless and helpless.

Don't:

- Let shame eat away inside you: it is never too early (or late) to deal with it and whatever has caused it. Sweeping it under the carpet will create an underlying tension that will affect your relationship with yourself and others close to you.

- Keep an incident of abuse (especially sexual abuse) secret – *especially* if someone has asked you to do so.

- Blame yourself or allow anyone else to blame you if you were abused. No one deserves to be abused and taking the blame will prevent you from healing. It is important that children also understand this.

Homeopathic treatment
The homeopathic suggestions are first-aid measures only, to help with acute situations. If you are carrying a deep sense of shame about yourself – especially if it relates to sexual abuse – it is essential you seek professional help.

- *Aurum metallicum (Aur.)* See also p. 269.
  Shame in those with a strong sense of duty. They blame themselves for what happened, feeling they have done something wrong, suppressing angry feelings and sinking into a depression because of this.
- *Ignatia amara (Ign.)* See also p. 298.
  Shame with feelings of numbness and a sense of constriction on the chest, of not being able to get enough air in. They blame themselves and feel guilty, as if they had done something wrong.
- *Nux vomica (Nux-v.)* See also p. 317.
  Feels shame and anger, wants to hit back and may even do so – either verbally or physically or both.
- *Opium (Op.)* See also p. 321.
  Shame with lingering shock, blames themselves and sinks into a sluggish state they can't climb out of.
- *Staphysagria (Staph.)* See also p. 341.
  Shame with indignation: especially after sexual abuse. Feels angry, humiliated and resentful, especially towards the perpetrator of the abuse; i.e. blames others, not themselves.

SHOCK

Shock is the emotional reaction we experience to a sudden, un-expected event, such as an accident, an injury (or witnessing a disaster or accident, even at second-hand on television) or a traumatic event such as a bereavement or a burglary. It is also the first reaction to many emotional stresses. Common symptoms include feeling shaken and scared, or numb if the shock was severe (with, say, a threat to life) and we are having difficulty accepting or understanding what happened. Some people rally in a frightening situation, helping others to cope, and then suffer from delayed shock once the emergency has passed. Others fall apart, and can even become hysterical and out of control.

Happy events such as childbirth or even marriage can also be a shock at least initially, and can leave people feeling disorientated and 'ship-wrecked'! Bad news can be shocking, however we receive it: perhaps you remember opening a letter, answering the phone or opening the door to learn something unpleasant, shocking or sad, that left you upset for the rest of that day – or even longer.

Dental and medical treatments, in particular any surgery, can leave people shocked – emotionally and physically – and this can slow the healing process if ignored. The diagnosis of an unexpected illness can cause many people to panic as they struggle with catastrophic fantasies. Overworked, busy doctors may skimp on information, forgetting how vulnerable patients are to medical terminology. The words 'tumour' or 'pre-cancerous' for example, may cause people to become literally speechless with fear.

Our shock response is an inbuilt safety measure, the fight-or-flight instinct where the body is flooded with adrenaline as a response to fear. This gives an energy boost for dealing with a difficult and/or dangerous situation. After that danger has passed we need to deal with the effects of this response so that we don't become ill. People who have experienced repeated shocks in their lives are more vulnerable to this type of emotional stress.

If the shocking event was particularly distressing then the response can be correspondingly severe and cause Post Traumatic Stress Disorder (PTSD). This syndrome occurs after an event that is outside the range of normal human experience such as sexual abuse, a natural or man-made disaster or the witnessing of violence. People become detached, not wanting to think about the event, finding it difficult to remember parts of what happened and losing interest in their everyday lives. They can suffer from many symptoms including: flashbacks (with pictures and feelings intruding unexpectedly), nightmares, irritability, a persistent jumpiness, chronic fearfulness, anxiety, insomnia and an inability to concentrate. Depression can develop if this state festers and isn't acknowledged or healed. People with PTSD always need professional help, from a psychotherapist trained in working with this particular disorder.

Do:
- Take shock seriously. Shock can't be seen (there's no blood) but can be as serious as a physical injury. Your nervous system and your emotions are under severe strain – now is not the time to have a cup of sweet tea and carry on as if nothing has happened.
- Breathe – shock causes us to tense up. Try it out next time you have to brake suddenly to avoid a car or bicyclist pulling out unexpectedly in front of you. You may feel frightened, angry and break out in a sweat – all at once! Take a single, slow, deep breath immediately after the shock has occurred and as you breathe it out you will feel a sense of release.
- Take some physical exercise – the more vigorous the better – to discharge the adrenaline caused by a fright and help you to relax.
- Relax after a shock in the ways that work for you.
- Ask a friend or neighbour to stay with you until a bad shock has passed – overnight if necessary. You don't have to go through this stressful time on your own.
- Get some help if you realize that you are suffering from delayed shock or from Post Traumatic Stress Disorder.
- Get any information you need to take the edge off, say, a shocking diagnosis: go back to your doctor (with a friend for support if possible) and ask the questions you weren't able to ask at the time.

Don't:
- Pretend you are all right when you aren't.
- Put your head in the sand over a situation that needs some action. Get information, get support, get reassurance – the sooner the better.

Homeopathic treatment
Homeopathic remedies will help with acute shock. The sooner you prescribe the better, but if you suspect that you are suffering from the more serious PTSD then you will need to seek the help of a homeopathic practitioner. If a reprimand or a disappointment, for

example, is at the root of a shock reaction, especially in children,
then you will need to take that into account when prescribing.

- *Aconitum napellus (Aco.)* See also p. 255.
  Acute shock with great fear and trembling. There may be a fear of
  death because the situation was so serious.
- *Arnica montana (Arn.)* See also p. 265.
  Delayed shock. Denies anything is wrong. After an accident may
  insist they are all right.
- *Belladonna (Bell.)* See also p. 273.
  Shock with great restlessness. Frightened, looks terrified (like
  Aconitum napellus) but may also be very angry at what happened.
- *Borax venata (Bor.)* See also p. 276.
  Shock, mostly in nervous babies who become jumpy and hard to
  'put down'.
- *Calcarea phosphorica (Calc-p.)* See also p. 281.
  For fear, depression and exhaustion following on from hearing
  unpleasant (unexpected) news. Becomes restless and dissatisfied.
- *Carbo vegetabilis (Carb-v.)* See also p. 284.
  Shock with collapse. Breaks out in a cold sweat and feels faint.
  Craves fresh air and feels better for being fanned.
- *Gelsemium sempervirens (Gels.)* See also p. 297.
  For shock after bad news with trembling. Becomes dazed and
  confused and doesn't know what to do next. May try to hide
  feelings.
- *Ignatia amara (Ign.)* See also p. 298.
  For shock after hearing bad news. With numbness and a desire to
  be alone. Hides feelings.
- *Opium (Op.)* See also p. 321.
  Shock with stupor. May feel a great fear (like *Aconitum napellus*)
  but sinks into a dream-like state which they can't snap out of.
- *Stramonium (Stram.)* See also p. 344.
  Shock with fear and nightmares. Usually caused by a terrifying
  situation.

TRANSITIONS

Many of life's transitions are physical stresses but because they can evoke such strong emotions, and because everybody experiences them to some degree, I have included them here.

A transition is a change in our lives over which we have little, if any, control. At birth we leave the warm, sheltered environment of the womb and make our first journey into the world; at each stage of growth we make physical, emotional and social changes that take us from sitting to walking, from being at home to going to school and so on; at puberty we move from childhood to adulthood; in our twenties or thirties (very roughly) we make decisions about work and sex and what we are going to do with our lives; in our forties or fifties we experience a mid-life transition which eventually takes us into a vulnerable period of aging – and that final transition, our dying.

Transitions can take place suddenly, sometimes unexpectedly (like some births or deaths) or they can take place over months and years (like some puberties or menopauses). Some can pass by almost unnoticed with very little fuss or trouble, and others can be lingeringly difficult. Some people can find themselves going through more than one transition at a time, for example puberty *and* parenthood, thereby experiencing an increased stress load. A transition is like any other journey on life's long road. It can be interesting, overwhelming, boring or hard work. It can run smoothly or be a rough, bumpy ride. There are no 'right' ways to make these journeys and it is by understanding these transitions better that we are able to move through them more easily and hopefully enjoy them, even celebrate them. Children, especially young children, are particularly vulnerable to transitions because of the range of feelings and physical changes that can assail them without their having a language or a framework within which to understand or express them.

There are also minor daily transitions: the change of pace and demands from work to home and back again. Working parents can find these transitions especially difficult as they let go of the mantle of 'parent' to rush to work, taking on a work personae for a certain length of time and then back again. Women experience monthly transitions leading up to their menstrual periods, and for some these can be very disruptive.

Transitions are catalysts for change because in order to move forward we have to let go of something. This can evoke feelings of helplessness and fear, especially a fear of the unknown. With each transition there is an ending: the ending of a pregnancy with birth; the ending of a relationship with divorce or death; the ending of childhood with adolescence; of fertility with menopause and so on.

Some people experience a sense of loss or regret with a major life change: someone who has reached retirement without achieving their career goals and women who have reached menopause may mourn the loss of their fertility – and will need to do so in order to embrace their post-menopausal freedom fully. Couples who have been unable to have children may find it especially hard to come to terms with this time in their lives. Men can experience a mid-life crisis (sometimes called a male menopause) in their forties and fifties as they appraise their achievements – and their failures.

A transition is always stressful, to some degree, because it usually involves physical and emotional changes which need adapting to and integrating, and is affected by our inherited strengths and weaknesses as well as our cultural and social backgrounds. There's an assumption that because we are biologically programmed to go through these changes, we should be able to do so without great difficulties. If only this were true! Unreal or idealistic expectations of, say, loving parenthood or having a carefree adolescence, are often at the root of a stressful transition. This is common after childbirth, with new parents chasing their tails as they try to come to terms with *their* reality, with the overwhelming number of changes that have come their way, contrasting sharply as they often do with the images that abound in the media.

Our health *is* affected by the passage of time through our lives, from conception all the way through to death. There are different adjustments and challenges, physical and emotional, which are particular to each age. Whilst there *are* normal developmental signposts that provide markers on our path, each person varies, each stage will affect each person differently, each person will find their own health affected in different ways. Transitions don't have to be painful and difficult, but they can be, with some stages bringing new or additional responsibilities and others asking of us that we let go of things or people that we don't feel ready to say goodbye to.

These transitions give us an opportunity to take stock: to look back and see how far we have travelled, to assess our achievements and our hard times; to look forward and reassess our goals, our hopes and dreams for the future, to make plans which take into account any updated expectations. In the present we can use them as an opportunity to make lifestyle changes, to make necessary adjustments to work and/or relationships.

Do:
- Build an awareness of transitions into your life and the lives of those close to you. Remind yourself that this is a staging post, to put it into perspective, especially if you are going through some difficult changes.
- Focus on what *is* happening to you – your body, your thoughts, your feelings – not on what *should* be happening to you or on stereotypes that you may have picked up from the media or your culture. Be wary of doctors, parents or even a critical inner voice, that tell you what you should be feeling or how you should be behaving at this time in your life.
- Be kind and considerate towards yourself, and compassionate if the changes become difficult to cope with, especially if others in a similar position have 'sailed through'. Being hard on yourself will only add insult to injury and make your transition more difficult.
- Take appropriate action to maintain or improve your health. Slow down if necessary, to provide an opportunity to integrate the changes, however mundane. Stop for a cup of tea on the way home to think through work problems in order to let them go so that you can arrive home without your mind racing. Or add something challenging into your life if your transition has left you feeling empty and bored, after, say, your retirement.
- Consider marking your transition with a 'rite of passage' – a ritual, celebration or ceremony – that is meaningful to you. You may want to be alone, for an hour or a weekend, to think and

write, or just be. You may want to throw a big party and invite everyone you know or gather certain important friends and/or relatives around you for a more intimate dinner.

- Get information and/or reassurance about what you are going through. Not knowing can be the biggest stress of all.
- Use this transition as an opportunity to take stock. Use the challenges that *your* life change throws up for you to explore your relationships with yourself and the world (including those close to you), your beliefs, your health – your life! To let go of the past and contemplate the future whilst embracing the 'here and now'.
- Make a 'time line'. Draw a long line on a large piece of paper. Put your birth at one end of the line and 'now' at the other end and fill the bits in between with important and significant events from your life. Add in some words (or even pictures) that represent how these events affected you, both then and now. Add in any illnesses or periods of ill health. As you look back down that line, try to get a sense of what has shaped you, what has made you who you are. Children love to do this too.
- Help your children to understand and adjust to changes in their lives. This can be a struggle with adolescents but it is still worth trying. Be tolerant of those who are going through tough times, without making a doormat of yourself.
- Be patient – some transitions go on for years. It's not over until it's over!

Don't:
- Ignore the signals that your body is giving you about the transition you are going through.

Homeopathic treatment
Homeopathy can help those whose health has been affected by a major life change. The remedies below are very general, and as such, should only be used if they fit with what you are going through. You may want to cross-reference this section with another, like loss for example, in order to find a remedy more suited to how you feel. If you don't find one that matches, seek the advice of a local homeopath for a constitutional prescription to help ease the passage of this transition.

- *Anacardium orientale (Anac.)* See also p. 259.
  Identity crisis at any age. Discontented, gloomy and anxious. Feels isolated and separate. Finds it hard to integrate the new energy, new feelings. Tries to cut off and hardens up.
- *Arsenicum album (Ars.)* See also p. 266.
  Finds change difficult. Worries about the future, their health, and fears death (especially in the elderly, the very sick, and the dying).
- *Baryta carbonica (Bar-c.)* See also p. 271.
  Emotional immaturity at any age (from birth through to old age). Children are late developers, slow to 'grow up' (emotionally and/or physically). The elderly can regress back to childish scattiness.
- *Calcarea phosphorica (Calc-p.)* See also p. 281.
  Generally dissatisfied and discontented. Nothing is right. A physical growth spurt causes a general depletion.
- *Lycopodium (Lyc.)* See also p. 305.
  Finds reality too much. Bright mentally but becomes allergic to responsibility, to work, to family duties. Generally lacking in confidence, they become indecisive and anxious.
- *Natrum muriaticum (Nat-m.)* See also p. 310.
  Sad about letting go of the past. Dwells on memories, idealizes them. Becomes unhappy and discontented. Keeps feelings hidden inside.
- *Pulsatilla nigricans (Puls.)* See also p. 330.
  Has difficulty separating, at any age, from those they are dependent on – although typically it is the child who finds it hard to grow up and leave home. Clings to family, or familiar territory. Feels lonely and isolated. Fine at home but shy in the world.
- *Sepia (Sep.)* See also p. 334.
  Overwhelmed with work, and hormones. For puberty, menopause and childbearing years. Becomes sluggish and indifferent to loved ones.
- *Sulphur (Sul.)* See also p. 345.
  Self-obsessed and idle. Adolescents (at any age!) who become dirty, dreamy and discontented. They make many plans, but do nothing.

UNCERTAINTY

Uncertainty is always stressful and can make you feel as if you are living in a sort of vacuum, putting your life on hold (or a part of it) whilst you wait: not knowing what is happening to your body when you are ill; not knowing what is happening to those close to you when you can see something is going on but they won't say; not knowing what is happening at work when a threat of redundancy is talked about; not knowing what is going to happen next in your life until you get your exam results, and so on. There are some situations that are desperately painful, for example, when a child leaves home without saying where they are going and the family is left not knowing, for months and sometimes for years. It is a tragedy if someone close to you goes missing and can be worse than a bereavement as there is always the chance that they may be found, which can put those who are waiting into a painful limbo.

Even everyday uncertainty, such as getting stuck in traffic without information, or when the train stops unexpectedly in a tunnel for half an hour, can be stressful; the uncertainty of being unemployed can have devastating repercussions on families and communities; those with relatives or friends in the forces have to get used to waiting, but when the posting is to a war-torn area those periods of uncertainty are harder to live with.

Uncertainty fills us with a complex mixture of feelings: worry, fright, frustration, anger, confusion and powerlessness. Helplessness may be particularly difficult to live with, especially for independent types who like to be in control, or it may bring up painful childhood memories of feeling powerless. Waiting without knowing how long the wait will be, or without knowing what the outcome will be, for oneself or for others, can be an unbearable strain. Most people can handle almost any situation, however difficult or painful, as long as they have some idea what is happening.

People respond to uncertainty according to their personalities: stoical types tend to take it in their stride, others become frightened that something dreadful is going to happen and some worry themselves silly.

There is a myth that you shouldn't worry or be upset if there is nothing to worry or be upset about. Often you *know* something is not as it seems, that information is being withheld or, worse, that you are being lied to. If such a situation does not resolve, you may doubt your own feelings and lose your trust in others, or yourself.

Do:

- Identify areas of uncertainty in your life, whether they are at home, at work or at school, with people or things.
- Explore your choices for dealing with any situation where you are waiting and make a decision about the position you are going to take. This will help you to feel that you are active rather than passively waiting for something to happen to you.
- Listen to those inner feelings. They may be accompanied by an apparently irrational anxiety but there will be *something* you can do to alleviate the situation for yourself.
- Remember, information is power. If you feel you need information in any situation then do what you can to get it.
- Find out if there is a way you can get information quicker than waiting for it to arrive in the mail. You can usually telephone to find out the results of an exam, a medical test or a job interview, or to find out how a sick relative is, but think through the consequences of asking for information if you can't then talk it through fully, i.e. with the results of medical tests. And consider how you need to give information to others, especially to children, and try to do it in a way that is age-appropriate so as not to frighten them or create unnecessary anxiety.
- Ask those close to you to take your feelings into account if you find not knowing particularly difficult to handle. For example, to ring home if they are late so that you are not pacing the carpet imagining all sorts of blood-and-guts scenarios.
- Ask yourself what is the worst that can happen in an uncertain situation so that you can face it. And look at what you would do if the worst came to the worst. It won't always be that bad but sometimes it is, in which case you will need to get all the information and/or support that is available.
- Get philosophical in situations where there is nothing you *can* do. Sometimes we have to just wait and see – there's actually nothing

to be done except acknowledge that this is a difficult time. Distract yourself and try to get on with your life.

● Fight like fury if you feel instinctively that something can be done and it won't be unless you make it happen.

Don't:
● Let an uncertain situation fester on in your life. Any action you take will enable you to feel you have some measure of control over what is happening.
● Put your life on hold whilst you wait for an uncertain situation to resolve.

Homeopathic treatment
Use one of the remedies below only if you have a clear picture and can match it, otherwise seek the advice of a homeopath.

● *Argentum nitricum (Arg-n.)* See also p. 262.
Anxious and hurried. Feels out of control and hates it. Incredibly anxious about what may happen.

● *Arsenicum album (Ars.)* See also p. 266.
Concerned for self with anxiety about the future. Fears for own welfare, especially own security, particularly financial.

● *Calcarea carbonica (Calc-c.)* See also p. 277.
Concern over others with great anxiety about anything and everything but especially about the future. Fear that something bad will happen. Feels like they are going crazy and tries to hide it.

● *Causticum (Caust.)* See also p. 286.
Pervading sense of gloom, that something bad is going to happen.

● *Gelsemium sempervirens (Gels.)* See also p. 297.
Anticipates the worst. Dreads anticipated ordeals/bad news. Feels anxious about being out of control.

● *Phosphorus (Phos.)* See also p. 325.
Uncertainty with fear and anxiety about what will happen, often centred around others' welfare.

WORRY

Worry, or anxiety, is bad for your health! It is an emotion that serves little purpose, because worry in itself achieves nothing, although short term anxiety can be beneficial in that it alerts the sufferer to an issue that requires resolution: it may signal a need for a change in pace, additional support, more study or training, or even a break.

Those who are shy are often anxious, as are those who are exceedingly conscientious and perfectionist. Anxiety can be mild to severe depending on the situation and your own tendency to get wound up. Typical symptoms that accompany it are tension, restlessness, nervousness, loss of appetite, sleep difficulties, sweating, difficulty concentrating, a racing pulse and, eventually, fears and phobias. If acute anxiety isn't attended to, ill health may result: it isn't the exams that made you sick but the days or weeks before them when you became increasingly uptight, stopped eating regularly and couldn't sleep.

Anxiety may develop into a full-blown panic attack, in which you may find it difficult to breathe, experience palpitations and even chest pain. If you start to feel faint because you are panicking and breathing too fast (therefore taking in too much oxygen and hyperventilating) then the following steps will help you to cope:

- Stop what you are doing and sit down wherever you are – even on a pavement or a supermarket floor. This is less stressful than fainting and possibly hurting yourself if you fall awkwardly.
- Breathe *slowly* into your cupped hands or a *paper* bag if you have one, to decrease your oxygen intake and increase your carbon dioxide intake. This will make you feel better immediately.

If you are always anxious in certain situations which occur frequently then you may be suffering from deep-seated, chronic anxiety, for which it is important that you don't self-prescribe. You will need to seek the advice of a professional homeopath and possibly a counsellor trained in stress management. Seek help if your anxiety is accompanied by weight loss (because you may have an hormonal imbalance) or obsessive thoughts, or if it follows drug or alcohol withdrawal.

Do:

- Take your anxiety about an event or situation seriously as it will give you information about how stressful it is for *you*. Use this information to plan a strategy for dealing with both the situation and your anxiety so that your health doesn't suffer.
- Be honest with yourself about how well prepared you are for an up and coming event such as an exam, interview or driving test. Is your anxiety telling you that you need to do some more ground work, preparation and/or revision? There's nothing more worrying than knowing, deep down, that we've left everything until the last minute and it'll be a matter of chance if we succeed. Some people are luckier than others!
- Be honest with others if you are a worrier. Make sure those close to you come home when they say they will, or ask them to telephone you to put your mind at rest. It isn't good for your health to stay up all night waiting for the hospital to call when your teenager missed the last bus home, decided to sleep over with a friend, and forgot to phone you. If others complain that you are being over-protective you can tell them how stressful it is for you to worry needlessly.
- Write your worries out in full. Especially if it is the middle of the night and you can't sleep. Break your problems down into their component parts and list them down the page. Then trouble-shoot: take each problem and list the action/s needed to deal with it as well as a date and time for each one. You'll find there is surprisingly little you can do at 3.00 a.m. to solve any of your worries.
- Do something, however small and 'easy', to get you going, to give you a sense of achievement and boost your self-confidence: tidy your room or your desk or both! It's remarkably easy for anxiety to get out of hand if you can't find anything. Or worse, if you start to lose things.
- Consciously think about something else.
- Take a glass of warm or cold milk last thing at night – calcium can help anxiety. Add a spoonful of honey for a soothing drink.
- Work out what's the worst that could happen (both fact and fantasy) and talk it through with a tried and trusted friend to put it in perspective. For example, if you don't get this job, or you

have to sit the exam again, it is not the end of the world. Remind yourself of the things in your life that *are* working.
- Do something nurturing or fun to take your mind off your worries. You'll be amazed at how much better you'll feel if you can have a good belly laugh or a tender moment reading a bedtime story to a young child.
- Help your child to understand their own worries and to deal with them so that they don't affect their health.

Don't:
- Isolate yourself and think you have to deal with a stressful and anxiety-inducing situation on your own. It isn't healthy for you.
- Wind yourself up further by sticking to the thing that is making you anxious and becoming more and more inefficient.
- Put your head in the sand by saying 'it'll be all right on the night'.

Homeopathic treatment
The following remedies are for some common anxiety-producing situations. If you find a remedy that works for you then you can use it again in similar circumstances.
- *Aconitum napellus (Aco.)* See also p. 255.
  Anxious and fearful. Suffers from a panic attack in a crowded place where they cannot easily get out.
- *Ambra grisea (Ambr.)* See also p. 257.
  Anticipatory anxiety in those who are shy and easily embarrassed. Dreads the pressure of performing in front of others – at an interview, oral exam, social event, etc.
- *Anacardium orientale (Anac.)* See also p. 259.
  Extreme anticipatory anxiety with difficulty concentrating in those with low self-confidence and a fear of failure.
- *Argentum nitricum (Arg-n.)* See also p. 262.
  Acute anticipatory anxiety with restlessness, before an exam, an interview or for stage fright. They get so wound up that they may even forget everything when the ordeal comes.
- *Arsenicum album (Ars.)* See also p. 266.
  Anxious, restless and fussy. Dislikes being in a situation where they aren't in control. Increasingly fussy and critical when anxious.

- *Calcarea carbonica (Calc-c.)* See also p. 277.
  Terrible worriers, particularly about their health. They worry about catching an infection, especially if there is one going around.
- *Gelsemium sempervirens (Gels.)* See also p. 297.
  Anxious and sluggish. Seize up both mentally and physically, becoming almost literally paralysed with anxiety – dull and dopey – especially before an exam or a public-speaking event.
- *Kali phosphoricum (Kali-p.)* See also p. 301.
  Nervous exhaustion after a period of anxiety, especially with worrying about relatives.
- *Lycopodium (Lyc.)* See also p. 305.
  Anxious and lacking in self-confidence. Dread taking on new things (jobs/interviews), exams (including driving tests), public-speaking or acting. Irritable and indecisive but when the time comes they shine.
- *Natrum muriaticum (Nat-m.)* See also p. 310.
  Anxious socially. Hates parties and gets wound up before an event where there are going to be lots of people.
- *Nux vomica (Nux-v.)* See also p. 317.
  Anxious and irritable. A difficult work period with many worries causes irritability and exhaustion.
- *Silica (Sil.)* See also p. 338.
  Anxiety with poor self-confidence in bashful but strong-willed people. Gets wound up about public speaking, exams and interviews because they don't believe they can perform well enough.

PHYSICAL STRESSES

INTRODUCTION

The maintenance of our general physical health is dependent on many factors: the old axiom 'You are what you eat' is simply not true, as it stands. Each person is a complex package shaped only in part by what they eat. While an adequate diet is important, so too are our needs for exercise, rest, relaxation and sleep. A poor diet and lack of sleep can and will affect our health, but so can other physical stresses such as chemicals (from the environment, medications and food) and external factors such as the weather, physical injury and illness.

When stress became popular as an emotional concept, physical stress faded into the background. In our excitement over a new way to understand disease some forgot about the basics. Just as it is a mistake to ignore or discount emotional or mental stresses (including those that occurred a long time ago), it is also a mistake to ignore or dismiss physical stresses when you are assessing your stress load and looking at ways to deal with it.

Some of the case histories in this book deal with complaints that are the result of physical stress alone: a baby who suffers from difficult teething (page 48); an infant who is unwell after a fall on the head (page 49); a child who is vulnerable to cold, wet weather (page 50); the effects of pollution on one man's lungs (page 55); mercury poisoning from dental treatment (page 58) and a fracture in an elderly woman (page 70). Some stories bring to life situations where emotional and physical stresses are intertwined: the emotional *and* hormonal changes of adolescence (page 53) or menopause (page 62) and exhaustion from the emotional *and* physical demands of a young family (page 60).

There is so much advice now on how to live a 'stress-free life', so many books, so many things to *do*, it is easy to become overwhelmed, to feel there simply isn't time to do it all, to fit it in. It is important to put this advice in perspective. We can avoid or eliminate some stresses like unnecessary medication, coffee and alcohol, but we may be stuck with others – with pollution, for example, if we are living in a city, or even the weather! In these instances we need to work out ways to minimize their impact on our health.

In this section there is a lot of common sense advice for you to pick and choose from, to experiment with integrating into your life. It may be helpful if you think of all these words as a buffet rather than as a complete meal – a buffet that you can keep coming back to. If you try something and like it, then keep it on your menu. But if it doesn't taste right, you don't have to have it again!

I know a woman who swims for an hour every morning. The rest of her life is filled virtually to the brim with work and family. She says that she could feel guilty that she doesn't do more for herself, but swimming means a lot to her: she has a blissful hour every morning to herself. This balances out the demands of her family; her physical body feels wonderful after the exercise (which is important because her job is sedentary) and she has found her own way to relax and meditate as she swims, thereby helping her to get in touch with herself, to solve problems and give her mind the relaxation it needs to do a mentally demanding job.

ENVIRONMENTAL STRESSES

We live in an increasingly complex world where, if you believe everything you read, hear, or see on TV, you are vulnerable to attack from a vast, invisible army of chemicals contaminating the air you breathe, the water you drink and the food you eat.

Individual susceptibility to these stresses varies enormously. A strong immune system (a healthy vital force) can handle exposure to most environmental stresses, but some people can become sensitive to a particular stress through a prolonged exposure. Those with poor health, with inherited weaknesses or chronic complaints – especially those on orthodox medication – are more vulnerable to environmental stresses. Many people with a subtle low-grade poisoning experience a lowered level of vitality with non-specific symptoms of weakness, fatigue and general malaise as well as an increased susceptibility to acute and/or chronic illness.

Chemicals

Runaway technology has meant that industrial chemicals are flooding our environment at an alarming rate which is increasing each year. The majority of these chemicals are not tested for either ecological or health effects and are being increasingly implicated in the rise of chronic diseases. The chemical industry produces toxic products, by-products and waste, all of which need manufacturing, transporting, using and disposal. All of these activities involve people.

Poisonous dioxins, phenol compounds and organochlorines are spreading through the environment at a worrying rate. Chemicals in cosmetics, toiletries, paints, cleaning materials, glues, clothing, household and garden insecticides, and fumes from plastics, rubbers, foam rubber mattresses, pillows and carpet underlays are causing a variety of side effects for some of the humans who use them – from skin complaints and asthma, to infertility and cancer.

Many fabrics are treated with chemicals to be fire, moth and mould resistant as well as shower and wrinkle proof. Some of these chemicals, such as dieldrin which is used to moth-proof woollens, are highly toxic and are known to affect the liver and nervous system. People who experience headaches and exhaustion when shopping (and/or a sense of disorientation) aren't necessarily stressed out at the thought of spending money!

Cosmetics and toiletries

The skin is our largest organ and we need to treat it with special care and respect. Our lungs have a surface area the size of a tennis court which makes them particularly vulnerable to fumes and sprays. In addition, the wisdom of some of our so-called modern toiletries needs questioning.

Antiperspirants (for armpits or feet) block the pores of our skin and inhibit one of the natural cleansing processes of the body. Perspiration is one of the body's ways of eliminating waste and cooling down. Simply blocking off the problem from the outside can create another problem for our inner organs to deal with. Deodorants (which don't stop you sweating, they just cover up the smell) are a more sensible option together with more frequent washing.

Suntan lotions and sunscreens protect against sunburn, and skin cancer, but need using discriminately as the chemicals are absorbed into the body (where they are transported to the liver for disposal – or more worryingly, for storage). They also enable us to endure something we ordinarily could not do and recent statistics show a higher incidence of certain skin cancers in those who are staying in the sun by using masses of sunscreen creams. It is more sensible to use adequate clothing and a hat as a protective measure – and to avoid the sun altogether during the hottest parts of the day.

Cosmetics are a minefield! Make-up can irritate the eyes, nose and skin. Nail varnishes and nail polish removers, many hair sprays, dyes and perms give off toxic fumes and other toxic chemicals which are absorbed through the skin. Formaldehyde is added to many air-fresheners, spray starch and mothballs as well as many cosmetics and toiletries. Petroleum-based products (which can cause skin irritation and rashes) are added to many cosmetics, deodorants, soaps, bubble baths and shampoos. Colognes can burn the skin if worn outside for prolonged periods in bright sunshine and some perfumes and eaux de toilettes can actually cause sensitive people's throats to close up.

Our buildings

Buildings that are centrally-heated, draught-proofed, with blocked-up chimneys and double-glazed windows that are rarely opened can cause gases such as formaldehyde and carbon monoxide to build up. Many office buildings and shops (including supermarkets and shopping malls) have the added problems of poor lighting, exposure to chemicals from asbestos (some older buildings), plastics, fabrics, flooring and cleaning materials, flickering fluorescent bulbs, static electricity and air-conditioning which causes moulds, dust, chemicals and bacteria to be continuously recirculated. This can stress the healthiest immune system.

Tinted glass and low frequency fluorescent lighting can increase feelings of tiredness and may cause headaches. Normal fluorescent lighting does not have the same light spectrum as daylight and it will not, therefore, help your body clock to set itself. If you are working only in fluorescent lighting during daylight hours you can end up in a permanent state of jet lag. If you cannot work by a window or do not have access to daylight then get 'daylight spectrum' fluorescent light bulbs (or tungsten lighting) installed. If you have a lunch-break, do take it and get outside, even in poor weather.

Chemical stresses at work

People at risk from chemical toxicity include dentists (mercury in amalgam vapour), car mechanics (oils, petrol and fumes), miners (dusts), construction workers (dusts and chemicals), painters and decorators (paints, varnishes, wood preservatives and glues), plumbers and printers (lead), hairdressers (perms and dyes), farm workers (insecticides, pesticides and other chemicals), anaesthetists (gases), office workers (computers, photocopying machines, paper-correction fluid and glues), cleaners (sprays – especially insecticides – and cleaning fluids, drivers (exhaust fumes), to name but a few.

It is important to ask yourself what chemicals you are handling or inhaling at work. What are the side effects (that you know about) and might they be affecting you? Can you take protective measures (with a mask, gloves, etc.)? Can you get support and/or information from your health and safety officer?

What to do?

Just knowing what is commonly but invisibly poisonous can help us to make some simple alterations to our lives: to eliminate the poisons, to significantly reduce them or to find healthier alternatives. While some alternatives cost more, many will cost less. If you suspect that you are suffering from a chemical sensitivity – at work or at home – find out as much as you can in order to explore your options for dealing with it. Your local Environmental Health Officer is a mine of information about these matters. In addition, you may need the support of, say, your doctor to get appropriate help, for example with suspected mercury poisoning from amalgam fillings that may be leaking. Think twice and take advice before undergoing costly treatments such as amalgam filling replacements as this 'solution' can stress your body significantly in the short term and needs planning for.

An ionizer can help if you suffer from sinus congestion or a weak chest; a humidifier is useful for those who suffer in centrally-heated houses; an air purifier is worth considering if you live in a polluted area and know that it is affecting your health, i.e. you are well when away from home in an unpolluted enviroinment.

Get informed: read books, check out your local whole food shop for non-toxic, natural alternatives – they are not necessarily more expensive, join an organization that is committed to helping us clean up our environments. Harass your chemist, builder's merchants, garden centre and hardware store for products that are not tested on animals and are risk-free to humans.

As a matter of course, it is wise to use commonsense measures when handling chemicals. Read the instructions carefully and take the health warnings seriously. Make sure you have adequate ventilation if you use a chemical that gives off fumes. Dry-cleaning solvents, paint strippers and varnishes should be used outside or with ventilation. Always wear a mask when dealing with toxic fumes – in particular gloss paints, paint strippers, varnishes and some oven cleaners.

Take your own state of health into account when exposing yourself to chemicals and avoid the ones you have control over. For example, if you have asthma or any chronic chest complaint then it is sensible to avoid sprays of any sort – in the house or garden – and additional, unnecessary chemicals that give off toxic fumes, such as perms and hairsprays.

Explore natural alternatives such as vinegar and newspaper for cleaning windows, lemon juice for burnt pans and bath stains, bicarbonate of soda to clean sinks and basins and borax as a water softener for washing clothes as well as for cleaning toilets.

Metals
All metals are toxic in surprisingly small amounts, affecting especially the nervous system, the liver and the kidneys. In large amounts some can be fatal – in particular, arsenic and lead.

- **Aluminium** is thought to be a contributory factor in the development of Alzheimer's disease and can cause unpleasant symptoms including severe constipation. It is commonly found in small amounts in food cooked in aluminium pans, antacids (for indigestion), many cosmetic preparations including antiperspirants and some talcum powders.
- **Arsenic** is highly toxic in large quantities, causing severe

vomiting, diarrhoea and prostration. In small amounts the symptoms are more insidious with anaemia, chronic exhaustion and depression developing over time. It is used in the manufacture of some dyes, paints, wallpapers and medicines, many household and garden pesticides.

- **Cadmium** affects the body's enzyme activity and one of the early signs of toxicity is high blood pressure. It is found in water and some foods such as oysters, some instant coffees and teas, canned foods and soft drinks – and cigarette smoke. Industrial sources include insecticides, rubber tyres, dyes, plastics and solder.
- **Lead** can cause anaemia, nerve damage, learning difficulties in children, an increased susceptibility to infections and depression. It is found in exhaust fumes (and foods exposed to fumes), some old paints, water from lead pipes and cigarette smoke. If you have lead water pipes into your house then – especially first thing in the morning – run your water for a few minutes, until it changes temperature, to avoid drinking or cooking with water that may have small quantities of lead and cadmium dissolved in it.
- **Mercury** poisoning has been well recorded: common symptoms include mouth ulcers, recurring infections and depression. Many fish are now found to be contaminated from waters polluted with mercury (an industrial by-product). Mercury is used in dental amalgam – leaking fillings are another common physical stress for some people, but especially for those with poor health. Some countries are banning or limiting the use of amalgam in fillings. Alternatives are available, although they are more expensive and need a high degree of skill to install.
- **Nickel** – many people are allergic to the nickel in some jewellery, especially costume jewellery, developing rashes on the ears, on fingers or around the wrist.

Airborne stresses
- **Carbon monoxide poisoning** is unfortunately common – on average fifty people die in the UK every year of accidental poisoning from faulty gas appliances (gas, solid fuel, coke, paraffin) or cars with internal leaks. Aching and exhaustion, headaches, nausea, dizzy spells, exhaustion with heaviness,

especially in the legs, are all indicators of carbon monoxide poisoning. The regular servicing of all gas appliances is vital – especially those using butane. They must all be ventilated adequately, with a vent, chimney or open window.

• **Crop spraying** affects our health, and contaminates air, water and soil. Ask your local farmer to let you know when they are spraying crops so that you can shut the doors and windows of your home if, for example, you suffer from asthma.

• **Dusts** from brick, stone or plaster affect peoploe who are exposed to an unusual amount at a vulnerable time, causing coughs, catarrhs and sinus problems. House dust and its little helper, the house dust mite, have been implicated in a wide range of respiratory complaints.

• **Electricity** is thought to affect some people adversely – mainly from high voltage lines. The detrimental effects of excessive electromagnetism are still being researched but in order to reduce exposure it is sensible not to be too close to an operating electrical appliance: for example, move your bedside electric clock away from your head; sit well away from your television and turn your electric blanket off at the plug before you get into bed.

• **Exhaust fumes** from cars, buses, motor bikes, etc. contain lead, sulphuric acid, nitrous oxide and carbon monoxide as well as other active chemical agents. Exposure can cause headache, sleepiness, ear, nose and throat irritations along with psychological symptoms such as mental confusion, paranoia, anger and even loss of reasoning. Children in pushchairs and cyclists are especially vulnerable. Consider travelling a quieter, less polluted way to work or school; changing your work schedule to avoid travelling during the rush hour; moving if you live on a busy street and know or suspect that car fumes are affecting your health.

• **Fibre glass** insulation causes tiny airborne splinters of fine glass to be released when it is unrolled. These can lodge under the skin causing an unpleasant rash, or in the lungs where they can cause pain, a cough and even bleeding.

• **Moulds** can cause chronic bronchitis, exhaustion, a lowering of the immune system and a wide range of allergic reactions. If you live in a damp area, or a damp house, and your health is poor then consider moving or treat the damp in your immediate environment.

- **Pollens** increasingly affect those who suffer from hay fever and asthma. This rise in sensitivity to tree, grass and/or flower pollens is thought to be due, in part, to a general increase in chemicals in the environment.
- **Radiation:** background radiation comes from the earth, the atmosphere, buildings and even food. Low levels of radiation are produced by microwave ovens, television sets and computer monitors. The average person receives far more radiation from the environment than from dental and medical X-rays, which account for about a quarter of our total exposure. Radiation in excess stresses the immune system, affecting bone growth, fertility and, in areas where there have been serious radiation leaks (from reactors), is associated with an increase in cancers and abnormalities in babies.

  Newer computers emit lower radiation and have screens to reduce radiation further, but as the majority of the rays come from the back of the machine make sure you are at least 3–4 feet from the back of someone else's computer. Keep your screen an arm's length from your face; use a protective screen, don't spend longer than four hours a day in front of it – and take frequent breaks.
- **Smoke** from fires, factories and power stations, and cigarettes produce carbon monoxide and certain chemicals, some of which are highly toxic, depending on what is being burnt. Some people are sensitive to smoke, experiencing a tight chest or a cough on exposure.

Waterborne chemicals

Our tap water may be free of bacteria but it can contain traces of chemicals which have been used in the processing, such as chlorine and aluminium, as well as copper and lead from plumbing and, in some areas, fluoride. Water filters remove some metals but may also extract valuable trace minerals. Some of our lakes, rivers and seas are now so contaminated with bacteria and chemicals that it is sensible to check that it is safe to bathe/swim.

- **Chlorine** is used in public swimming pools as a disinfectant. This stings mucous membranes, especially the eyes, and can cause

skin rashes, fatigue, asthma, fainting or dizziness and stomach pains.
- **Fluoride** has been implicated in some cancers and dental problems in areas where there has been compulsory fluoridation of the water supply.

Other chemicals
- **Chlorine** is used in the manufacture of bleaches, disinfectants, antiseptics and paper-making. The bleaching of paper involves the use and production of many toxic chemicals such as dioxins which affect the liver, suppress the immune system and have been implicated in some cancers, birth defects, sterility, miscarriages and skin diseases.

  The pollution involved in the production and disposal of household paper products (toilet paper, tissues, kitchen roll, disposable nappies, tampons, sanitary towels and writing papers) is worrying, especially those which use non-biodegradeable plastics in their manufacture, i.e. sanitary towels and nappies which have polypropylene barriers.
- **Formaldehyde** is used extensively in the production of building materials, such as chipboard, concrete, plaster and glues, dyes, fabrics (including furnishing fabrics, vinyl, some leathers and carpets), toiletries (antiperspirants, tanning agents, germicidal soaps, some shampoos, disinfectants) and foam rubbers. Exposure can cause asthma, dermatitis, nausea, headaches, tiredness, irritation of the mucous membranes and throat disorders. It is the major agent responsible for the burning and streaming of eyes from inner city smog.
- **Phenols** are toxic chemicals used in the production of herbicides, insecticides (aeroplanes departing from insect-rich countries are sprayed with insecticides immediately before take off and many public places such as hotels and theatres are regularly sprayed), detergents, petrol, resins, nylon and polyurethane. Phenols affect the liver and the nervous system.

Homeopathic treatment
Homeopathy can help by clearing out the effects of chemical stresses either directly, or through constitutional treatment. If you suspect

that you are subject to some sort of chemical poisoning seek expert advice. Having your full case history taken by a competent homeopath can bring to light an offending chemical that you are unwittingly 'proving' (see page 26).

You can use specific remedies to deal with the effects of chemical stresses. For example: mixed pollens for hayfever that comes on when the flowers bloom; dusts in potency if *Silica* hasn't helped; a particular hair dye or perming agent or a paint or chemical (such as formaldehyde) where a specific poisoning can be identified, and so on. This is known as isopathic prescribing rather than homeopathic, and while it can be extremely effective, it is also a bit hit or miss. The medicine that is used is the toxin or chemical or pollen itself, which has been prepared by homeopathic methods i.e. diluted and succussed (see page 28) to a certain potency (usually the 30th). But since most of these substances have not been proved (that is, tested on healthy people) they cannot be prescribed according to the homeopathic Law of Similars, because there is no symptom picture against which they can be matched. Their use is more haphazard than matching symptoms from the provings with those experienced by a patient, but there are times when they can be successful, especially when all else has failed. You can order these specific remedies from the homeopathic pharmacies direct and if they do not have them in stock they can make them up provided you can send them a small sample of the substance.

There is a limit to what you can do to treat yourself for the effects of an environmental stress. You can self-prescribe on minor or occasional environmental stresses – the following remedies are those that I have found useful. There are many others and you will need to seek the advice of a homeopathic practitioner or pharmacist if the one you are interested in is not listed here.

- *Acid sulphurosum (Ac-sul.)*
  Ill effects of exhaust fumes: severe headache with ringing in the ears; constipation; persistent choking cough; feeling of tightness in the chest with difficulty breathing.
- *Alumina (Alu.)*
  Ill effects of aluminium or lead poisoning. Common symptoms include: slowness; sluggishness; dizziness; pallor, frequent (dry) coughs and colds; dry, itchy skin; constipation; joint pain; heaviness and weakness of arms and legs.

- **Arsenicum album** (*Ars.*) See also p. 266.
  General sensitivity to chemicals. Tendency to colds, coughs and
  sore throats. Pale, anxious, exhausted and restless.
- **Bromium** (*Brom.*)
  Ill effects of dust. Dry cough worse for taking a deep breath. With
  hoarseness and sore throat.
- **Cadmium sulphuratum** (*Cad-s.*)
  Ill effects of cadmium; of radiation. Burning pains in stomach
  with nausea and salty taste in mouth. Vomiting with cold sweats.
  Sleep apnoea (stops breathing in sleep and wakes with a start).
  Nose chronically blocked.
- **Carbo vegetabilis** (*Carb-v.*) See also p. 284.
  Ill effects of carbon monoxide poisoning, gas/coal/charcoal
  fumes, exhaust fumes. Sluggish, heavy and trembly. Very pale.
  Body feels cold (although head may be hot) and feels better for
  cool air or being fanned. Heavy headache with nausea, burping
  and dizziness. Choking cough.
- **Carboneum sulphuratum** (*Carbn-s.*)
  Ill effects of gas/coal/charcoal fumes. Sleepy, dizzy and trembly.
  Cold sweats with general weakness. Heavy headache, irritating
  cough and difficulty focusing the eyes.
- **Causticum** (*Caust.*) See also p. 286.
  Ill effects of lead. Indigestion, pains in joints with stiffness and
  general exhaustion.
- **Chlorum**
  Ill effects of chlorine. Catarrh, headache and acid stomach.
  Difficulty breathing with feeling of constriction in the chest and
  the throat.
- **Cuprum metallicum** (*Cupr.*)
  Ill effects of copper. Violent cramps anywhere in the body.
  Nervous trembling with exhaustion. Stomach ache with diar-
  rhoea or constipation. Hoarse cough.
- **Electricitas** (*Elect.*)
  Ill effects of electricity. Anxiety with fear and restlessness. Terrible
  headache with dizziness. Palpitations with nervous trembling.
  General exhaustion and stiffness.
- **Hepar sulphuris calcareum** (*Hep-s.*)
  Ill effects of mercury. Generally sensitive to chemicals. Low pain

threshold. Tendency to abscesses anywhere. Catarrh, coughs, sore throats. Cuts are slow to heal. Feels the cold intensely.

- *Ignatia amara (Ign.)* See also p. 298.
  Ill effects of smoke, especially tobacco smoke, in sensitive people. Common symptoms from small amounts include: the shakes, headache, indigestion and insomnia (with very light sleep).
- *Lycopodium (Lyc.)* See also p. 305.
  Ill effects of aluminium. Constipation with hard, knotty stools. Bloating with rumbling and flatulence. Discomfort is better for passing wind.
- *Mercurius solubilis (Merc-s.)*
  Ill effects of mercury. Generally sensitive to chemicals. Exhaustion with heaviness and internal trembling. Depressed, apathetic and restless. Sore throat, cough, colds, thrush, abscesses with swollen glands. Profuse, smelly sweat with increased saliva, smelly breath, metallic taste in mouth and mouth ulcers.
- *Niccolum (Nicc.)*
  Ill effects of nickel. Itchy rash from jewellery containing nickel. Itching is not relieved by scratching.
- *Nitricum acidum (Nit-ac.)* See also p. 314.
  Ill effects of mercury. Generally sensitive to chemicals. Mercury poisoning causes severe sore throat and mouth ulcers.
- *Opium (Op.)* See also p. 321.
  Ill effects of gas/coal/charcoal fumes. Drowsy and looks terrible – drugged. Sluggish (mentally and physically). Hot and sweaty.
- *Petroleum (Petr.)*
  Ill effects of exhaust fumes. Headache, nausea, dizziness, and vomiting. Head feels heavy and aches. Feels worse for fresh air and when getting up from sitting or lying.
- *Phosphorus (Phos.)* See also p. 325.
  Ill effects of electricity. These types are generally sensitive, especially to electrical charges – those that come before or during a storm as well as from high voltage power lines/electric shock.
- *Plumbum (Plb.)*
  Ill effects of aluminium; of exhaust fumes. Cramps in legs. Constipation with small black stools or watery diarrhoea. Numbness and stiffness of limbs. Heaviness with weakness. Depressed and dull. Anaemia, cuts slow to heal.

- **Radium bromatum** (*Rad-br.*)
  Ill effects of radiation. Exhaustion with great sleepiness. Sleeps a lot but doesn't feel refreshed. Headache, aching in back, joints and muscles. Itchy rash. Depressed and irritable.
- *Silica* (*Sil.*) See also p. 338.
  Ill effects of inhaling fibre glass or dust, causing a cough, catarrh, sinusitis or sore throat. Silica aids the body's efforts to expel the dust or fibre glass. Generally sensitive to some chemicals.
- *Spigelia* (*Spig.*)
  Ill effects of smoke, especially tobacco smoke. Common symptoms include: toothache, neuralgic headache, palpitations, dry, irritating cough, pains in the chest.

EVERYDAY STIMULANTS AND SEDATIVES

Alcohol, caffeine, sugar, spices and tobacco are all strong 'medicines', and can be harmful either in excess or to those who are sensitive to them. People are adding them into their lives in ever-increasing quantities, especially when overstressed. Some people use caffeine (coffee or tea) to get going – to switch themselves on in the morning; more caffeine as well as sugar, cigarettes and even spicy foods to keep them going and prop up their worn-out nervous systems during the day; and then alcohol to enable them to shut down – to switch off at night. Apart from depleting the body of the vitamins and minerals necessary to combat stress, these habits are stressful in themselves.

Alcohol
In small quantities alcohol may be good for you: red wine has been hailed as an aid to digestion and is said to reduce the risk of heart disease. In excess it is toxic, affecting the liver and brain – causing vomiting and unconsciousness. If you experience headaches, diarrhoea, catarrh, irritability (or any strong physical or emotional symptoms) when you drink alcohol, you are sensitive to it. If you suffer from hangovers after even a small amount of alcohol it may be the sugars, the chemical additives or the yeasts that are to blame.
  Alcohol has a primary sedative effect and a secondary stimulat-

ing effect. That is why some people feel sleepy if they drink too much too quickly and why others who are drinking over a period of time become wound up. As a sedative, alcohol can numb emotional as well as physical pain which is why some people turn to it when they are depressed or upset.

Some people drink to drown their sorrows, to gloss over emotional stresses they don't want to face. Some people drink out of habit, increasing their consumption over the years, almost without noticing it, until they find they can't do without it. Some may begin drinking earlier and earlier in the day and may even conceal the evidence of their habit from those close to them. There are those who drink on an occasional basis but to such excess that they leave a trail of destruction that is hard to explain – and deal with.

While alcohol can be enjoyable – in moderation (and even on the odd occasions in excess) – its addictive properties are well known. Alcohol addiction is a painful, distressing, destructive and tragic condition. People who retreat into an alcoholic haze can end up losing everything that matters to them: their families, their jobs, their homes, their self-esteem, and even their reason to live.

Tea and coffee
Tea and coffee are potent stimulants, containing caffeine in varying quantities depending on their strength, as well as many other active ingredients. Long term excessive tea and/or coffee abuse can result in chronic fatigue, premature aging and even depression.

Caffeine stimulates an artificial energy rush to keep us going. Unfortunately, it also masks the symptoms of tiredness, so that people who drink more coffee when they are tired can end up completely exhausted. It is more sensible to reduce it and deal with the underlying stresses and get more sleep, than to keep pumping in the caffeine and creating physical problems that will take longer to deal with.

If you become shaky, experience palpitations or find it difficult to sleep if you have tea or coffee late in the day, then you are probably sensitive to the caffeine content. Some people can drink ten cups of strong coffee a day with no effects; others find that one cup sets off anxiety, palpitations and the 'shakes'. They will often find their health improves when they cut it out.

It is sensible to cut out caffeine, especially when overstressed, or drink it in moderation and only in the first half of your day, or when you need to prop yourself up on, say, a long drive. The endless drinking of tea or coffee, in the work place or at home, may simply be an unquestioned habit. Habits are comforting, reassuring rituals in themselves – part of our social and cultural fabric. Unfortunately they can contribute to unhealthy stress or even be one of the unhealthy stresses that is causing ill health.

Tea or coffee that is brewed in an aluminium pot or kettle is doubly poisonous because small amounts of the metal are leaked into your drink.

Many people have turned to decaffeinated tea and coffee, thinking they are healthier. Unfortunately, not all the caffeine is removed, and traces of the substances used in the decaffeinating process may remain.

It is tempting to replace tea or coffee with herbal infusions but many herbs are strong medicines: some are natural stimulants, others are sedatives. If taken in excess they can make you feel unwell. I know people who have unknowingly 'medicated' their babies with daily doses of chamomile tea, turning a happy, contented baby into an irritable, colicky one who won't sleep at night (see *Chamomilla*, page 289). Fruit teas are unlikely to cause unpleasant symptoms because they are made mostly of peels and berries.

Sugar

Sugar has been implicated in a wide range of chronic diseases from irritable bowel syndrome to hypoglycaemia and diabetes. Some experts believe it is a bigger culprit than fat in coronary heart disease (because it causes increased blood levels of cholesterol, triglyceride, uric acid, insulin and cortisol). It contributes to (or in some cases causes) hyperactivity in children. It is fattening, rots our teeth and white sugar has no nutritional value, i.e. it contains no vitamins or minerals.

Soft (fizzy) drinks can affect the formation of healthy bones – because the high phosphorus content affects calcium absorption. They are so high in sugar that they distort the taste buds of young children who demand more of them to accommodate their habit. Babies who are drinking these products in lightweight plastic bottles are running the risk of serious dental cavities as well as jaw malformations if they carry them around sucking on them constantly.

Excessive sugar intake in any form is bad for you. Some 'natural fruit' drinks for children with no 'added' sugar have a fructose content that is four and a half times higher than sugar. Fructose isn't made from fruit, but is a commercially refined sugar which is thought to be more harmful than sucrose. Of all the sugars, glucose is thought to be the least harmful.

Hidden sugars in processed foods need additional salt to make them palatable. This combination of unnecessary sugar and salt – as well as the excessive use of animal fats, and of course chemical additives, is thought to be the major stress factor in the diseases of the so-called civilized world.

Even the so-called health food market is guilty of adding sweeteners, usually in the form of honey, corn syrup, maple syrup or concentrated fruit juices, to a variety of products. Many so-called wholefood cereals actually have a higher sugar content than those found at your local supermarket.

To reduce your sugar intake you will have to increase your detective faculties. Do your own research at the supermarket – sugars are listed by the milligram on most foods under the carbohydrate content. There is about a teaspoon of sugar in each 5g. I conducted my own research by listing a typical day's diet for some British children – a bowl of cereal, a carton of Ribena, baked beans on toast, three biscuits (cookies), a bowl of tomato soup, a can of Coca-cola, a fruit yoghurt and a small chocolate bar. After I had done my sums I came to the shocking conclusion that this child was eating the equivalent of a kilo of sugar over a week.

Chocolate

Chocolate contains caffeine, theobromine (a heart stimulant) some vitamins and minerals as well as a small quantity of a chemical substance which is produced by the brain when we are in love (or euphoric). It is thought that this substance is, in part, responsible for its addictive properties by stimulating the pleasure hormones in our brains. It is a deeply seductive and complex stimulant (caffeine combined with theobromine and a high sugar content) and cravings can get out of hand if people rely on it, instead of real food, for frequent energy lifts.

Spicy foods

Some people turn to spicy food for a stimulus when they are overstressed – or understressed. Pepper – whether it is black pepper, chilies or cayenne pepper (in Tabasco sauce) – is a stimulant that can pep us up when we are feeling jaded.

If you turn to spicy foods to keep you going or indulge excessively in them then your digestion can be affected – and your temper as irritability is a common side effect. Peppers are notorious for causing digestive problems – diarrhoea, stomach aches, heartburn and wind.

If you find that you are more irritable than usual after lunch or if you have difficulty sleeping after an Indian or Chinese meal then it may be the spices that are to blame.

Tobacco

Cigarette smoke contains a frightening number of chemicals, including high levels of formaldehyde, cadmium and 43 carcinogens (discovered so far). It is a mystery how some people who smoke stay healthy. Tobacco is simultaneously a stimulant and a relaxant, as well as being an appetite suppressant which makes it an interesting drug, especially for women, who are turning to cigarettes in increasing numbers. There is no doubt that smoking is bad for your health – the arguments are well known: it causes cancer, heart disease and emphysema. It is a complicated drug providing relief from stressful emotions such as anxiety, depression and anger – although the mechanics of this are not fully understood.

Many people yo-yo between stopping and then starting again, sometimes out of carelessness. The rituals involved in smoking should never be underestimated – they are a powerful, motivating force in many smokers' lives. Now that smoking has become an anti-social activity, people who smoke perceive themselves as outcasts which, perversely, can reinforce their desire to continue.

Homeopathic treatment

If your intake of everyday stimulants or sedatives is simply a (bad) habit picked up from friends, family or the media and you have a strong constitution, then you might want to try cutting down or even stopping altogether for, say, forty-eight hours. If you grind to a halt, feeling exhausted, headachy and even depressed then you are overdoing it – whether your addiction is to chocolate, diet cola, tea, beer, wine or cappuccinos.

Alcohol and cigarettes are complex and insidious habits, or addictions that many people need help with in order to give up successfully – to enable them to identify and deal with the underlying emotional stresses in their lives that led to the addiction in the first place.

Use the following homeopathic remedies to help you to deal with the side effects or even withdrawal symptoms when giving up a stimulant or a sedative, to help your body to rebalance and give your flagging nervous system a boost. Or use them for those occasions when you unwittingly overdo it.

- *Alumina (Alu.)*
  Ill effects of tea (especially if it is brewed in an aluminium pot/ kettle). Sluggish (mentally and physically) and exhausted. Wants to lie down but resting doesn't help. Severe constipation. Itchy, dry skin.
- *Argentum nitricum (Arg-n.)* See also p. 262.
  Ill effects of sugar/sweets (including acute effects from an unaccustomed overdose). Craves sweets and sweet things in any form. Eats it straight from the bowl when desperate (and no one is looking). Common symptoms include: diarrhoea or diarrhoea alternating with constipation; bloating; explosive flatulence and stomach ache.
- *Caladium (Calad.)*
  Modifies tobacco cravings and can help to stimulate a dislike for smoking. Use when wanting to give up – in a low potency over several days.
- *Calcarea phosphorica (Calc-p.)* See also p. 281.
  Ill effects of soft drinks. Appetite lost in those (especially children) who have had too many soft drinks. Pale, thin, tired and discontented. Common symptoms include: teeth decay, diarrhoea, stomach aches.

- *Chamomilla (Cham.)* See also p. 289.
  Ill effects of caffeine. Insomnia, restlessness and great irritability. Common symptoms include: nausea, headache, stomach ache, diarrhoea.
- *China officinalis (Chin.)*
  Ill effects of tea. Nervous exhaustion, anaemia and despondency in tea drinkers. Become sensitive to light, smells and noise and easily upset. Common symptoms include: headache, nosebleeds, nausea, indigestion, bloating, diarrhoea and flatulence, insomnia with unrefreshing sleep.
- *Chocolate (Choc.)*
  Ill effects of chocolate. Irritability, especially at home; difficulty concentrating. Common symptoms include tiredness, headaches and bloating.
- *Coffea cruda (Coff.)* See also p. 293.
  Ill effects of caffeine. 'Wired-up' after too much caffeine (coffee or tea or soft drinks). Overexcited and emotional. Sensitive to smells and noise. Restless and unable to relax or sleep (sleep is very light).
- *Ignatia amara (Ign.)* See also p. 298.
  Sensitive to caffeine. Common symptoms from small amounts include: the shakes, headache, indigestion and insomnia (with very light sleep).
- *Lycopodium (Lyc.)* See also p. 305.
  Ill effects of sugar/sweets. Craves sweets and sweet things, especially chocolate. Appetite poor, is full up after eating only a little. Anxious and irritable. Very bloated and windy.
- *Nux vomica (Nux-v.)* See also p. 317.
  Ill effects of any stimulant/sedative -- either the acute effects (children are wound up and irritable from unaccustomed junk food after, say, a party), or longer term (after subsisting on coffee, alcohol and spicy foods to get through a difficult work period). Irritable – especially after giving up smoking. Palpitations and the shakes from too much caffeine. Common symptoms include: tension, exhaustion, headache (especially a hangover headache) and insomnia.
- *Opium (Op.)* See also p. 321.
  Ill effects of alcohol. Acute alcohol poisoning with or without vomiting. Drowsy and looks terrible – drugged. Sluggish

(mentally and physically). Hot and sweaty.
- *Staphysagria (Staph.)* See also p. 341.
  Ill effects of tobacco. Stimulates an aversion to tobacco in those who smoke to suppress hurt or anger. After stopping smoking angry feelings burst out unpredictably – feels like a volcano waiting to happen.
- *Sulphur (Sul.)*
  Ill effects of alcohol; of sugar/sweets. Flatulence, indigestion and diarrhoea after beer (which they love) and sometimes after whisky.
- *Sulphuric acid ((Sul-ac.)*
  Ill effects of alcohol. Debility with internal trembling, with a craving for stimulants. Impatient and irritable – does everything on the run. Common symptoms include heartburn, diarrhoea and piles. Helps to modify craving for alcohol.
- *Tabacum (Tab.)*
  Ill effects of tobacco. On stopping smoking deals with withdrawals. Common symptoms include: nausea, dizziness, feeling 'spaced out' or ungrounded.
- *Thea*
  Ill effects of tea. Nervous exhaustion, palpitations and indigestion in tea drinkers. Feels 'spaced out'.

FOOD

Food provides essential building blocks for a healthy and active life. As natural 'omnivores' it is important that we humans eat as varied a diet as possible, as this is the one that is most likely to provide us with the wide range of nutrients that we need. Food provides essential building blocks for a healthy and active life, but food does not nourish the physical body alone.

Food is only one factor, among many, that shapes and determines the quality of our health. Our ability to digest and absorb the nutrients from the food we eat is as, if not more, important than what we eat. We bring our emotional bodies to each and every meal – as well as our social and cultural histories: these can be reassuring ways to remember who we are and where we have come from. We can attempt to change our physical relationship with food but we may put some of the other benefits at risk.

An inadequate diet, especially at crucial times in our lives, can be a severe stress in itself. And unhealthy stress (emotional or physical) can play havoc with our eating patterns which, in turn, increases our stress load, creating a vicious cycle that is hard to break. Careful attention to diet during emotionally or physically stressful times will go a long way towards balancing out those stresses.

If we are to believe everything we read, we should cut out all fat or salt, eat no meat, never combine carbohydrate and protein in the same meal (or always do so), eat only raw foods – and so on. Be careful about following a diet that excludes major food groupings (like fats) or any diet that doesn't fit with what nourishes *you*. Some of these turn out to be either problematical or even dangerous. Some who have excluded fat from their diets are now thin but suicidally depressed, and their children are found to have a wide range of worrying physical and developmental problems.

People on strict diets – whatever the reason – find themselves excluded from social occasions which involve food. Food is often a focus of cultural rituals from weddings to religious festivals, and is one of the commonplace ways we demonstrate our care for others. Children with chronic catarrh are sometimes advised to cut out dairy foods by well-meaning health care professionals. This can make visiting friends almost impossible. Think carefully before you buy into someone else's idea of what they think you should be eating, and decide whether the stress of eliminating a food is going to outweigh any possible benefits.

Camp fires

When overstressed, many people lose their appetites, skip meals and develop habits like having only one meal a day. Missing meals, especially breakfast, is an unhealthy habit, particularly for children, those who are physically active and those who are under emotional stress.

Metabolism is the process whereby your body produces energy from food. It is a fascinating drama in which virtually every organ and system of the body has a part to play. Think of it as a camp fire which you feed with logs (food) to produce heat (energy). This energy is measurable in the blood in the form of blood sugar (glucose), and needs constantly replenishing (every 3–5 hours) in order to stay alert and productive. Your brain and nervous system need a constant supply of glucose (via the blood) to function adequately. People who are naturally skinny have faster metabolisms than those who gain weight easily and burn their food at a slower rate.

Blood sugar levels rise after a meal and decrease gradually – during which time you begin to feel hungry. If you ignore those hunger pangs your blood sugar levels drop. A cup of tea or coffee at this point makes us feel better temporarily, by stimulating the release of adrenaline into the body. This suppresses the appetite and so the cycle begins. Adrenaline is an outmoded, emergency resource designed to help us run away from dinosaurs. Whilst it helps to raise energy levels (for a short time), the stimulation of adrenaline on a habitual, daily basis is a recipe for disaster, causing a wide range of physical symptoms from palpitations and anxiety to chronic fatigue.

Sugar can also provide quick energy, causing our blood sugar levels to rise dramatically, and to plummet just as dramatically a short time later. Many people have some more sugar at this point. This yo-yo-ing of blood sugar levels is disastrous for our health and should only be done in an emergency, otherwise it will lead inexorably towards exhaustion and ill health. When a sugar enters the body, insulin (from the pancreas) is released to deal with it. This leads to a release of adrenaline to offset the insulin effect. It has been described as similar to accelerating very fast and then doing an emergency stop. It is just as wasteful and wearing on the body. The pancreas and adrenals become tired and sluggish. Eventually the pancreas stops being able to produce insulin, which is when diabetes – by and large an avoidable disease – is diagnosed.

When we go to sleep at night all our bodily processes slow down, including our digestion, which is why it is unwise to go to bed on a large meal. Our camp fire damps down and when we wake in the morning we have dying embers. People who have tea and coffee and miss breakfast are throwing dried leaves on their fire. It will burn brightly for a moment and then go out! As it will do every time we miss a meal.

Some people have fast metabolisms, i.e. their camp fires burn quickly and need feeding sooner or more often than those with a slow metabolism. Experiment to find out what suits you best. Some people thrive on 'grazing' – eating 5–6 small meals a day (finding a large meal lies heavily on the stomach and makes them tired), others do better on three main meals. Some people need a snack before going to bed – a glass of milk, a bowl of cereal or a piece of toast – finding it easier to get sleep and sleeping more deeply with a 'full tummy', especially if their evening meal was three or more hours before bedtime.

Eating little and often will prevent that feeling of tiredness that occurs after a meal eaten once your fire has gone out, even if it is something light and easy to digest like fruit or yoghurt. It will also, especially during times of high stress, help your energy levels remain high and ensure that your body is not running on adrenaline. Many people really can revolutionize their energy patterns, almost overnight, simply by attending to their own camp fires on a more regular basis.

Dentists advise against snacking as they believe the saliva cannot readjust to fight the bacteria that attacks teeth but one solution is to brush (and floss) after every meal.

Food that is metabolized and used as energy is not stored as fat. It is the extra unnecessary food that is stored as fat, especially heavy foods eaten late in the day when our metabolic processes are slowing down. Shifting the bulk of your food consumption to earlier in the day (to breakfast and lunch) ensures that it will be converted more efficiently into energy.

Weight loss, weight gain

Those who are understressed or bored may turn to food for comfort, to fill the empty spaces in their lives. A constantly over-loaded digestive system and weight gain can be serious stresses in themselves, more especially if they are accompanied by a lack of physical activity as this puts a strain on the heart and the circulation – and can lead to obesity. Children are just as vulnerable as grown-ups to over-eating when under- or overstressed. Excessive weight gain in infancy (up until about the age of two) lays the groundwork for a battle with weight control that can last a lifetime.

Research suggests that a sure way to gain weight is to follow a diet – especially a fast weight-loss programme. Repeated dieting has been implicated as a bigger risk factor in coronary heart disease (the biggest killer in the UK) than being slightly overweight. Your metabolic rate is reduced when you go on a diet – your body adapts to a decreased intake of calories which may not provide you with adequate nutrition.

It takes twenty minutes for your mind to receive the message that your stomach is full – if you bolt your meal it is much easier to over-eat, to continue eating when you don't really need to.

A low metabolic rate is sometimes caused by a hormonal imbalance and you will need to seek the advice of your doctor if you suspect there is a medical reason for your weight gain. Sudden (and sometimes gradual) weight loss can be a symptom of (sometimes serious) ill health. It may be due to emotional stress which has resulted in eating less, or poverty, a religious fast, or obsessive pre-anorexic behaviour. If you don't know why your weight has changed, or you do know and you have no control over it, then it is time to ask for help.

Fasting – hailed as a cure-all by some – is an effective technique which stimulates the body's intrinsic self-healing abilities but it doesn't suit everyone. A proper fast involves eating nothing and drinking only water in order to give the digestion a complete rest and encourage the body to detoxify. This can be a potent process causing a variety of symptoms from fevers and headaches, to diarrhoea and catarrh. If you want to try it do get yourself some expert help – from a fully qualified naturopath who can monitor your progress and help you through any healing crises that occur. Many people find that a day on fruit (not a real fast) and water with lots of rest is wonderfully rejuvenating.

Healthy eating

Keep a diary for a week of what you eat and drink and the times you do so. Include tobacco, alcohol, and any medications you may be taking (prescribed or otherwise). Note the gaps between meals and whether they coincide with feeling tired, manic or grumpy. Add in any physical symptoms such as indigestion or insomnia and notice whether they coincide with when or what you eat or drink. Notice also what foods you are eating at every meal (or most meals) and whether there are any important foods missing from your diet. You

will notice patterns you were not previously aware of and be able to
make useful adjustments to your eating habits.

- A varied diet with a little of everything is most likely to contain
  the wide variety of nutrients that you need. Include some of the
  main food groups everyday: carbohydrates (your main source of
  energy) in the form of potatoes, rice, pasta, grains; protein
  (responsible for the growth and repair of all cells of your body);
  fat (another source of energy and storage for certain vitamins);
  fibre (responsible for removing waste and toxins from the body);
  vitamins and minerals (responsible for the healthy functioning of
  all the body's systems).
- The World Health Organization tells us that we need to eat about
  a pound in weight (400 g) of fruit and vegetables a day – about
  five portions. A portion translates as: a single piece of medium
  sized fruit, a cup of small fruit (berries or grapes), two heaped
  tablespoons (or equivalent) of vegetables, a small bowl of salad
  (you will need more lettuce, cucumber or tomato because they
  are largely water), a glass of fruit juice (one per day). A recent
  Which? report came up with the alarming figure that one in four
  of secondary school children in the UK eat no fruit or vegetables.
- Fresh whole-foods contain more of the vitamins and minerals
  essential for health. Refined carbohydrates, such as white bread
  and sugar, provide 'empty calories', i.e. carbohydrates without
  vitamins or minerals which are metabolized faster than products
  made from whole grains. Processed foods (like biscuits and most
  commercial cereals – including supermarket mueslis) are high in
  fat, sugar and salt.
- Shop around for additive free foods in order to reduce your
  'chemical' intake. The numbers listed on labels are confusing and
  misleading. Some are relatively harmless like E140 (chlorophyll)
  or E322 (lecithin). Others are known to cause side effects which
  range from mild to severe. E102 (tartrazine – a yellow/orange
  food colouring) is known to cause hyperactivity, insomnia and
  allergic skin symptoms such as urticaria in children. E250
  (sodium nitrite) and E252 (saltpetre) have been shown to cause
  cancers in animals. Sulphur dioxide (E220) is used as a
  preservative in many products and can cause coughs and
  asthma.

- Consider buying organic foods where possible, especially meats and dairy products. The increasing numbers and quantities of chemicals (growth promoters, hormones, antibiotics and other medications) used in the factory farming of animals is worrying. Vegetables and fruit grown organically are free of chemical residues from fertilizers, insecticides, etc. They often taste better and are beginning to come down in price because of demand.
- Awareness of your fat intake as part of an overall picture is valuable, but tackling cholesterol as a road to lasting health would be like polishing your car to keep it going. Eat less fat if your diet is high in it, or more if you have cut it out. Choose healthy fats like cold-pressed vegetable oils (olive and safflower are the best) and don't cook them, or if you do, keep the temperature low and for a short period of time. Cut down on saturated fats and cross margarine off your shopping list – it is a highly synthesized food containing unhealthy fats and needing chemical additives to make it palatable.

  Although our cholesterol levels are genetically determined, a high fat diet plus smoking and a lack of exercise increases our risk of high blood pressure, heart disease, diabetes and weight gain. As we get older that risk automatically increases. If we are emotionally overstressed the risk factor begins to go through the roof. But equally, a long term fat-free diet can cause dry skin, vaginal dryness in women, hormone imbalances, aching joints and fatigue. Women have higher fat requirements than men or they can tolerate higher levels without risk because they have a hormonal (oestrogen) protection.

Allergies and sensitivities
Most people with so-called allergies are simply suffering from a food sensitivity. Very few people are genuinely and severely allergic with a serious physical reaction such as diarrhoea and vomiting from say, garlic, nuts, shellfish or cow's milk. An allergy manifests itself in serious symptoms which may need immediate medical attention, whereas food sensitivities cause symptoms which are more of a nuisance, like catarrh. They can be unpleasant, like colic in babies, or they can develop into a chronic complaint such as irritable bowel syndrome or migraines.

Sensitivity and allergies are usually a symptom of an underlying chronic condition. Allergic reactions are a part of the body's defence mechanism therefore those who are overstressed (especially from environmental stresses), whose bodies are flooded with adrenaline and other hormones on a regular basis, can develop a food sensitivity.

Common allergens include dairy products, wheat, yeast, corn, citrus fruit and eggs. Also, any food or foods that are eaten frequently can be the culprit, for example, chocolate or soya (in oil, soya sauce, tofu and many other products). I know one mother whose child's chronic catarrh disappeared overnight when she eliminated orange juice from his diet. Beware of allergy, or cytotoxic testing – it is not 100 per cent accurate and is not available on the NHS.

If you suspect that you have become sensitive to something you eat then you might want to try an elimination diet. Eliminate one major foodstuff at a time and do your research carefully in order to avoid all sources. There is milk in some form in most baked and many processed foods. Yeasts are also difficult to avoid because many foods contain yeast moulds, including bread, mushrooms, wine, vinegar, soy sauce, cheese, coffee, tea and canned fruit juices.

If you feel better, if your symptoms clear up, then it is worth continuing to avoid the food you have eliminated for a further two weeks. You can then reintroduce the suspected culprit for several days in a row. If your symptoms return eliminate it again but for longer this time – at least several months – re-introducing it from time to time to check whether you are still sensitive. You can develop a food intolerance at any age. And then grow out of it again.

Some foods may trigger latent viruses. For example, recent research in the US has shown that foods high in arginine such as chocolate, nuts and gelatine can bring on an attack of herpes and, similarly, foods such as seaweeds which are high in lysine, can retard them.

Don't be disappointed if the results aren't immediately clear. Some food sensitivities are triggered by combinations and if this is the case you will need to talk your difficulties through with an experienced practitioner.

Removing one stress-induced allergen can lead to another taking its place. Homeopathic treatment can help by addressing the underlying cause or causes, including inherited factors, i.e. allergies that run in the family.

Supplements
It is nutritional madness to take supplements instead of eating. A poor diet and expensive supplements will not make you healthy. Research has shown that fresh fruits and vegetables are packed with compounds known as 'phytochemicals'. They have never seen the inside of a vitamin bottle for the simple reason that they have only recently been identified by scientists. They are thought to be part of a plant's protective mechanism, and there is growing evidence that these protective properties are passed on to humans. It is hard to replicate the health-preserving qualities of fresh foods.

There are times when vitamins can be beneficial, when our nutritional needs are increased, or when illness or a poor diet is depleting our bodies of essential nutrients. Those who will benefit include pregnant and breast-feeding women, smokers, those on certain medication (including the contraceptive pill and antibiotics), those on restricted diets (for whatever reason), vegans, alcoholics, people with certain chronic diseases, those convalescing from an acute illness, those exposed to environmental pollution, and those suffering from stress.

Vitamins are essential for the metabolic processes -- they act as spark plugs, as catalysts which regulate the process of metabolism. It is with their help that proteins and carbohydrates are converted into energy. Unfortunately, it can take a long time for the signs and symptoms of a vitamin or mineral deficiency to appear.

It is possible to over-dose on supplements, especially the minerals and the fat soluble vitamins. Vitamins and minerals have complex relationships with each other, so that an excess of one can cause an imbalance in another. It is quite a minefield. A good multi-vitamin and multi-mineral will meet most requirements, but if you decide to take a single supplement i.e. iron, then do find out (from a good book or a nutritionist) the best and safest way to take it, balancing it out, if necessary, with other vitamins or minerals.

Take them as you would a homeopathic medicine, for shortish

periods of time, stopping when there is an improvement and starting again if your symptoms return. Take them for two to three weeks at a time, have a week off, see what happens and then start them up again if necessary. If they aren't helping or you aren't sure whether they are, then don't carry on taking them without professional advice.

Before embarking on long term or massive doses it is prudent to seek the advice of an expert (ask your doctor for a referral). While vitamins are a useful and powerful tool in restoring and retaining health, always ensure that the apparent need for them is not masking a deeper problem. Above all, get expert advice from a nutritionist about the correct dosage, about whether you really need to take them and how you might obtain the same nutrients from your food.

Homeopathic treatment
There really is a limit to what homeopathy can do if your basic requirements for food are not being met. Trouble-shooting and problem-solving in this area of your life will be more rewarding than taking medications – even homeopathic medicines.

However, if you suffer from food allergies or an eating disorder or if you are having difficulties eating a balanced diet because of other stresses then you will need expert help. Don't treat these yourself. Seek the advice of a nutritionist if you are on a limited diet of any sort, and are under emotional stress.

The following remedies are to help you with ordinary, everyday, occasional stresses around food such as loss of appetite, food poisoning, temporary sensitivities and the results of over-indulging, especially in junk foods.

- *Alumina (Alu.)*
  Ill effects of junk/processed foods, especially in babies/children who have had trouble with formula milks (even soya milk formulas) and/or bottled or tinned or packet baby foods. Common symptoms: severe constipation with no urge to go and large, hard (or soft) stools; lack of vitality; general sluggishness; frequent colds and coughs; dry skin.
- *Antimonium crudum (Ant-c.)*
  Ill effects of over-eating; from acidic foods (including sour fruits

and wine). Digestion is affected. Becomes sluggish, sleepy and iritable. Tongue is coated white. Common symptoms: disordered stomach; belching, diarrhoea and nausea.

• *Arsenicum album* (*Ars.*) See also p. 266.
Severe food poisoning after eating bad meat or drinking bad water. Common symptoms: simultaneous vomiting and diarrhoea; diarrhoea (burning pains after stool) with exhaustion and cold sweat; nausea; frequent, violent vomiting – vomits smallest quantity of anything eaten or drunken, feels faint after.

Ill effects of ices. Dislikes ice cold anything and when under stress can suffer from indigestion, nausea or diarrhoea from iced drinks or foods (including ice cream) and sometimes fruit.

Loss of appetite in anxious, restless types who are fussy, picky eaters.

• *Calcarea carbonica* (*Calc-c.*) See also p. 277.
Ill effects of milk. Diarrhoea (sour-smelling) containing undigested food in teething infants from milk/dairy products.

Slow metabolism, puts on weight easily. Big appetite, which is lost in times of stress, for example, in teething children.

• *Carbo vegetabilis* (*Carb-v.*) See also p. 284.
Food poisoning. With severe bloating, flatulence and diarrhoea from rotten eggs, fish, vegetables or meat.

Ill effects of over-eating; eating fatty rich foods. Digestion is weak. Indigestion (bloating, stomach pains and belching) and uncomfortable flatulence which is better after passing wind.

• *China officinalis* (*Chin.*)
Ill effects of fruit. Digestion is slow, everything (but especially fruit) turns to gas. Very bloated – passing wind doesn't relieve discomfort. With painless diarrhoea.

• *Lycopodium* (*Lyc.*) See also p. 305.
Cannot fast; has to eat little and often otherwise loses appetite. It returns after beginning to eat but then feels quickly full up, i.e. after only eating a small amount. Prefers hot foods/drinks.

Digestion is slow, becomes easily bloated with gas (with loud rumbling) and suffers from acidity (with sour belches) and heartburn. Feels better for passing wind.

Ill effects of flatulent foods (beans, cabbage, onions etc.); of shellfish, which causes vomiting and diarrhoea.

- **Magnesia carbonica** *(Mag-c.)*
  Ill effects of milk; of junk/processed foods. For sickly babies or
  children who have difficulty digesting milk. Green, sour-smelling
  diarrhoea with bloating and rumbling in tummy, heartburn and
  nausea. Children brought up on processed foods are sluggish,
  anxious, irritable – they love meat but won't eat vegetables.
- **Magnesium muriaticum** *(Mag-m.)*
  Ill effects of milk. Colic and constipation (or diarrhoea) in restless
  babies who are having difficulty digesting milk. Sweat and stools
  smell sour. Stools are passed with difficulty, are hard and knotty.
- **Natrum carbonicum** *(Nat-c.)* See also p. 308.
  Ill effects of milk. Weak digestion in sensitive types. Difficulty
  digesting milk with indigestion, nausea and diarrhoea.
- **Natrum muriaticum** *(Nat-m.)* See also p. 310.
  Ill effects of salt; of bread/wheat. Too much salt or too many
  wheat products causes constipation and digestive upsets.
- **Nux vomica** *(Nux-v.)* See also p. 317.
  Ill effects of junk foods; of over-eating. Bilious after overindul-
  ging in everything, but especially the wrong foods at the wrong
  times, usually under mental and emotional stress. Digestion
  slows down with heartburn, indigestion, flatulence and constipation. Appetite is affected, feels hungry but doesn't want to eat –
  except foods that are likely to further stress the digestive system.
- **Phosphorus** *(Phos.)* See also p. 325.
  Ill effects of fasting. Thirsty, hungry people with a fast
  metabolism who don't put on weight, however much they eat –
  when healthy. When depressed, sick or stressed they can become
  easily hypoglycaemic or begin to gain, especially if over-
  indulging in salt, sweets and chocolate. Eating increases the
  appetite with hunger again soon after eating.
- **Pulsatilla nigricans** *(Puls.)* See also p. 330.
  Food poisoning after rotten meat, especially sausages, with
  diarrhoea and vomiting.
  Ill effects of fatty/rich foods; of ice cream. Finds fat in any form
  difficult to digest (including fried foods, pastry and fat meats like
  pork) with nausea, indigestion and heartburn with belching.
- **Sulphur** *(Sul.)* See also p. 345.
  Ill effects of fasting. Fast metabolism – needs to eat often

otherwise can lose appetite although eating something can bring it back again. Feels especially hungry mid-morning, typically around 11 a.m. Always thirsty, (with or without an appetite) for large quantities of liquid, often water. (Thirsty children who dislike meat and eggs, but love sweet things and are often too busy/restless to eat.)

• *Veratrum album* (*Verat.*) See also p. 351.
   Food poisoning. Simultaneous vomiting and diarrhoea that is much worse for eating fruit, and may even have been caused by it.
   Ill effects of fruit in those who crave fruit, causing diarrhoea.

ILLNESS

Once our bodies have become stressed to the point that they have produced symptoms of illness then that illness in itself can be an additional stress – especially if we do not take appropriate care of ourselves. We need to understand the place of illness in our lives and work with it in order to minimize its potentially stressful impact.

Illness is often seen as a bad thing, an inconvenience (preventing us from working), as something which has come, uninvited, from the outside (i.e. bacteria or viruses) and which must be eliminated so that we can carry on with our lives uninterrupted.

Those who have subscribed to 'new age' theories have added a new stress to struggle with: the idea that we can be as well (or as ill) as we want to be, that if we are ill we have an attitude problem. That if we can only mobilize our will (which only happens if we want to, of course) then we can choose to be well.

The idea that illness is solely caused by external agents, that it is a bad thing and must be destroyed, is as silly as the idea that we create our own reality and therefore our illness is our own creation too. Both attitudes are an oversimplification.

Our bodies are a miracle of intelligent complexity. Our susceptibility to disease is complex, involving many factors: our inherited strengths and weaknesses; our cultural and family histories; our life experiences, encounters with illness and injury, beliefs and attitudes;

our psychological make-up; physical strengths and weaknesses; environmental and work factors; living circumstances (including adequate sanitation and good nutrition) – and finally, luck.

Illness is part of our human condition. It isn't necessarily good or bad. It doesn't only come from the outside, and neither are people capable of making themselves ill just by thinking the wrong thoughts. However, you might want to use your illness to think about the things in your life that you wanted to alter anyway: to motivate you to make lifestyle changes, to reduce unhealthy stresses: to change your diet, to exercise and/or sleep more, to introduce a meditation or relaxation programme, to do some emotional or spiritual spring-cleaning, rework your social life, to have more fun (or less!)

Acute disease

Acute disease is self-limiting; in other words, given time, it will usually clear up of its own accord. An acute disease has three stages: the incubation period, when there may be no symptoms: the acute phase, when the recognizable symptoms surface; the convalescent stage, when a person usually improves. Ordinary, everyday acute diseases include colds, childhood diseases or food poisoning. Depending on the disease, and on the age and constitutional make-up of the patient, some acute illnesses can be a severe stress, for example, flu in the elderly, and some, like meningitis and endocarditis, can be life-threatening.

Chronic disease

Chronic disease such as arthritis, cancer, heart disease, AIDS, multiple sclerosis and chronic fatigue syndrome (ME), are more deep-seated than acute diseases. They usually develop slowly, continue for a long time and are often accompanied by a general deterioration in health. The development of the disease does not take a predictable course; neither is it possible to say for how long it will last.

Chronic disease is stressful. Sufferers often find that every area of their lives is affected: sleep, appetite, energy and moods. People who are house- or bed-bound, in hospitals or even hospices, may feel lonely, isolated and frightened, more especially if they have few or no visitors.

Pain
Pain is stressful, and it comes in all shapes and sizes. Emotional stress can cause physical pain which is not necessarily serious in itself but can be an additional worry. Just knowing that we are not seriously ill at a time like this will help us to bear emotional stress more easily.

Acute pain, such as pain after surgery or dental work, can cause tension and can interfere with healing. This is where homeopathy is so effective – at alleviating pain and speeding healing.

People with long term chronic pain become worn down and debilitated with the effort of dealing with suffering. It can seriously limit us, rippling out into every area of our life, causing sleeplessness, difficulty resting or exercising and lead to emotional symptoms such as anger, hopelessness and depression.

The more sensitive we are to pain the more of a strain it will be. Some people have naturally low pain thresholds – this is a card we are dealt along with our constitutional make-up, something we may have to come to terms with, rather than fight against in the erroneous belief that we can 'cure' ourselves of it, or have to be brave and bear it.

Pain is one of our body's protecting mechanisms. It is a warning sign, a signal from our body that something needs attention. Minor pains such as headaches, back ache and stomach aches may be alerting us to the need to address a physical or emotional stress in our lives. Taking pain killers and carrying on as if nothing is happening is only appropriate as a short term measure, or if we know that the stress was minor and temporary. The cause of pain needs identifying in order for it to be dealt with effectively.

Suppression
The 'alleviation' of a disease or of symptoms of disease without taking the whole person into account can lead to a more deep-seated illness developing. For example, some children whose earache has been 'successfully' treated with antibiotics develop glue ear and hearing loss. Homeopaths call this suppression – where a complaint has been successfully treated but has led to a more serious or chronic condition developing. Illnesses which result from suppression are beyond the scope of the home prescriber as treatment often involves

the return of an original complaint and this needs careful management for a successful outcome.

Developmental milestones

We are more susceptible to illness at those times when our bodies are going through major physical changes – from infancy through to old age. They can pass by almost unnoticed or they can be rough passages, highlighting weaknesses that need attention. Physical and emotional pressures increase during these times as our hormones adjust to the next stage of growth – and these can be very stressful. Puberty does not happen overnight and can be, like menopause, a protracted process – or one that happens without much fuss. Inherited factors, nutrition, difficulties at home or school and personality all have their part to play.

Some children have difficulty teething – suffering great pain from sore, swollen gums, as well as producing colds, coughs, earache, diarrhoea, mood swings and sleeplessness with every tooth that comes through. These same children will often have a difficult time second time around when their adult teeth arrive. And then again when their wisdoms erupt – or try to.

Some children suffer from growing pains in their bones or muscles or joints. Growth spurts occur throughout infancy and childhood, and these can be painful and exhausting. Adolescents can grow at an impressive rate, causing a type of arthritis that they will, eventually, grow out of. However, it is often painful enough to prevent them from playing sports as it occurs commonly in the knees and spine.

It is beyond the scope of the home prescriber to deal with serious complaints that come on during these times, for example difficult or delayed menstruation, sexual dysfunction, arthritis during adolescence or the menopause, etc. However, constitutional prescribing has an excellent track record for helping those who become stuck, healthwise, during one of these changing phases of their lives.

Caring for yourself when you are ill

How you look after yourself when you have an acute illness will, in part, determine how well and how quickly you recover. There are times in our life when we are more vulnerable to illness than others. Children starting school often contract more illnesses as their immune systems adapt to a new environment; adolescents, pregnant, nursing and menopausal women, the elderly – especially if eating poorly – are more vulnerable.

Rest is essential: don't use your 'sick leave' as an opportunity to do the spring cleaning or a 'little' gardening. Our metabolism slows down when we rest and sleep, which allows the cells of our bodies to focus on repairs and renewals. And don't plan on going back to work until you are fully recovered as it is easy to relapse during convalescence.

Drink plenty of fluids such as water (hot or cold), herb teas appropriate to your complaint, fresh fruit juices, hot lemon and honey. Eat lightly: soups, porridge, stewed or fresh fruits and yoghurt. Cut out all caffeine, alcohol, sugar (including squashes and soft drinks) as these are stimulating and will interfere with the healing process.

Be cautious about taking antibiotics for an acute illness. Viral illnesses do not respond to antibiotics and, in addition, increasing numbers of bacterial illnesses are antibiotic-resistant and need to be treated specifically. Ask your doctor whether antibiotic treatment is appropriate for your illness, and whether it will make any difference to the course of your recovery.

Caring for sick children

Acute illness in childhood, especially in infants, can be frightening for parents – and for their children. Sick children need reassurance if they are frightened; comfort if they are in pain; distraction from an itchy rash; sponging down if they are too hot – and so on. Many parents love this nurturing time when their chldren are willing and eager to cuddle up to them. Explain clearly (even to a baby) what is wrong and say how long the illness is likely to last. The sound of your voice is comforting to them – and to you!

Don't take sick children out or have a lot of visitors. Encourage them to rest: make up a bed on the sitting room sofa in the daytime so that your child doesn't feel shut off from family life. Keep excitement levels down and encourage quiet activities such as reading, drawing, playing board games, watching a little television (too much is over-stimulating) and listening to the radio.

Children who are sickening for something can become more

demanding and regress temporarily, sucking things, even wetting the bed, sometimes before the physical symptoms of the illness (rashes, swollen glands, etc.) appear. Be patient, this will pass once they are on the road to recovery.

If you are a parent nursing one child after another through a childhood illness engage the help of neighbours, friends or family to step in occasionally so that you can rest or get out to shop or recharge your batteries.

A word about fevers
A fever is a helpful and necessary part of the process of healing in any illness, especially an acute illness. Some people 'throw' high fevers and look, as well as feel, very ill, therefore giving cause for concern, but they may be ill for a shorter time and often recover sooner than those whose temperature is lower for longer. A high temperature generally indicates that the body's defence mechanism is fighting an infection and temperature variations indicate how it is coping. Attempts to control a fever artificially with paracetamol, or even with homeopathic medicines, are likely to confuse the body's natural efforts to heal itself.

Small children who develop a fever, especially infants under six months old, must be watched carefully because they are vulnerable to becoming quickly dehydrated. Delirium and tantrums sometimes accompany high fevers, and, although these are distressing, they are not dangerous.

Never give aspirin of any sort during or after a childhood illness as this can cause serious complications, especially in children but it makes sense for adults who contract these illnesses to avoid it too. Use paracetamol only in an emergency, where the temperature rises above 104°F (40°C) and/or to alleviate pain.

Homeopathic treatment
Homeopathic treatment and appropriate care during the acute phase can help to prevent complications developing in the convalescent stage. It is not the purpose of this book to go into the homeopathic treatment of acute diseases themselves, but to guide you to prescribe on any minor weakness remaining as a result of an acute illness.

Some people do not recover from an acute illness: symptoms

remain and become chronic (long term) for example, swollen glands, depression and exhaustion after a flu, or a cough after a chest infection. A professional homeopath should always be consulted in these instances.

It is in the convalescent phase that many people find they do not recover as well or as quickly as they had expected. Perhaps the illness has been stressful enough to affect the nervous system, or a loss of body fluids – through sweating, bleeding, diarrhoea or vomiting – has been exhausting. If you feel low and exhausted after an illness then homeopathic treatment can help you to recover your former equilibrium.

There are a few remedies below to help with illnesses that surface as a result of teething or growing pains in children. Homeopathy can help with a physical milestone that is proving a bumpy ride, but in most instances you will need to consult a professional homeopath who can take your whole picture into account.

- *Calcarea carbonica (Calc-c.)* See also p. 277.

   Difficulty teething in good-natured children who become cranky when teeth are coming through – and get frequent coughs, colds and even diarrhoea at this time.

- *Calcarea phosphorica (Calc-p.)* See also p. 281.

   Convalescence: with loss of appetite, anaemia, headaches and exhaustion with heavy, weak feeling in legs. Discontented and sluggish. Feels the cold, especially draughts.

   Difficulty teething. Teeth are slow to come through and accompanied by coughs and colds.

   Growth spurt/growing pains; children suffer from growing pains (in the back and/or knee joints) during a growth spurt. Adolescents who grow a lot suffer from joint and back pains.

- *Carbo vegetabilis (Carb-v.)* See also p. 284.

   Convalescence: especially after a childhood illness or a chest infection or any illness with a loss of body fluids. Irritable, sluggish and low in vitality. Slightest exertion is exhausting, may be too tired to eat. Head feels heavy.

- *Chamomilla (Cham.)* See also p. 289.

   Teething infants/children suffer from terrible pains and tantrums.

- *China officinalis (Chin.)*

   Convalescence: after an illness with loss of body fluids. Anaemia, headache and/or nervous exhaustion with profuse sweating on exertion and during sleep. Feels faint and may have a ringing in ears. Pale face with dark rings around eyes. Has difficulty sleeping. Despondent and apathetic.

Appetite lost in sick or convalescing people. Feels hungry but doesn't want to eat and then the appetite returns after eating only a mouthful. Doesn't want cold food/drinks, feels better after hot food/drinks.

- *Gelsemium sempervirens* (*Gels.*) See also p. 297.
Convalescence: feels completely exhausted after flu or any illness with high fever, aching joints and swollen glands. Heaviness and trembling with exhaustion. Apathetic and depressed. Thirstless.

- *Kali phosphoricum* (*Kali-p.*) See also p. 301.
Convalescence: nervous and muscular exhaustion worse for the slightest physical exertion. Sensitive and jumpy. Sweats easily with slightest exertion. With head and backache and insomnia.

- *Phosphoric acid* (*Pho-ac.*) See also p. 323.
Convalescence: after an illness with fluid loss. Faint and tired. Nervous exhaustion worse for slightest exertion. Looks pale with dark rings around eyes. Sweats easily. Apathetic and uncommunicative.

Growing pains. Growing pains during a growth spurt with exhaustion and apathy afterwards.

- *Phosphorus* (*Phos.*) See also p. 325.
Growing pains; puberty. Growing pains during a growth spurt and exhaustion afterwards. During puberty children grow a lot, become jumpy and easily frightened and suffer from nosebleeds.

- *Pulsatilla nigricans* (*Puls.*) See also p. 330.
Convalescence: children (or even adults!) regress emotionally and become clingy after an illness (especially measles). Catarrh, cough, eye and/or ear problems linger with or without swollen glands.

- *Silica* (*Sil.*) See also p. 338.
Teething difficulties in shy, skinny children who develop slowly. Teeth come through slowly and with great difficulty. A remedy that is useful for those experiencing difficulty with second or wisdom teeth that are slow to erupt.

INJURY

Any injury to the body can be stressful – whether it is caused by an accident, a physically demanding event such as childbirth or a marathon, or is unintentionally the effect of a dental or medical intervention, especially a surgical procedure.

Accidents and injuries

Some people are accident-prone because of an inherited weakness, because they are moving too fast for their bodies, because they do not pay enough attention to their surroundings in certain situations, because they ignore (or do not know) safety guidelines or because they are involved in a high risk activity. Some people (especially children) are always falling on their heads, others have ankles that sprain easily, some have a terrifying ability to crush their fingers in doors or to break bones. Accidents often happen when our ability to concentrate and our judgement is affected – when we are upset, tired or even hungry, or under the influence of alcohol or certain drugs (in particular anti-histamines, anti-depressants and recreational drugs).

Identifying the cause of a tendency to have accidents and dealing with it can help with preventing them. In addition, basic safety measures (for adults and children) exist to prevent many everyday accidents: wearing seat belts in the car, helmets at all times on motorbikes and bicycles, reflective clothing and lights when cycling at night.

Sports injuries are an area where a little prevention goes a long way. Warming up, adequate training, good equipment and some sort of supervision in the beginning all help to prevent accidents. Athletes who undergo particularly stressful activities such as marathon running and climbing need to get a full medical check-up periodically to ensure that they are strong and healthy (especially their hearts).

Accidents at work are often the result of failing to follow safety procedures or being bored or tired: find out where your job places you in terms of risk factors. Make sure you have any necessary training and confidence in your capabilities to handle physical stress at work.

The sorts of injury that result from physical violence at work are unfortunately common in some professions i.e. social workers, probation and prison officers, police and publicans. Prevention in these professions is complicated and involves some sort of training as well as back-up support.

Use a combination of commonsense and skill to deal with injuries. Take a basic first aid course with the St John Ambulance Brigade or the Red Cross so that you can deal with the practicalities of accidents confidently.

Act quickly, listen to your instincts and always seek medical advice after a serious accident or injury, especially if it involves a child, even if it is just to get some basic reassurance. Serious cuts and falls, deep splinters, injuries to the head, back and eyes, burns and animal bites all need medical attention.

An accident may be over in seconds, or minutes, but the time needed to recover can be disproportionately long. Take as much time as you (and your body) need in order to rest, recover and heal from a physical injury. If you don't, you may be left with a weakness that makes you vulnerable to reinjury. Build up your physical strength gradually if you have suffered a broken bone, for example. Use homeopathic medicines to speed the healing, and consult a physical therapist, an osteopath or chartered physiotherapist, to aid that process.

Medical interventions

Many medical tests and treatments – well-intentioned and important though they may be – involve an injury to the body. Tests such as blood tests, cervical smears, certain X-rays, i.e. any investigative practice and treatment (including minor surgical procedures or major surgery) involve something being done to the body which can hurt. The effects of this potential hurt can be minimized if medical professionals are gentle, efficient, skilled and kind. And if the patient is well prepared.

In order to make an informed decision, you will find it helpful to ask some or all of the following questions.

- Why do you, or why does your doctor think you need this test, treatment or surgery?
- What are the pros and cons of this particular intervention?
- How exactly is it carried out and what will it involve?
- Who will be carrying out the procedure and how experienced are they?
- How long will it take and will there be any after effects?
- What medications are involved, both during and afterwards and what effects might they have?
- How long will you need to recover afterwards?
- Are there any risks involved and what are they?
- What may happen if you don't have this procedure, i.e. what other options do you have?

Don't get fobbed off at this point by well-meaning but harassed doctors. Ask if you have some time to play with so that you can seek alternative treatment if you want to try and avoid surgery, for whatever reason. You will need to make a decision that is right for you – one that may be different to someone else's in a similar position. Don't be rushed into making a choice and don't forget that you can ask for as many second opinions as you need in order to make a decision that is right for you. As patients, we do deserve to be treated in a respectful, gentle and non-patronizing way. If you haven't consented to a medical intervention where you are able to, it is regarded as a common assault from a legal point of view.

Your understanding of what is going to happen to your body and your acceptance of that, as well as your trust in the medical professionals who are carrying out the procedure will help you to handle the experience better and your body to heal faster afterwards.

Take a companion with you if you are anxious and a list of questions so that you don't forget anything. It is useful to take notes as study after study has shown that we remember only a small percentage of anything our doctors tell us.

While medical professionals cannot give cast-iron guarantees as to the outcome of any procedure, they do have a responsibility to answer your questions and to give you any information you decide you need to make your decision, so that you can be an active participant in your own health care. If you so wish. If it is too stressful for you to know what is going on, if you have an implicit faith in your doctor and are happy for them to get on with their job, then don't feel pressured into making an 'informed choice'.

Think ahead and prepare yourself for situations where you know you are going to feel tense and/or anxious. Any operation that involves a cut into the body or routine treatments such as a dental procedure, a gynaecological examination, an episiotomy during childbirth, can be unpleasant. Ask professionals to be gentle with you and to work at a pace that is comfortable for you. In some instances we can say if we are experiencing pain or discomfort and ask for a break or for a slowing down. Take a friend or partner with you or ask the nurse to hold your hand.

Some decisions are particularly difficult. The decision, for example, to undergo fertility treatment can lead to one intervention and/or treatment after another, spanning many years. Whilst they have been consciously and carefully agreed to, the physical impact can be, at times, hard to cope with. You will want to consult a professional homeopath to help you with this type of physical stress.

Homeopathic treatment

Start by identifying which part of your body has been injured and how that has affected you. The following are first aid remedies for common situations, for the stressful effects of common injuries to the body occurring after an accident or a medical or dental procedure.

- *Aconitum napellus (Aco.)* See also p. 255.
  Shock after injury. Anxious, frightened and trembly after an injury. This is one of the first remedies to take to deal with the shock before working out what to take for the stress itself. Give before a general anaesthetic where there is great anxiety, especially a fear of death, to reduce the stressful impact of any surgical procedure.
- *Apis mellifica (Ap.)* See also p. 261.
  Severe reaction to an insect bite (especially a bee or wasp sting). Bite is swollen, shiny and inflamed. It stings or burns and itches and is sensitive to touch and to heat.
- *Arnica montana (Arn.)* See also p. 265.
  Head injury. Bruises. Injury to bones; to muscles. Shock after injury including delayed shock with bad dreams relating to the incident. This is our greatest accident and injury remedy. It reduces swelling from bruising to muscle tissue whether it is a head injury,

a bruise to any part of the body, dental treatment or surgery. Give immediately after a head injury and watch the egg disappear in front of your eyes. Give after a fracture, a sprain or immediately after any surgical procedure to bring down swelling and begin the healing process.

- *Arsenicum album (Ars.)* See also p. 266.
  Burns with blisters caused by heat or chemicals. Great anxiety with burning pains that are better for heat.
- *Bellis perennis (Bell-p.)*
  Injuries to glands e.g. a breast or testicle. Bruises. Injuries to muscle. Bruised soreness which doesn't respond to Arnica calls for this remedy where there is deep bruising after childbirth or especially after abdominal surgery. It is useful for lumps or bumps that remain after the bruising has disappeared. It is called for in any injury to a gland where a lump remains.
- *Bryonia alba (Bry.)*
  This is for any injury to a joint or bone (including whiplash) with great pain that is worse for the slightest movement, and better for pressure and for heat.
- *Caladium (Calad.)*
  Insect bites (especially mosquitoes and midges) itch and burn maddeningly.
- *Calcarea phosphorica (Calc-p.)* See also p. 281.
  Injuries to bones: fractures that are slow to heal after the swelling and acute pains have cleared.
- *Calendula officinalis (Calend.)*
  Incised wounds. Promotes the speedy healing of any cut or wound whether it is after an accident or surgery or childbirth. The wound is painful, sometimes out of proportion to the injury.
- *Cantharis vesiticatoria (Canth.)*
  Burns with blisters caused by fire or scalding liquids. The burning pains are better for cold bathing or cold compresses.
- *Causticum (Caust.)* See also p. 286.
  Serious (third degree) burns with blisters caused by fire or chemicals. Pains are severe.
- *Conium maculatum (Con.)* See also p. 295.
  Injuries to glands i.e. a breast or testicle that become lumpy and

feel stony hard. The injured area is sensitive, painful (with stitching pains) and may tingle and feel cold.

- **Hepar sulphuris calcareum** (*Hep-s.*)
  Cuts/wounds become inflamed, are painful to touch with sore, splinter-like pains.
- *Hypericum perfoliatum* (*Hyp.*)
  Injuries to nerves and nerve-rich parts of the body – to eyes, fingers, toes, spine, especially to the coccyx. This remedy helps damaged nerves to heal and prevents inflammation (sepsis). Pains are severe and shoot up (or down) nerve pathways.
  Incised wounds with great pain. Whiplash. Bites or stings.
- *Kali bichromicum* (*Kali-bi.*)
  Deep burns of any sort that are slow to heal, that become inflamed, are painful and leave scars.
- *Ledum palustre* (*Led.*)
  Bruises. Injury to muscles with discolouration, especially to eyes. Incised wounds. Bites. This remedy helps prevent inflammation and sepsis, after a wound (especially a punctured wound i.e. from a nail or knife) or a bite from an insect or an animal. Wounds feel cold (inside) but the pains are soothed by cold bathing or cold compresses.
- *Natrum sulphuricum* (*Nat-s.*)
  Head injuries. Headache and sensitivity to light after a head injury, with or without depression.
- *Opium* (*Op.*) See also p. 321.
  Shock after surgery, or after injury with the images of the incident recurring during the waking hours.
- *Phosphorus* (*Phos.*) See also p. 325.
  Ill effects of an electric shock. Becomes frightened and easily startled.
- *Ranunculus bulbosis* (*Ran-b.*)
  Injuries to nerves and to joints with great stabbing or shooting pains worse for the slightest movement. Cannot find relief from pain in any position.
- *Rhus toxicodendron* (*Rhus-t.*)
  Injuries to joints. Whiplash. Injuries to the tendons/ligaments of any joint with sore, aching pains that are better for heat. With stiffness that is worse for rest but the pains are worse on

beginning to move after sitting or lying.
- *Ruta graveolens (Ruta.)*
  Injuries to bones; to joints. To the periosteum or covering to the bones i.e. to shins, knees or any bony area thinly covered with muscle. Pains are sore and bruised.
- *Silica (Sil.)* See also p. 338.
  Helps to expel splinters. Injuries to bones: fractures that are slow to heal. Cuts/wounds are slow to heal. Also for wounds that become inflamed with pus or where scars break open after they have healed up.
- *Staphysagria (Staph.)* See also p. 341.
  Incised injuries/wounds are incredibly painful after an accident, surgery, dental treatment, etc. The pains are stinging, smarting or tearing and worse for touch.
- *Stramonium (Stram.)* See also p. 344.
  Shock after surgery. Feels terrified, looks frightened. Has nightmares and difficulty sleeping. Sometimes babies (and mothers) need this remedy after a frightening and difficult birth.
- *Symphytum (Symph.)*
  Injuries to bones with pain; to eyes. Fractures are very painful with sticking pains.

MEDICATION

Conventional medicines can and do save lives, and deal with diseases that were formerly beyond the scope of orthodox doctors. But the over-use of orthodox medications (both prescribed and over-the-counter), especially for minor complaints, is becoming an increasing concern. People are often surprised when they add up their overall medication intake.

I am concerned that we should use drugs sparingly, or not at all in certain situations, in order to ensure they are going to work when we really need them, and to preserve the health of our immune systems. Apart from the benefits of many prescribed drugs, they are also stressful to some degree, from over-the-counter purchases such as aspirin (causing stomach aches and even bleeding) and paracetamol (causing liver damage – increasingly a concern in children) to prescription sleeping tablets (causing dependency) and steroids (causing immune system weakness).

All medications are chemical stresses and are toxic to some degree, even when they are alleviating symptoms. Different medicines affect different organs and systems of the body, but to a certain extent the liver, bowels and kidneys are involved in dealing with most chemicals that enter the body – with 'fighting' them, with detoxifying or getting rid of them, or with storing them. Chemicals may cause side effects and these will vary from person to person, depending on the strength of their general vitality and any particular weaknesses. One person may suffer from diarrhoea and nausea after antibiotic treatment, another from depression and exhaustion. Mostly these side effects pass and the patient recovers. Some, however, are left with symptoms they didn't have before which they offer up for further treatment. So people who may have wanted to avoid unnecessary medication find themselves taking one prescription after another. Or worse, one prescription on top of another.

People who are cautious with their own health often find it more difficult to resist a 'pill for every ill' when it comes to their own children. Whereas they may have avoided unnecessary medication for themselves they can end up giving their children one course of antibiotics after another for minor coughs, earaches and even colds.

Many ordinary medications are simply relieving symptoms – and in the long term may mask more serious illnesses since they do not deal with the underlying complaint. For example, pain-relieving drugs like aspirin and paracetamol alleviate pain without dealing with the cause of the pain, just as coffee masks tiredness, not providing real energy. If you are taking, say, antacids on a regular basis then you need to get a thorough check-up to find out what is causing your indigestion.

Think carefully before agreeing to a course of antibiotics, especially if you know or suspect your infection is viral in origin i.e. if you have a cold, cough or flu. Over-prescribing, the increasing resistance of bacteria to antibiotics, partly because of the massive use of these drugs in farmed animals, and rapid mutation of bacteria are making the development and long term 'success' of antibiotics a race against time. You need to save them for when you might really need them.

As well as masking symptoms many medications can increase your load by adding chemicals to an already weakening body.

Decongestants give only temporary relief, and cause a complicated sort of dependency whereby the congestion becomes worse on stopping them. Laxatives cause the bowels to gradually lose their strength and ability to work naturally, as well as making it difficult for you to absorb essential nutrients from your food.

Corticosteroids have been acclaimed as wonder drugs because of their efficacy in reducing inflammation and allergic reactions. The large numbers of steroid drugs available to doctors (and therefore to patients) has coincided with a decrease in the efficacy of antibiotic treatment. This has meant that these drugs are being routinely prescribed for many infections, inflammations and rashes. Their side effects are many and complex, the most serious include a compromised immune system, osteoporosis, retarded bone growth in children, delayed healing of wounds and thinning of the skin.

Illegal drugs have a strong effect (which is why people use them) and therefore all have the ability to seriously undermine and ruin the health. Some turn to drugs (like alcohol) to meet a short term need, to help them cope better: to lift depression, to provide more energy, to dull physical pain, to escape emotional pain. The price – drug addiction (and a compromised immune system) – is devastating, to the user and those close to them.

Supplements – vitamins, minerals, aromatherapy oils and herbs – can have adverse effects if they are taken in excess, especially if they are not needed. Make sure you get expert advice if you are taking any supplement in the long term, especially in megadoses.

Oral contraceptives and hormone replacement therapy tampers with hormones and their natural functioning. Many women do not find them to be problematical, but some find they suffer from a wide range of problems, such as migraines, depression, weight gain and low energy, which do not go away when they stop taking them. As with all other medication side effects, these are mostly beyond the scope of the home prescriber to deal with homeopathically.

A word about vaccinations
Vaccinations are stressful to the immune system – that is how they work. Childhood vaccinations are often administered in a worrying cocktail to young infants whose immune systems are still developing. Homeopaths regularly see children who have never been well since a particular vaccination or vaccination programme, suffering from recurring coughs, colds, earaches and sore throats or more serious complaints such as asthma, eczema and behavioural problems. Many homeopaths will give useful advice on how to vaccinate so as to minimize the side effects – and can sometimes suggest alternatives. For example, the homeopathic alternative to the flu vaccination (*Occilococcininum*) will prevent a flu from developing or make it a milder illness.

Wait until your baby is at least three months old (breast-fed babies have a natural immunity that lasts at least three months) or has started on solids to have them vaccinated. Proceed cautiously if there is a history of allergies, asthma or eczema on either side of your baby's family. Ask your doctor to administer each inoculation singly with a couple of weeks in between. If there is a problem with one of the vaccinations you will know which one it is. Seek homeopathic treatment for a child who has reacted badly to a vaccination, with a high fever, distress or more serious symptoms or if minor symptoms don't clear up quickly.

Leave at least six weeks between your inoculations for any foreign travel, but especially for travel to high risk countries, to allow any effects to wear off well before your trip. Think carefully before planning a trip to a high risk country (where inoculations are necessary) if you suffer from chronic illness of any sort.

Start with your own research
Research has repeatedly shown that at least a third of all prescription medications are not taken and/or are not taken correctly. Use the following guidelines to help you avoid the 'medical treadmill', to use orthodox medications sparingly, if possible, and wisely, and to begin to take an active interest in the medications that are prescribed for you – or those purchased over the counter at the pharmacy.
• Start by listing the contents of your medicine cabinet and note

which you take on a regular basis, which you take occasionally and which you take once in a blue moon. Put to one side the ones that are out of date, and rather than throw them away, take them to your pharmacy for safe disposal.

• Get a book that lists the side effects of all drugs and go through your list one by one, noting common side effects and whether you have experienced them. You may be surprised to find, for example, how a steroid ointment for a minor skin complaint that you had been using on a daily basis will affect your skin in the long term; or how your stomach aches may be a side effect of the anti-inflammatories that you had been taking for headaches.

• Keep track of all the medicines that you use: the dates you take them, whether they work, what side effects you experience. Build up a picture of what works for you and what doesn't. This will help you identify patterns of drug use – and abuse. Many people are shocked to find that they are taking up to 40 aspirin a month, or six courses of antibiotics in a year, or a combination of medications which adds up to a pharmaceutical cocktail about which relatively little may be known. Women who are taking oral contraceptives or hormone replacement therapy, for example, need to keep track of their medication intake as their chemical stresses can add up rather quickly.

• Explore alternatives (herbal, homeopathic, kitchen cupboard, aromatherapy, etc.) to boost your immune system and to deal with minor illnesses without recourse to strong medications. For example, a combination of garlic, vitamin C and the herb echinacea have been found to help with viral illnesses.

Prescription medications

The days when a patient enjoyed an exclusive, continuous relationship with his or her general practitioner are passing. It is more likely that he or she will see one of a group practice, the one that is available on that particular day, someone with whom they may not be familiar. The doctor may have to rely on sketchy notes and whatever information is presented in the five or so minutes allotted. This represents a breakdown in what has been, for many patients, an important healing relationship. It leaves doctors functioning more as technicians than healers and means that many of their prescriptions will focus on physical symptoms alone without taking the person into account, and especially any underlying stresses. It is reasonable to ask your doctor at least some of the following questions when presented with a prescription:

- What has been prescribed and why?
- What common side effects might you experience? It isn't commonly known that side effects can surface at any point during treatment, not just at the beginning. And those same effects may not clear up of their own accord once the medication has been stopped. Some common medications i.e. antihistamines, can cause drowsiness and make driving and operating machinery a risky business.
- Are there alternative medications to those chosen?
- Do you really need this prescription – and if so, why? This may seem like a redundant question but the bottom line is that many patients expect a fast relief of symptoms, expect a prescription and expect it to work. Many doctors find it difficult or time-consuming to explain that a patient's illness is acute and will clear up in its own time whether they prescribe or not. They say that the flu takes a week to be cured with antibiotic treatment and it takes seven days with bed rest and plenty of fluids!
- Is there anything you can do to avoid or minimize potential side effects? For example, to take live yogurt alongside antibiotics to help your bowels. Those on strong medications, such as chemotherapy for cancer, will find it especially beneficial to take at least some practical measures to help their bodies deal with the chemical onslaught. Support groups are usually especially helpful in this regard.
- What practical measures can you take to help you deal with your complaint? For example, to use steam for sinus infections and the croup.
- Will this medication interact with any other drugs you are currently taking?
- Can you reduce any other medication (even temporarily), or stop them until you have finished with the one being prescribed, especially if it is for an acute illness?

- Is there a danger of addiction or dependency, i.e. with sleeping tablets, anti-depressants etc?
- Can alternative medicine help you with your current complaint – and will your doctor support you choosing to try an alternative method alongside orthodox medicine or even instead of it? Especially if you are in a 'high-risk' category with regard to chemical toxicity, i.e. if you suffer from kidney or liver disease, a compromised immune system or if you are pregnant or breast-feeding.
- Will anything affect this medication? For example, alcohol and caffeine are not recommended whilst taking certain medications.
- Do you have to finish the course? Can you stop after, say, five days of a ten day course of antibiotics? (And if not, why not?)
- Can you adjust the dose yourself i.e. reducing and stopping the medication without consultation with your doctor, for example, with sleeping tablets, anti-inflammatories or oral contraceptives? And then take it on an as-and-when-needed basis?
- Do you need to consult your doctor before stopping or reducing the medication? For example, steroids and some medications – for epilepsy, diabetes, heart, thyroid and asthma – should either never be reduced or stopped or can only be tapered off under medical supervision.
- What might happen if you don't take the drugs you have been prescribed? Some doctors are adopting a wait-and-see policy for minor complaints and supporting patients who choose, for example, TLC and alternative medical treatments over antibiotics for their children – or themselves.

Doctors do vary in the drugs they prescribe. If you are concerned you can always get a second (and, if necessary, a third) opinion in order to get the reassurance you need that your medication is both appropriate and necessary. Your pharmacist can advise you about the drugs you have been prescribed, and can sometimes recommend less toxic alternatives, or give advice about how drugs interact and how you can minimize the possibility of side effects.

Homeopathic treatment

The following remedies are to help you over the immediate, acute side effects of a few common medications. There are many more –

you will need to consult a homeopath who can evaluate your whole picture in order to prescribe effectively. In any case, you must consult your medical practitioner before reducing or stopping any prescribed medicines. The homeopathic solutions should be taken for a short period of time only to help you recover your vitality and encourage your liver and kidneys to detoxify. If you do not notice an immediate improvement then you will need to consult your doctor or a professional homeopath.

- **Adrenalin (Adren.)**
  Ill effects of local anaesthetic. Wired up and shaky after a local anaesthetic at, say, the dentist.
- **Alumina (Alu.)**
  Ill effects of antacids; of laxatives. Constipated and sluggish.
- **Cadminium sulphuratum (Cad-s.)**
  Ill effects of radiotherapy; of chemotherapy. Constant nausea, with or without vomiting. Diarrhoea, exhaustion and chilliness.
- **Calcarea carbonica (Calc-c.)** See also p. 277.
  Ill effects of aspirin. Stomach aches, nausea and constipation.
- **Cortisone (Cort.)**
  Ill effects of steroids. Changeable moods, difficulty concentrating, headache, dry skin, bloating and water retention.
- **Nitricum acidum (Nit-ac)** See also p. 314.
  Ill effects of drugs in general. Sensitive to all medications, especially antibiotics. Becomes irritable and exhausted.
- **Nux vomica (Nux-v.)** See also p. 317
  Ill effects of drugs in general, of laxatives, of antibiotics, diet pills, sleeping tablets, etc. Tired and irritable and liverish.
- **Opium (Op.)** See also p. 321.
  Ill effects of general anaesthetic. Spaced-out, cannot come-to after surgery – falls asleep constantly. Constipated and sluggish.
- **Phosphorus (Phos.)** See also p. 325.
  Ill effects of general anaesthetic. With vomiting. Feels shocked by the anaesthetic and upset.
- **Pulsatilla nigricans (Puls.)** See also p. 330.
  Ill effects of the contraceptive pill/HRT; from iron tablets. Depressed and weepy. Periods are irregular and problematical. Constipated.

- **Radium bromide** (*Rad-br.*)
  Ill effects of radiotherapy; of x-rays. General lethargy; aching (like flu) all over the body. Itchy skin rashes. Cuts/wounds are slow to heal.
- **Sepia** (*Sep.*) See also p. 334.
  Ill effects of the contraceptive pill/HRT. Depressed, exhausted and irritable. Periods are scanty and painful.
- **Silica** (*Sil.*) See also p. 338.
  Ill effects of vaccination. Sick after, with colds and coughs.
- **Sulphur** (*Sul.*) See also p. 345.
  Ill effects of drugs in general; of vaccination. Becomes restless and difficult. Suffers from fevers and infections.
- **Thuja occidentalis** (*Thu.*)
  Ill effects of vaccination. Frequent colds and coughs which are worse in cold, wet (damp) weather.

PHYSICAL STRESS AND STRAIN

Physical fitness is essential to our general health – it actually enables us to deal more easily with all sorts of stresses, both physical and emotional. The older we get the more important it is that we are physically active – we are always building the health for our future in the present and it is never too late to start!

The human body needs to move, to maintain the strength of muscles and bones as well as the flexibility and mobility of muscles, nerves and joints. Exercise is as important for babies and children as it is for adults, for pregnant women, the elderly, the disabled and the chronically ill. Taking the major joints through a full range of movements on a daily basis will help to keep them supple (neck, shoulders, elbows, wrists, upper and lower spine, hips, pelvis, knees and ankles). Using gravity is important for the health and strength of our bones. Some people say you should be on your feet for about two hours a day to encourage healthy bones. Even people who aren't mobile, including those who are wheelchair- or bed-bound, need to exercise to maintain the strength of their bones.

Engaging in regular vigorous activity stimulates the metabolism and the immune system and can be immensely energizing. In addition, it will maintain the strength and health of your heart and your circulation and ensure a boost of oxygen to all your muscles and organs.

A sedentary life is a problem, at any age. Those who are vulnerable are the naturally sedentary who dislike exercise in any shape or form; those who are depressed; people who have a physical problem (such as low thyroid); those addicted to television; who drive to work; who have sedentary jobs; the sick and the disabled. A sedentary lifestyle has many physical repercussions; the circulation slows down, the arteries clog up, the muscles lose their resilience and bones lose their strength and decalcify.

We all have different exercise requirements to balance out the way we live. Rest and relaxation are not the only antidotes to emotional and physical stresses. A person who leads a sedentary life may well feel tired at the end of the day but the last thing they need is physical rest for whilst the brain is exhausted and the body may *feel* exhausted, it will only become more sluggish if it isn't exercised and thereby set up a vicious cycle that is hard to break.

At the other end of the spectrum, some people feel quite literally euphoric after exercising. This is because endorphins are released which get taken up by morphine-like receptors in the brain. The feeling is not unlike taking drugs and those who become accustomed to an exercise high can feel irritable or withdrawn when they don't exercise, i.e. when these endorphins are no longer being released. Exercise can become addictive, and, like any addiction, can be some people's way of avoiding dealing with emotional problems or difficulties in their own lives. If you suspect that you are an exercise 'addict', give yourself some time off and see what feelings surface, whether, for example, you become depressed. If you do then it will be healthier to deal with the emotional stress or underlying problem rather than keep on 'running' away from it.

Do you need some exercise?
If you answer yes to one or more of the following questions (without having a complaint such as asthma or a heart condition as an excuse) then you may want to think about making exercise a priority.
- Do you get out of breath on stairs or a hill (especially when walking up at a normal walking pace)?

- Do you have to use your arms to lever yourself out of a chair?
- Do you have stiff joints, especially after you have been sitting or lying down for a while?
- Do you have difficulty opening jars?
- Do you feel physically tired – too tired to exercise?
- Are you physically inactive?

What is the underlying cause of your inactivity? It is important to find out if you have an undiagnosed medical problem before embarking on an exercise programme if you have answered yes to any of the above questions.

Keep a diary of your physical activities for a week. Note how much time you spend on your feet, how long you walk each day, whether you engage in activities that involve twisting and stretching, how much 'vigorous activity' you have in a day, how much lifting.

Make physical activity a part of your life, not something you have to make an effort to go somewhere and do. Incorporate it into what you already do and do it a bit more, i.e. run for the bus, walk to work or to the station or get off a bus or train a stop early and walk the rest of the way!

Be creative with how you add more exercise in – use your stairs at home, just run up and down them on rainy days or if you are stuck inside with a sick child or at a sitting-down job. Get a dog, or walk a friend's or neighbour's. Get a bicycle or a skipping rope. Make a social occasion of it – swim, walk, run, go bowling or dancing with a friend. Take a child to a playground and have fun with them – don't just stand there and watch! Be creative about the housework or boring tasks like filing, mowing the lawn or washing the car: put on some music (use a personal stereo if your task is noisy!) and make it enjoyable. Watch a child do a boring household chore: many will use it as an opportunity to play.

Protecting yourself from strain

When doing anything physical it is sensible to organize your body so that there is minimal strain. It is stressful to spend long periods of time with muscles tensed, shoulders hunched or your body (or even a part of your body) twisted or crouched awkwardly.

A little preventative action goes a long way. It is an investment you won't regret. If we put our bodies under unnecessary strain on a regular basis it is only a question of time before they complain, and then it can be much more time consuming to get them strong again than if we had taken things easier in the first place.

Learn to relax your body in your everyday life. When standing don't lock your legs, relax your knees enough to feel them bounce a little, and let the muscles in your legs and up into your buttocks soften a little. Shift from foot to foot if you are having to stand for periods of time or bounce up and down gently. If you are unable to make big movements, then relax your muscles and wiggle your toes.

Keep your spine straight. Try the following exercise when sitting or standing; slump gently, relaxing your shoulders and breathing deeply and evenly, then imagine a cord attached to the top of your head pulling your head upright until your spine feels straightish with a nice little curve in the small of your back, your shoulders, buttocks and leg muscles relaxed and your breathing unaltered.

Take care of your lumbar curve (your lower back should gently curve in, but not too much). Check out your seating at home, at work and when driving and put a little cushion in the small of your back so that it is nicely curved. If your back slumps when you sit (or stand or lie down) then you will be more vulnerable to lower back strain and, therefore, pain.

Check your position when you are standing at a work surface such as in the kitchen or garage. Your surface should be 2"–4" (5–10 cms) below your elbows when they are bent. Most kitchen work surfaces have been designed for women of around 5' 4" high. If they are lower you will have to bend to chop or wash up – enough to strain your lower back. You can buy an extra washing-up bowl and invert it under the one you use to raise it up. Make sure your ironing board is high enough for you to iron without bending. If you are shorter than 5' 4" you may need a box or small stool to stand on to reach some surfaces comfortably.

Check your position when sitting at a computer or typewriter. Make sure your elbows and knees are at right angles so you can relax your shoulders, back and legs. In order to encourage your lumbar curve your hips should be at about 110°. This can take a bit of fiddling to get it right.

Your head should be upright and not consistently turned to one side or looking down (to write, answer the telephone, to work at a computer or any other machine) as this will strain your neck. Make sure computer screens are high enough and directly in front of you, i.e. not to one side so that you have to turn your head when you are working. Your eyes should be level with the middle of your screen so that you are not having to look down, which will strain your neck, eyes, head and shoulders. If you use a laptop computer, do not use it on your lap. Don't cradle the telephone between your ear and your shoulder.

Chairs (and toilet seats) shouldn't cut into your thighs when your feet are flat on the floor, especially if you have short legs (including children). Some people hold their legs (and buttocks and lower back) in tension with their heels off the floor to 'adapt' to high seating. Your feet should be flat on the ground with your thighs comfortably supported – they shouldn't end up with a line from the chair or stool (or toilet). You can raise your feet using a stool or telephone directory (or two!) if necessary.

Organize your work on a desk or work surface sensibly. You need to be able to get close to your work surface, without reaching out to work. If you have to reach out to get to a typewriter, keyboard, chopping board or anything else, you may strain your shoulders and your back.

Make sure that your work (keyboard, steering wheel, chopping board, desk) is central to your body. If it is out by even a few inches you will have to twist your whole body to work, drive or write etc. and this may stress your back, shoulders and arms.

Squat, kneel down (using a pad or cushion to protect your knees) or even sit instead of crouching or bending down awkwardly to do floor level jobs, i.e. when bathing children and brushing dogs, cleaning the bath or kitchen floor, weeding the garden, filling or emptying the washing machine, etc. When squatting you can rest one knee on the ground for balance, and then place your hands on your thighs to help push yourself up (keeping your back straight). Get a vacuum cleaner that is the right height so that you don't have to bend forward to clean.

Get into cars carefully, sitting down first then swinging both legs in and getting out by putting both feet on the ground first. It is possible to strain your back by putting one leg first.

Lift (children, sacks of concrete, anything – even relatively light things like bags of shopping) using your legs and arms, squatting right down, keeping your back straight and sticking your bum out (like weight-lifters or gorillas), and keeping the object you are lifting as close to your body as possible. This isn't elegant but it is good for your body.

Carry babies and infants close to your body and alternate hips so that you don't become 'lop-sided'. Lift infants and children in and out of buggies and cars very carefully – it is all too easy to strain your lower back. When carrying heavy shopping or work, spread your load in two bags and/or a back pack or use a shopping trolley, or carry a single heavy bag in both arms in front of you (like a baby). Learn how to lift (from an expert) if you are caring for the chronically sick, disabled or the elderly or if you are expected to lift at work.

Seek the advice of an Alexander Technique teacher or Chartered Physiotherapist if you want some expert help with changing unhealthy patterns of standing, sitting, lifting and moving.

Pay some attention to your mattress – it shouldn't be too soft nor too hard. When you lie down on your side your spine should make a straight line rather than curve. Sleep with one pillow if you lie on your back or have narrow shoulders, two pillows if you are broad-shouldered (to fill the gap between the shoulder and the side of your head). Too many or too few pillows can strain your neck.

If you wake with lower-back ache try sleeping in the 'recovery position': on your side with your underneath leg stretched out straightish and your top leg bent enough to give your lower back the curve it needs to prevent strain when asleep. Some people like to have a pillow under the top leg/knee to further reduce strain on the back.

Watch out for tight clothes, especially clothes that constrict your hips or your waist (including leggings and tight trousers) as these restrict your blood flow and the movements of your hips and knees. Bras that are too tight can impede breathing and affect the healthy functioning of your lymph glands.

Wear comfortable shoes that support your whole foot including your heel – too tight shoes, shoes with high heels, loose shoes (especially trainers with laces that aren't done up!) can all strain feet, legs and back. Get special inner soles if your arches need supporting, i.e. if your feet ache after standing for even relatively short periods of time. An orthopaedic surgeon or chiropodist will help if you have problem feet which are affecting your health or your posture.

Breathing is automatic: you cannot stop breathing even if you try! But a poor breathing pattern can be stressful as it involves a reduced oxygen intake and therefore supply to your body. Many people develop poor but adequate breathing patterns, mostly due to bad posture or emotional stress. We hold our breath if frightened, shocked, sad, tense, anxious, angry, excited or even when concentrating. If those patterns of shallow breathing are repeated, breath-holding can become habitual.

Imagine you have a couple of balloons in your chest that are filling with air each time you take a breath and emptying each time you breathe out. Allow this to happen rather than trying to make it happen, thereby causing more tension.

If you find it difficult to breathe, if your chest is tight or feels constricted because you suffer or have suffered from a complaint like asthma, seek the advice of a Chartered Physiotherapist, Alexander Technique teacher, cranial osteopath or even a singing teacher to retrain your breathing. If your breathing is shallow because of emotional tension then you may benefit from seeing a psychotherapist to release any repressed feelings.

If you learn how to breathe in conjunction with a relaxation technique and/or exercise programme, they will work well together and you will find yourself being able to relax more easily and more fully.

Exercise without strain

Be careful to choose exercise programmes which are appropriate to age and ability, which are going to energize and 'stretch' you rather than drain, or worse, strain you. Make it an enjoyable experience – you are more likely to stick at something if you want to do it. Join an exercise class or a gym if you know you won't do it on your own or get a group of friends together and hire a personal trainer. Be realistic and sensible – know your limits and stick to them.

Different types of exercise help in different ways: yoga and tai chi build flexibility; weight training builds strength; aerobic exercise builds stamina and burns off excess adrenaline and is therefore useful for those in emotionally stressful, sedentary jobs; good all-round exercise like swimming and cycling helps build strength, stamina and flexibility. For adults in a relationship active sex counts as it can stimulate the parts that other exercises fail to reach!

If you can't get out then exercise for ten minutes a day at home to warm up and loosen stiff muscles and keep them healthy.

Seek the advice of your doctor before embarking on an exercise programme, particularly if you have a sedentary lifestyle and are unfit or unwell (especially if you are on medication) or if you suffer from dizziness on exertion.

Protect your body from stress and strain when exercising by:

- Choosing your exercise carefully: jogging puts an enormous strain on joints, especially the knee joints, particularly if you are running on concrete (however good your shoes are). Your joints will grow old before their time and may need replacing – an expensive and painful procedure.
- Thinking carefully before taking up high-risk sports as you grow older.
- Getting some training if the sport or exercise you have chosen is new to you.
- Dressing appropriately – buy the best trainers (with supports) for any sport that involves running.
- Dressing warmly, at least to start off with, especially if outside in the cold. You can always take clothes off but a chilled muscle is difficult to relax.
- Warming up before you start. It is easy to strain a muscle that hasn't had a chance to stretch and flex.
- Starting gently, and building up gradually, especially if you have been sedentary.
- Taking breaks to stretch into the opposite direction, especially if you are bending or bending one way, for example, when playing golf or bowling.
- Being careful not to overdo it. Sprains and strains can take a depressingly long time to heal.

Dealing with strain
Once you have strained any muscle – whether exercising or DIYing or giving birth – it is important to take immediate action. The older we get the longer our bodies take to heal a sprained muscle or ligament (the elastic tissues which attach muscles to bones). Now is not the time to be stoical and carry on in order to prove how strong you are. If you carry on stressing a strained muscle it will take longer to heal, and you may have a permanent weakness as an added unwelcome bonus. Don't take pain killers and carry on (except as an emergency or a stop gap). Pain is your body's way of telling you to get help.

Rest is a priority, but don't rest a strained joint or back for too long. The muscles can stiffen and become weak alarmingly quickly, making long term recovery very difficult. You will need to start some gentle exercise as soon as any severe pain has eased.

You can use something cold – frozen peas, an ice pack or a cold compress – to relieve pain and bring down any swelling. Or heat to relieve aching or pain: a soak in a bath with Epsom salts water to draw out inflammation. Try heat *and* cold to find out which is the most soothing or comforting as this will also help you in your choice of remedy.

Repetitive Strain Injury
Any job that involves repetitive movements of small muscles, i.e. knitting, sewing, typing, etc., can also cause strain, but a different type of strain. Repetitive Strain Injury (RSI) is a relatively new disease syndrome which is becoming increasingly common in people working in offices and factories, especially those using computers, who are doing small, repetitive tasks. The body is held still and tense, in a poor posture, whilst intense activity is carried out on the 'periphery', usually by the hands or fingers. Intense effort is usually involved, to keep still and to do the task. The increased physical tension causes the muscles to be deprived of oxygen and the nerves that supply those muscles to be affected.

Common symptoms include a feeling of weakness in some muscles, pains which change place, nerve involvement (electric-shock type symptoms or 'jerking' of limbs), non-specific aches in joints, a feeling of swelling or burning or stiffness or numbness which is not observable or measurable (there is no actual swelling or heat, etc.).

Preventative measures are essential to keep RSI from your door. Once the nerves within muscles have been sensitized they can be hard to heal.

If you work at computers, you can alleviate some of the stress of this type of task by replacing the rubber diaphragm of the computer keyboard annually (or more often if you press hard) to give better shock absorption. Learn to touch type as typing with ten fingers means that the load is spread. When typing let your arms swing gently rather than holding them tightly next to your body. Get a wrist support for your keyboard to relieve tension in your arms. Take breaks to ease any build up of tension in your muscles. Get an antiglare screen to protect your eyes from strain.

Travel strain

Travel can be stressful – whether it is commuting daily to and from work or school, or a business or holiday trip. Many people are exhausted when they set off on their holidays, having worked up until the last possible moment and then spent all night packing and getting anxious about all the last minute things they have to do. Surveys have shown that almost half of international travellers are ill as a result of their trip. Arguably, some become unwell as a result of everything they were doing before their trip – we often work flat out, planning to relax once we are away, only to find ourselves grinding to a complete halt. Try starting your holiday twenty-four hours before you leave. This will give you time to begin to unwind, to pack unhurriedly and provide a calmer start to your break.

Pack with care. Heavy bags cause strained muscles, slipped discs and hernias. Take smaller bags and more of them if necessary. They really do have kitchen sinks in most countries now, although if you are going to Russia you are advised to take a bath plug! Travel light – leave the family size shampoo behind. Get some wheels for your luggage and use them, even for short distances, i.e. from the bus stop to the terminal. If you have a bad back ask other people to lift for you. Take appropriate clothing, considering the weather and your planned activities. For example, take good shoes (that have been broken in) if you are hill walking or hiking or planning to do some extensive sightseeing.

Long-haul travel that crosses time zones – especially by plane – causes jetlag. The stress of the journey itself combines with the confusion your body clock experiences as it adapts to local time. The more you can rest, and even sleep, the better. It is sensible to reduce your stress load whilst travelling: avoid alcohol and caffeine and drink plenty of water to prevent dehydration. Get up and walk around as much as you possibly can to keep your blood circulating and help prevent swollen ankles and feet.

For many the strain of the journey to and from work each day, in the rush hour, is enough to cause ill health, whether travelling by car or by public transport. Many people are choosing to earn less and travel less, and work closer to home or from home – or move closer to work. If you do have to commute, then explore working flexihours in order to avoid rush-hour jams. If you do get caught up in traffic, remind yourself that there is absolutely nothing you can do to get yourself there faster and regard this hold up as an unexpected gift of time when you can relax and think, or even daydream.

Homeopathic treatment

Homeopathy can help with strained muscles (from gardening, travelling, exercising, spring cleaning or having a baby!); it can also speed the healing of a sprained joint (ligaments) and help to strengthen weak joints that are vulnerable to strain. For chronic, long term strains it is advisable to seek the advice of a professional homeopath if the remedies below do not quickly help.

- *Argentum nitricum* (*Arg-n.*) See also p. 262.
  Voice strain, through singing or speaking. Voice becomes hoarse, or loses voice altogether, with or without a sore throat, in singers and public speakers who suffer from anxiety.
- *Arnica montana* (*Arn.*) See also p. 265.
  General physical strain after gardening, exercise, on long journeys or at high altitudes. Muscles feel sore and bruised and are no better for exercise. Travel weary. Stiffness and exhaustion after a long journey which is no better for getting up and moving about.

First stage remedy for all strains with swelling of bruised muscles.

Jetlag. Helps to prevent swelling if taken on a long flight. Take for a few days afterwards until sleep patterns get back to normal.

- *Bellis perennis (Bell-p.)*
  General physical strain is felt in muscles and joints after over-exertion. Useful where Arnica is indicated but hasn't helped as much or as quickly as expected.

- *Bryonia alba (Bry.)*
  General physical sprains to joints with severe, stitching pains which are worse for the slightest movement and better for complete rest. They are better for pressure: for lying on the painful part and for bandaging it tightly.

- *Calcarea carbonica (Calc-c.)* See also p. 277.
  Strained joints: ankles, hips, back, wrist. Also stiff necks. Strains (of wrist) are caused by lifting heavy weights awkwardly and do not clear up with *Rhus toxicodendron* or *Ruta graveolens*.

- *Carbo animalis (Carb-an.)*
  Strained joints, especially the wrist, from lifting – the joint then becomes vulnerable and unable to lift even relatively light things.

- *Coca*
  Altitude sickness with exhaustion and headaches.

- *Cocculus indicus (Cocc.)* See also p. 291.
  Altitude sickness. Jetlag. Feels faint, trembly and dizzy. Stiff and weak. Just wants to lie down and sleep but can't get to sleep. Feels hungry but doesn't want to eat. Worse for any exertion.

- *Gelsemium sempervirens (Gels.)* See also p. 297.
  Jetlag, especially if accompanied by anxiety or over-excitement. Trembles with exhaustion. Sluggish, body feels very heavy.

- *Ledum palustre (Led.)*
  Strained joints (especially ankles) with swelling and bruising. The pains are better for cold (compresses or being bathed in cold water) in spite of the painful part feeling cold to the touch. They are worse for movement and warmth and sensitive to touch.

- *Ranunculus bulbosus (Ran-b.)*
  Repetitive strain injury to arm/shoulder from sitting bent (sewing, writing, typing, playing the piano, etc.). Muscles of back are rigid and painful (especially between shoulder blades).

There is tingling in fingers and there may be shooting pains (in nerves) which are worse for movement and when lying down.
- *Rhus toxicodendron (Rhus-t.)*
General physical strain to muscles and/or joints (especially knees, wrists and ankles) with stiffness, trembling and weakness. Pains are worse for beginning to move, i.e. when first getting up after sitting or lying down. They are better for gentle exercise and then become sore with continued movement. They are also worse for continued rest, are not comfortable in any position. This causes the characteristic restlessness that is the keynote of this remedy. The pains are better for heat.
Strains to hips/back or any joints from lifting.
Repetitive strain injury with stiffness, aches and pains. Muscles go into spasm then twitch and jerk when at rest.
Travel weary. Stiff, restless and achy after a long journey. Getting up after sitting or lying down is difficult but after moving about a bit feels much better.
- *Ruta graveolens (Ruta.)*
Eye strain. Eyesight becomes weak and dim after prolonged close work (sewing, reading etc). Eyes ache and burn. They are worse in the evening and at night, in poor light and when trying to continue to work (for example, letters on a page may seem to run together).
Tennis elbow. Elbow feels sore, bruised and lame and is worse for any exercise.
Sprained joints, especially knees, wrists and ankles. Injured parts feel lame (standing and walking is difficult) and bruised and the pains are constant – there is no relief from even gentle exercise. They are also worse for pressure. Sprains are accompanied by a feeling of exhaustion.
Repetitive Stress Injury sometimes responds to this remedy where ligaments are involved.
- *Strontium carbonicum (Stront-c.)*
Sprained ankles with swelling which doesn't respond to *Arnica*. Stubborn sprains that don't respond to any other remedy.
- *Zincum metallicum (Zinc.)* See also p. 352.
Repetitive strain injury. Nervous system becomes irritated – the nerves are on edge. With exhaustion, restlessness and twitching

of muscles, especially at rest. Much worse for alcohol, especially
wine. Run down generally.

REST, RELAXATION AND SLEEP

We all need rest and sleep on a daily basis so that all of the cells of
our bodies can recharge themselves and carry out essential repairs.

Rest
Rest is different to relaxation in that it is something most of us do
automatically, often without thinking about it: a nap in front of the
television, a long, hot bath or shower, a dawdle in the local park, an
early night. A pet can help us to unwind – just playing with and
stroking a pet daily helps to reduce blood pressure and research has
showed that those who have pets have fewer colds and flus.

Pace yourself in your work by taking short breaks, especially if
you are naturally tense. If you wait until the end of the day your
tension levels may be so high it is hard to unwind.

Take mini breaks on an occasional basis. A few hours, half a day
or a whole day if you are feeling on edge. 'Time out' with no
schedules, no appointments (including social engagements), nothing to 'do'. Take off your watch, turn off the phone, just let the time
go. Eat when you are hungry and sleep or nap as and when you feel
tired.

Consider a longer break if you are seriously stressed and/or
exhausted, if your stress load has been considerable over a long
period of time. Spend a week or more in a place which is special to
you, where work or duties cannot 'get' to you.

Relaxation
Relaxation of mind and/or body involves an active, conscious effort
which is different to our passive state when we rest or sleep. A tense
person cannot relax simply by telling themselves to do so.
Structured relaxation is something, paradoxically, that you have to
do: a learnt skill that needs perseverance and regular practice for it
to work; an active process whereby you teach your body to let go of
tension, where chronically tense muscles are re-educated to relax

with the eventual aim that they can be relaxed automatically in everyday situations.

Symptoms of bodily tension include tense hands, clenched fists, tapping fingers and feet. These send negative messages to the brain because of the vast number of nerve endings in the extremities.

Tense people can lose the awareness that they are tense, because this state has become normal. Some people grip telephones and car steering wheels as if they were hanging on to something that was about to be taken away from them! Start with noticing where and how you habitually tense up. Then do it some more as you inhale – fully contract those muscles. As you breathe out let it go and stretch and then adjust your position until you find one where your muscles can relax. Organize your body to do repetitive everyday tasks in as relaxed a position as possible. You may need the expertise of an Alexander Technique teacher or a Chartered Physiotherapist to help you learn healthy ways to use your body.

There are many relaxation techniques available to help you to consciously relax, to let go of physical, mental and/or emotional tension. Consider exploring one of the following if you are finding it difficult to pace yourself, or to build quiet times into your life. You can learn these from books or seek out a trained teacher who can take you through the basic steps and help you iron out any problems or difficulties so that you can practise effectively. Check out local classes, ask your doctor or your local alternative practitioners what is available in your area. The following are all tried and tested methods of relaxation which affect the health of the whole body. They won't suit everyone so keep going until you find one that works for you.

- **Autogenic Training** involves specific mental exercises which can be practised anywhere at any time. These are designed to 'turn off' stressful responses and 'turn on' the calming rhythms associated with mental and physical relaxation.
- **Biofeedback** uses machines alongside a relaxation technique so that people can receive continuous feedback about how effectively they are relaxing, and also learn how a rise in their own stress levels (including anxious thoughts) can have physical repercussions.
- **Massage** relaxes muscles thereby improving circulation as well

as providing pleasure. In combination with aromotherapy oils it can be deeply healing and energizing (although some strong oils can counteract the effect of homeopathic remedies so keep them well apart).

- **Meditation** is now being taken up by many ordinary people who have discovered that its benefits far outweigh the inconvenience of finding twenty minutes once or twice daily to practice. Many religions include some form of meditation as the cornerstone of their daily practice. Some involve simply sitting and breathing, with some a mantra is repeated silently, others use chanting. Focused forms of meditation need to be learnt from a teacher.

   Some experts say that as little as twenty minutes meditating is the equivalent of two hours sleep. Meditating (or contemplating) enables the mind to experience an altered state of consciousness, a deeper, more relaxed awareness, without the effort associated with active thinking – a state that is different to the relaxation experienced at rest or during sleep. It provides the mind (especially one in over-drive) with an opportunity to slow down, and encourages a mental state of deep inner peace and calm.

   Research has confirmed that meditation enhances your health: people who meditate see their doctors less and spend much less time in hospital. People who meditate regularly sleep better, have lower blood pressure and less chronic illness. Benefits include improved concentration and memory, an increase in self awareness and an insight into the problems in one's life. It also aids mental clarity and creativity and fosters a spiritual awareness.

   It is important to build some reflective time into your life and children also benefit by learning to value this. Many people meditate in an unfocused way without knowing that is what they are doing when they slip into an ordinary, everyday daydream. If you are someone who finds it too easy to daydream, if meditating is an escape route for you from a stressful or a boring life, then unstructured meditating might not be for you. Seek out a teacher who could help you to harness your natural skills in a constructive way.

- **Music and song** are powerful therapies – sounds create vibra-tions which actually trigger the production of endorphins. The ancient Indian therapy of Ayurvedic medicine uses healing sounds to stimulate the body's organs and strengthen the immune system. If you love to sing and find it rejuvenating and relaxing, join a choir. Some people find that playing a musical instrument on a regular basis balances out the stress in their lives.

Music can evoke memories from the past – you can use it to help release feelings that are playing hard to get. For example, you feel depressed but haven't been able to cry. Play a piece of music that makes you feel sad and let the tears come.

Some classical music has negative associations: Beethoven has been found to increase depression, Chopin encourages day-dreaming and Wagner and certain military marches have been found to stimulate aggression and hyperactivity in children. The experts recommend Mozart or Gregorian chants to improve concentration and learning abilities.

- **Praying** is another way to find a quiet mind; for many people prayer has the power to take them out of themselves, to focus on a 'higher power'. It is calming to the soul, it helps people to reconnect with their spirituality, their inner light, providing strength – and faith. You don't need to belong to a church to pray. Search out prayer books from different faiths, and choose one or more that have some meaning for you, that make you feel connected, and say them on a regular basis. Or join a church, one that reflects your needs and beliefs, for a sense of community.
- **Self-hypnosis** is a state similar to sleep without a loss of awareness. Some people find it easy to learn and an effective way to relax as well as to make positive suggestions for changes in their lives, and even to assist with their own healing when they are ill. Studies have shown that hypnosis can significantly raise the white blood cell count (in those who are easily hypnotized). These are the cells that play an important role in our immune system. There are many relaxation tapes available (at most book shops) some of which have subliminal, hypnotic suggestions. Or you can record your own tape – this is best done with a trained hypnotist who can tailor it to meet your specific needs.
- **Tai Chi** and **Chi Gong** are forms of meditation using movement that originated from China and are designed to balance the

body's energies. They are useful for those who find it hard to sit still for even short periods of time. They use different movements which, once learnt from a teacher, can be made anywhere.

- **Thought control:** there are specific techniques for controlling so-called 'negative' thoughts. These are sometimes known as affirmations or positive thinking. They are a form of mental first-aid and are useful for reducing stress under certain circumstances. They are best done with the guidance of a counsellor who can help uncover the emotional stress that underlies the negative thought pattern. Simply 'stopping' a so-called negative thought or replacing it with a positive one, without dealing with the underlying cause or feelings, can be suppressive. Be wary of injuctions to 'smile' or 'think positive'. They may run against your natural rhythms of expression and create another, deeper tension, thereby causing more stress.
- **Visualization:** the imagination is a powerful tool for healing and for relieving stress. It involves the active dwelling on something delightful, peaceful and/or beautiful – a place or an image that is important or meaningful – which brings some of that healing energy into our inner life. Children are naturals and love to play with their imaginations. Grown-ups can recapture that skill and use it to take a mental break.

  Visualizations can be done before going to sleep at night, when travelling (unless you are the driver!), when lying in the bath (where the double treat of a hot bath and the visualization will help you feel wonderfully relaxed). Some people have found that it enhances their capacity to heal and use it alongside other medical treatments (orthodox and complementary) for chronic complaints such as cancer, AIDS and high blood pressure. A psychotherapist experienced in 'imaging' can help you work out a visualization specifically for your needs.
- **Yoga** originated in India, and is a system of physical, mental and spiritual exercises. The physical exercises (including structured breathing) were originally designed as meditation techniques and can be done separately. They involve gentle stretching and help develop and maintain physical flexibility, control, balance and poise. Many people use the physical exercises to start and end their day. Others have benefited from going more deeply into

the meditations. There are many different branches of yoga. Ask your local teachers what type of yoga they offer.

Sleep

A lot of healing happens when we sleep: the activity of the lungs and heart is reduced to a minimum; our body's temperature, blood pressure and pulse rate all fall and our muscles relax. This allows the cells of our bodies to carry out essential repairs, to grow and regenerate. Skin cells, for example, divide and grow twice as fast when we are asleep. This is why infants and children who are growing need more sleep and why the elderly often need less sleep.

We go through different cycles during sleep: as we fall asleep we are vulnerable to being woken by slight noises, then we slip into light sleep when noise doesn't usually disturb us. This is followed by deep sleep. These periods of deep and light sleep alternate (very roughly) about every two hours throughout the night.

Some people (snorers and asthmatics) suffer from 'sleep apnoea' – a condition whereby the breathing stops for ten seconds or more up to hundreds of times a night. This prevents them going into a deep sleep cycle. We need a certain amount of good, deep sleep to feel refreshed.

As we move between light and deep sleep (and vice versa) we dream. Dreams help us to process and digest the experiences of our day and allow us access to our deeper (unconscious) thoughts and feelings. People deprived of dreaming become irritable, depressed and even aggressive. Alcohol and sleeping tablets can cause dream deprivation by taking people straight into a deep sleep state, causing grogginess and the feeling that they haven't slept enough.

Our sleep requirements are thought to be genetically determined and whilst most adults need 6–8 hours per night, many can get by on less and others need more. Those who are consistently getting less than they need are courting chronic exhaustion. This doesn't happen overnight but in several stages.

At first we feel an ordinary sort of tiredness which can be dealt with fairly easily after, say, an early night, a lie-in or a nap. Meanwhile, it is possible to carry on working in spite of feeling like everything is a bit of an effort.

If ignored, this can develop into the next stage where rest and sleep is no longer refreshing. Many increase their caffeine, sugar or alcohol intake at this point and start eating badly, missing meals or cramming in junk food at erratic times. A day or weekend off at this point is necessary. If this isn't possible, then it is all too easy to spiral down into a deeply exhausted state where illness may be just around the corner. Many people keep on going, stopping only when a flu knocks on their door. We can avoid these acute episodes of ill health by simply taking to our beds when we are over-tired.

People with chronic exhaustion have seriously disturbed sleeping patterns, finding it difficult to switch off at night and/or waking in the night and not being able to get back to sleep, or sleeping lightly and restlessly. They become irritable, impatient and snappy and may even feel they are being picked on if others express their concern. They may not recognize that they are exhausted, may even feel that no one understands what they are going through. A real break (of a weekend or even a week) is necessary at this point.

Working shifts disrupts our biological clock (which sets our levels of alertness and tiredness) and affects our health and our ability to perform with potentially disastrous results, especially at work. Chronic diseases are higher amongst those who do shift work, and those with poor health find their problems aggravated by working shifts.

Those who are vulnerable to chronic exhaustion because of long or unsociable hours include politicians, long distance drivers, parents with small children, shift workers, air crews, doctors, nurses, factory workers and those caring for the sick at home. Many of these people work in a constant state of jetlag, feeling cut off, in a biological vacuum of fatigue.

Fatigue can lead to accidents and to human error. People who are chronically tired have been discovered to take 'micro sleeps' – they are to all intents and purposes awake, but they lose their concentration for a split second, with the blink of eye or even with their eyes open, and these losses can be dangerous if, for example, they are driving. The two hours before dawn are our most vulnerable, when we are most likely to have an accident if we are fatigued.

There are many ways we can stimulate alertness when tired: an interest in what is happening, a sense of danger, fresh air, turning the heating down or off, a snack (rich in carbohydrates to boost blood sugar levels), sound (the radio, a chatty companion or lively music), smells (aromatherapy oils can be effective), sucking mints or chewing gum (peppermint is a natural stimulant), or using the power of the imagination to summon up and replay interesting events in one's own life. Coffee simply masks tiredness (as aspirin masks pain). It is useful as a stop gap, as an emergency measure, but should not be relied upon, especially if other people's lives are dependent on your staying awake. The only cure for sleepiness is sleep. If you are driving, stop and nap – in a safe place with the doors locked if you are on your own.

A short sleep or nap can be enormously refreshing (alertness, productivity and even creativity are all increased) in the short term. The ideal length of time for a nap is 15–30 minutes (enough to energize you without feeling groggy) although some people find that a minute or two is enough to recharge their batteries. The best time to take a nap is 8 hours after waking and 8 hours before going to bed to fit in with your natural energy cycles (your body temperature dips around this time and people often feel tired when this happens).

It can take two or three weeks for your body to catch up on a sleep deficit or to adapt to a new schedule. Those working shifts should try to work at least three weeks at a shift before changing to a new one. Those who travel long distances should leave three weeks, if possible, between journeys. If your sleep has been disturbed you will need to make a conscious plan to re-set your body clock and get back to sleeping soundly and waking feeling refreshed.

- Plan on a minimum of eight hours sleep.
- Decide on a reasonable time to go to sleep and stick to it.
- Go to bed when you begin to feel tired rather than missing that moment and getting a second wind.
- Make sure your bedroom isn't too hot or too cold, has a good supply of fresh air and isn't too noisy (or wear ear plugs if it is).
- Make sure your mattress is firm enough to support you without being too hard and making you sore, that your bedding isn't too heavy (or too light).
- Take some evening exercise, especially if you are sedentary during the day.

- Don't take work to bed with you – make your bedroom a place where you go to relax and rest.
- Take a hot drink (not caffeine or alcohol) to bed with you, or a glass of milk.
- When in bed don't try to go to sleep. Allow yourself to relax: imagine your body is heavy and warm. Say the words 'heavy and warm' over and over. Repeat a soothing poem, a prayer or meditation mantra without putting any effort into it, or run through your day backwards starting with the present – most people find they fall asleep long before they reach the morning!
  If you go to bed and can't sleep, then read or listen to music for a half hour or so, or until you feel sleepy. If you still can't sleep then get up and trouble-shoot.
- Is there something on your mind that needs sorting out? If it isn't possible to talk about it then write it down. If you are having anxious thoughts write a 'worries' list and make an action column, writing everything you need to do as well as people to contact to help you. Keep a note pad by the bed so you can write down important thoughts that come into your head and won't go away. Getting them off your mind really can make a difference.
- If thoughts of work or worries persist, put the radio on to distract you. Or read for a while longer.
- How long is it since you last ate? If it is longer than three hours you may be hungry (this is especially true for small children), or it may be that you have adrenaline in your system stopping you from switching off. Get a light snack and a drink to help raise your blood sugar levels.
- If you do wake in the night and can't get back to sleep, get up and potter about: make a hot drink and take it back to bed with a boring book until your next natural sleep cycle comes along (up to two hours later).
- Ask your doctor to refer you to a sleep clinic (they have them at many of the major university hospitals) if nothing has worked.
  It takes some people a while to get going in the morning. This is because it actually takes our metabolism about half an hour to reach its waking-time levels. Giving yourself time to take things slowly until you feel fully awake is one way of working with your

metabolism. If you use caffeine to stimulate you before you are actually ready, your system will simply release adrenaline to make you feel awake (artificially).

Homeopathic treatment
Homeopathy can help you to relax if your muscles are tense and your nervous system is wound up. If you are finding it difficult to rest or sleep then it is essential that you identify the cause or causes before you think about taking a homeopathic remedy. If a physical stress – a sagging mattress, too much tea, coffee or alcohol or even hunger – is keeping you from sleeping then you will need to deal with these practical issues.

If you are caught up in a vicious circle of not being able to rest or sleep deeply because your sleep has been broken or disturbed then one of the remedies below will ease you back into a healthy sleep pattern.

- *Calcarea phosphorica (Calc-p.)* See also p. 281.
  Difficulty getting to sleep. Tension in neck and shoulders makes relaxing difficult. Difficulty sleeping after an illness or in growing children. Can't get to sleep before midnight and then feels dreadful and finds it hard to wake up in the morning, even after sleeping in longer than usual.
- *Cocculus indicus (Cocc.)* See also p. 291.
  Loss of sleep or disturbed sleep causes insomnia and dizziness. Feels anxious, especially about those they are caring for. Sleep is restless and unrefreshing, with anxious dreams or even nightmares.
  Appetite lost (feels faint and hungry) in those who have been deprived of sleep (through breastfeeding, nursing the sick or long distance travel). Nausea with empty feeling in stomach.
- *Coffea cruda (Coff.)* See also p. 293.
  Difficulty getting to sleep because of an overactive mind, excitement or too much caffeine. Cannot switch off. Sleep is light and full of vivid dreams.
- *Kali phosphoricum (Kali-p.)* See also p. 301.
  Difficulty getting to sleep from nervous strain, over-excitement, or after a period of intense work or study. Nervous exhaustion with an empty feeling in the pit of the stomach.

- *Nitricum acidum (Nit-ac.)* See also p. 314.
  Loss of sleep or disturbed sleep – especially from shift work – causes insomnia and irritability. Cannot get to sleep till the early hours (typically around 2 a.m.), then wakes feeling exhausted.
- *Nux vomica (Nux-v.)* See also p. 317.
  Loss of sleep or disturbed sleep – especially from overwork and mental strain or even too much caffeine – causes exhaustion, insomnia and irritability. Finds it difficult to get to sleep, in spite of feeling tired, sleeps lightly (with vivid dreams). Wakes in the early morning (typically around 3 a.m.) and can't get back to sleep. Drifts off into a deep sleep just before the alarm goes off and wakes feeling tense and exhausted. Complaints from a sedentary lifestyle. Becomes tense and unable to relax.
- *Sulphur (Sul.)* See also p. 345.
  Resulting from a sedentary lifestyle. Slumps and finds it hard to get motivated – to get up and go.
- *Zincum metallicum (Zinc.)* See also p. 352.
  Difficulty getting to sleep from a period of overwork or emotional stress. Feels run down, exhausted and tense. Sleep is light and unrefreshing. Restless legs which jerk on falling asleep and wake people up as they drift off.

WEATHER

The weather can affect our health and is worth taking into account when we are trying to make our lives less stressful. We vary enormously in our response to the weather and to temperatures in general. Some people are naturally warm-blooded and are aggravated by hot or humid weather. Others are chilly and are sensitive to the damp and the cold. And then again, some people love the damp, they feel better when it is raining and are happier in the cold and the wet. The effects can be general, for example, feeling a lack of energy in the heat or feeling heavy and sluggish on cloudy, overcast days. Or they can be acute, say, an earache after being out in a cold wind or a headache before a storm. Chronic complaints such as arthritis can be aggravated in the rain or in cold, damp weather.

Light, in particular sunlight, is instrumental in setting our body clock – through hormones which are light-sensitive. There are people who thrive in the sun, who feel enlivened and happy when the sun shines, and dull and depressed in the winter months when the sun goes into hiding. SAD, or Seasonal Affective Disorder, is the official label for a depression that surfaces during the short, cold, dark days of winter and disappears when the light and the sun return in the spring. Those with SAD might consider light therapy. Some hospitals, health centres and SAD support groups have 'sun boxes' for hire or loan which provide a bank of full spectrum lights to help stimulate those light-sensitive hormones in the winter months.

If you have an opportunity to take the weather into account when planning where you live, then do so. Some people move house in order to get away from a climate that has affected their health or the health of their children. This isn't always possible but it is worth weighing up the pros and cons of moving if your health has been badly affected by, say, a damp valley. Our homes have their own micro-climates too! Those with central heating and double-glazing may need to raise the humidity (with humidifiers or even bowls of water by radiators) to prevent dryness in themselves and their plants!

Plan your holidays carefully – if your health is aggravated by certain climates then avoid them if possible. If you feel better at the mountains or by the sea then go there when you can. If you suffer from SAD then take your annual holiday in the winter and go somewhere sunny.

Take commonsense precautions for dealing with the weather: warm clothing in the winter for those who feel the cold, waterproofs for those who are sensitive to the wet and sun hats for those who feel the heat!

If you suspect that the weather is affecting you then keep a diary which takes note of changes in the weather as well as changes in your health. You may find some connections that will help you select a homeopathic remedy to strengthen your vitality and make you less vulnerable to weather stresses.

Homeopathic treatment
If you fall ill with a cold or a flu, then do go back over the days preceding your illness and check if the weather was severe or had

changed rather than simply assuming you caught it because of a work or emotionally-related stress.

You can help yourself with homeopathic remedies for a variety of complaints caused by the weather. The following remedies cover both general and specific sensitivities. Make a note of which ones work so that you can use them again if a similar situation recurs.

- *Aconitum napellus (Aco.)* See also p. 255.
  Worse for cold in general, for getting chilled; sensitive to wind. This is the number one remedy for any complaints that develop after getting chilled in the cold and especially in a cold wind.
- *Agaricus muscarius (Agar.)*
  Ill effects of frosty, cold weather. Chilblains on hands and feet which are red, itchy and painful (burning).
- *Antimonium crudum (Ant-c.)*
  Ill effects of the sun. Excessively irritable from getting over-heated in the sun. Great weariness and sleepiness with diarrhoea.
- *Arsenicum album (Ars.)* See also p. 266.
  Sensitive to the cold; to wet weather; to swimming, especially in a cold sea and fall ill if chilled.
- *Baryta carbonica (Bar-c.)* See also p. 271.
  Complaints that develop during cold, wet (damp weather).
- *Belladonna (Bell.)* See also p. 273.
  Sensitive to getting head wet. This remedy is for those who develop an acute complaint with a high fever after getting their head soaked – in the rain, or even after washing their hair and going out without having dried it properly.
  Sunstroke: mildly delirious with fever (without sweating) and terrible, throbbing headache.
- *Bryonia alba (Bry.)*
  Ill effects of change in temperature or weather from cold to hot; sensitive to heat in general. For warm-blooded types who fall ill when the weather changes in the spring to warm, typically with a cold, flu or cough.
- *Calcarea carbonica (Calc-c.)* See also p. 277.
  Sensitive to damp, wet weather and to getting wet. For sweaty people who are easily stressed by these conditions.
- *Calcarea phosphorica (Calc-p.)* See also p. 281.
  Sensitive to wet weather and to draughts (developing a stiff neck).

- *Carbo vegetabilis (Carb-v.)* See also p. 284.
  Sensitive to heat in general and to humidity. Great sluggishness in these conditions.
- *Causticum (Caust.)* See also p. 286.
  Sensitive to cold, dry weather, to change in temperature or weather to dry. These are chilly people who feel worse when the weather changes to clear, dry and cold. They have a sense of release during mild, wet weather – both emotionally and physically.
- *Chamomilla (Cham.)* See also p. 289.
  For complaints in irritable types who are sensitive after getting chilled by a cold wind.
- *Conium maculatum (Con.)* See also page 295.
  For complaints that come with snowy weather.
- *Dulcamara (Dulc.)*
  Ill effects of a change in temperature or weather from hot to cold; sensitive to damp weather. For chilly people who, at such times, 'catch' colds and coughs and suffer from pains in their joints. Complaints (rheumatism, back pain) from sleeping in a damp bed or a damp house call for this remedy.
- *Glonoine (Glon.)*
  Sunstroke with violent, bursting, throbbing headache which is better for cold compresses and for firm pressure. Feels faint and flushed (face is red). Worse for any exertion and for heat. Appears dull and confused.
- *Hepar sulphuricum calcareum (Hep-s.)*
  Extremely sensitive to the cold; to cold dry weather; to draughts; to the wind. This is when they can easily develop a cough cold, earache or a sore throat.
- *Kali sulphuricum (Kali-s.)*
  Ill effects of a change in temperature or weather from cold to hot. Earache, coughs or colds which come with the first warm weather in the spring. Feels much worse for heat, especially stuffy heat, in any form and much better for fresh air.
- *Lachesis (Lach.)* See also p. 302.
  Sensitive to heat in general and to humidity. Cannot stand the pressure of external heat – they are hot enough already – and suffer from headaches and unpleasant sweating.

- *Magnesium muriaticum (Mag-m.)*
  For colds that come on after swimming in the sea.
- *Magnesium phosphorica (Mag-p.)*
  For earaches and headaches that develop after bathing or swimming in cold water. Pains are much better for heat and hot compresses and for pressure.
- *Mercurius solubilis (Merc-s.)*
  Super-sensitive to extremes of temperature, to heat and cold. They prefer a moderate temperature – a change of two degrees either way will make them feel worse, especially when they are ill.
- *Natrum carbonicum (Nat-c.)* See also p. 308.
  Sensitive to heat in general; to storms; to the sun, to extremes of temperature. They feel worse generally from excessive heat and particularly after exposure to the sun .– when they will suffer from headaches. They are sensitive to storms and will get headaches beforehand. They also find extremes of temperature difficult to handle. Ill effects of sunstroke, once the acute symptoms are over: feels tired and heavy, worse for the slightest exertion, head feels heavy and aches.
- *Natrum muriaticum (Nat-m.)* See also p. 310.
  Sensitive to heat; to the sun. They dislike hot weather and always feel worse for the heat of the sun, sometimes suffering from headaches, exhaustion and cold sores from extended exposure to the sun itself or from sea air.
- *Nitricum acidum (Nit-ac.)* See also p. 314.
  Extremely sensitive to the cold; these people develop colds, earaches and terrible sore throats when chilled.
- *Nux vomica (Nux-v.)* See also p. 317.
  Extremely sensitive to the cold; to cold dry weather; to draughts; to wet weather and to the wind. These types 'catch' cold easily, especially if chilled in a draught or a wind. They are much better for warmth and love the warm weather.
- *Phosphorus (Phos.)* See also p. 325.
  Ill effects of any change in temperature or weather. Lively, sensitive types who need the sunshine to feel fully alive. They become depressed in the dark, cloudy days of winter and brighten up in the spring. They can also predict storms coming because they invariably get a headache.

- *Pulsatilla nigricans (Puls.)* See also p. 330.
  Sensitive to heat in general and the sun; to getting wet, to getting feet or head wet. These are warm-blooded types who wilt in the sun and any stuffy heat – in or outdoors. They are also sensitive to getting wet, however, and will go down with an acute illness if drenched in the rain, or if their head or feet get wet.
- *Rhododendron (Rhod.)*
  Affected by cloudy weather and by thunderstorms. Very sensitive to changes in pressure, especially those that precede a storm. Joint pains, back ache and headaches are worse then.
- *Rhus toxicodendron (Rhus-t.)*
  Ill effects of bathing in cold water; of a change in temperature or weather from hot to cold; of cloudy weather; of damp, wet or foggy weather; to swimming in cold water; to getting wet; to the wind. This remedy is for those who are sensitive to the cold – even eating an ice-cream on a hot day can make them sick. They become depressed in the dark, cloudy days of winter and typically they suffer from many rheumatic or arthritic symptoms from the cold or damp in any shape or form.
- *Sepia (Sep.)* See also p. 334.
  Sensitive to frost and snow (and cold); to sea air; to getting wet. These types feel generally unwell in the cold as well as suffering from colds and coughs.
- *Silica (Sil.)* See also p. 338.
  Ill effects of change in weather or temperature from hot to cold. Sensitive to cold weather; to draughts; to wet weather; to getting feet wet; to wind. They suffer from frequent colds, earaches and coughs during the cold, winter months – especially if they go out without a hat or a scarf.
- *Sulphur (Sul.)* See also p. 345.
  Ill effects of change in temperature or weather from cold to hot. Sensitive to heat in general. Hot, restless, sweaty types who can't sleep or think in the heat, who are always better for fresh, cool air.
  Sunstroke: hot, thirsty feverish (with profuse sweating), dizzy and headachy. Skin is uncomfortable, is sore and itchy and worse for washing and for heat – with diarrhoea and restlessness.

HOMEOPATHIC
REMEDIES

ACONITUM NAPELLUS (*Aco.*)
Monkshood

Emotional state
Anxious with fear; before an exam/interview, etc. *Excitable. Fearful:* claustrophobic; in a crowd; of death. *Panic. Restless. Screaming* with the pain. *Sensitive* to pain.

Emotional stresses: fear; shock; worry.

This is a remedy for sudden shock that is accompanied and/or followed by fear and anxiety. The shock is significant, affects the whole system and can occur after surgery, an injury, an accident or even witnessing an accident, the type of shock that is now called post-traumatic stress syndrome. A life-threatening event such as an earthquake can bring on an *Aconite* state, as can a less severe situation such as a bad storm if there is a feeling that one's life has been threatened. Fear of death – however irrational it may seem – is an indication for giving *Aconite*.

After the shock there can be fear and even panic attacks in crowded places or in enclosed spaces. The sensation of panic comes on suddenly and is accompanied by restlessness and palpitations. It can also appear at night, typically on waking, and is often accompanied by a fear of, or a feeling of, suffocation.

People who need *Aconite* are distressed and restless, look shocked or even terrified, and may have staring, glassy eyes. They are tense and excitable, and can have outbursts of anger, with children throwing tantrums. If physically ill, there is a sensitivity to pain which causes great anguish.

Aconite can be given at any time after emotional stress (if the typical emotional state is present), unlike physical stress when it needs to be given within the first twenty-four to forty-eight hours. It may be needed *before* a stressful situation, an exam, a visit to the dentist, childbirth or even a plane flight, where there is great anxiety with fear or panic – especially of dying.

General state
Appetite: likes cold drinks. *Expression* anxious; frightened. *Eyes* sensitive to bright light. *Face* red. *Onset of pain/complaint* – sudden. *Pains* burning; unbearable; with screaming or moaning. *Sweat* hot; on covered parts of the body. *Taste in mouth* bitter. *Thirsty.*
Better for fresh air.
Worse at night; for touch.

Physical stresses: cold in general; cold, dry wind; getting chilled; shock after injury.

Complaints needing *Aconite* come on suddenly and strongly, often at night. After a shock or a walk in an unexpectedly cold wind (and getting chilled), the sufferer is fine on going to bed but wakes around midnight (usually just before) with a cough, fever or earache. This remedy works best at the beginning of an acute illness, within the first twenty-four to forty-eight hours.

There is a general sensitivity to pain, which is intolerable and drives sufferers to despair – children typically scream or moan. Teething babies throw high fevers, sleep restlessly and bite their fists furiously.

There is a resentment of interference, a not wanting to be touched because it makes them feel generally worse. There is sweating with thirst, a flushed face – especially with the fever – and a general anxious restlessness because it is hard to get comfortable and movement aggravates the complaint.

Complaints are generally worse at night and better for lots of fresh air. The thirst is for cold drinks, usually water, which is the only thing that doesn't taste bitter.

Aconite is also useful for injuries and wounds that won't stop bleeding (including after surgery) especially if shock is also present.

Typical physical complaints are:
- Common cold: with sneezing, headache and/or inflamed eyes.
- Cough: dry, barking, short, tickling; breathing fast; with hoarse voice; first-stage croup.

- Cystitis: pains pressing.
- Earache: with fever; pains unbearable; external ear is red.
- Eye inflammation: eyes dry, red; aching and burning; sensitive to light.
- Fever: dry, burning heat; worse at night; better for uncovering; heat alternating with chills at night.
- Headache: pains burning, bursting, pressing, throbbing.
- Insomnia: with anxious, vivid dreams; restless sleep.
- Palpitations: with fear; worse at night, in a crowded or enclosed place or out in an open space.
- Period problems: period is late after a shock or getting chilled.
- Retention of urine: in babies or children, from a shock or a chill.
- Sore throat: pains burning, stitching.
- Toothache: pains tearing in good teeth (after a chill).

AMBRA GRISEA (*Ambr.*)
Ambergris

Emotional state
Anxious: before an exam/interview, etc. *Depressed. Dull/confused. Easily embarrassed. Forgetful. Lacks self-confidence. Sensitive* to music. *Shy.*

Emotional stresses: embarrassment; worry.

These are sensitive, inhibited, introverted types who feel things strongly, who are emotional, but who find it difficult to express these feelings because of their own innate shyness and poor self-confidence. Because of this a pressure cooker situation can develop. They can have hysterical outbursts from time to time as the pressure builds up and has to find an outlet. If they do it is usually an overreaction to some relatively minor situation.

They find social situations excruciating because they don't know what to say or do, and become easily flustered and embarrassed, and will blush furiously if engaged in conversation. They become tongue-tied, especially with people they don't know and can even stutter and cough with nerves.

They avoid public speaking and suffer from anticipatory anxiety any time they are called on to speak in front of others – at an interview or oral exam. They may get so wound up that they break down with a physical complaint before the event.

They become haunted by memories of 'performing' badly, even in passing conversations, and then endlessly relive the embarrassment in their minds.

Children (especially adolescents) who go through a bashful stage, suffering from exam nerves and difficulty in concentrating and revising, may benefit from this remedy.

Music affects them deeply, making them tremble, cry, or giving them palpitations. Because of this they may avoid listening to it.

They have a fear of failure and in adults, the embarrassment of a failure leads to them losing self-confidence and becoming emotionally worn out. They become nervous, fidgety and twitchy.

The loss of one or more important people, usually relatives, in someone who is generally sensitive can cause depression. If the typical *Ambra grisea* symptoms are also present then this remedy will help them through their bereavement.

General state

Pains constricting.

Better for cold drinks; for the removal of pressure.

Worse for company; for conversation; in the morning on waking.

These types are embarrassed by their bodies, finding it impossible to pass a stool or urine if anyone is within earshot.

Physically they suffer from all sorts of 'nervous' symptoms such as palpitations, insomnia or a cough, many of which are worse after socializing, especially the insomnia.

This is a useful remedy for elderly people who are worn out and suffer from dizziness, insomnia, coughs and digestive troubles. They have a tendency to lose weight under stress because they lose their appetite.

They can suffer from twitchy legs and numbness of the arm lain on in bed at night.

When stressed emotionally, typical physical complaints include:

• Cough: dry, nervous; coughing fits; with belching; worse at night,

in company, for talking.
- Dizziness: in the fresh air; in the morning on getting up; has to lie down.
- Exhaustion: worse in the morning in bed.
- Headache: constricting, shooting or pressing pains.
- Heartburn: with nausea; with belches; better for burping.
- Insomnia: sleepy in the evening; sleepless after going to bed; restless sleep (wakes frequently); anxious dreams.
- Palpitations: from music or strong emotions (not expressed).

ANACARDIUM ORIENTALE (*Anac.*)
Marking nut

Emotional state
Angry. *Anxious:* with fear; before an exam/interview, etc. *Concentration difficult. Domineering. Forgetful/memory weak. Isolated. Lacks self-confidence. Morose. Suspicious. Vindictive.*

Emotional stresses: transition; worry.

Anacardium is for those suffering from nervous exhaustion as a result of over-study or exam nerves. It is also useful for those who are experiencing an identity crisis with inner suffering at any age. For example, adolescents who are struggling to discover themselves can find it a painful process, and can suffer a great deal, if they cannot resolve the inner conflict. There are two opposing forces inside, an intense inner conflict that produces the sensation of being pulled in two directions. A sense of inferiority or low self-esteem develops, and with it anxiety and indecision. They will even say they feel 'in two minds'.

On the one side they feel worthless, and are constantly trying to prove themselves because of their fear of failure. If this isn't healed another side will develop as a result of an inner split. An inflexible, bad-tempered, hard-hearted side. They become suspicious and vindictive without remorse for their actions. Their anger can surface in the form of outbursts in which they swear compulsively.

As the tension builds inside they harden up in order to try and cope and end up feeling as if they are living in a dream. A sensation of unreality and isolation increases and they become exhausted. Once worn out they become confused, their memory fails and they can't remember what they have read. They become absent-minded and apathetic and don't want to work.

General state
Face pale with dark rings around eyes. *Pains* constricting; cramping; pressing. *Sensation* of a band or a plug. *Senses* weakened. *Symptoms* one-sided. *Taste in mouth* unpleasant (putrid).
Better for eating (both during and after).
Worse for fasting; mental exertion.

There is a lack of physical as well as mental power. The senses (taste, sight, hearing, smell and even touch) are diminished. Eating provides some relief, both generally and specifically with some of the physical complaints below.

The pains are typically pressing or cramping and there is often a feeling of constriction, like a band around a single part of the body (a joint or the head, stomach, etc.). Another strange sensation is that a body part is 'plugged up', for example, the rectum in constipation.

Typical physical complaints as a result of stress include:
- Back ache: feeling of pressure on the shoulders; back stiff.
- Constipation: with inactivity of the bowels and ineffectual straining and a sensation that the rectum is 'plugged up'.
- Cough: worse at night.
- Cramps: in calves, worse when walking or on getting up from sitting; writer's cramps in the hand.
- Exhaustion: with trembling.
- Headache: pressing pains; sensation of a band around the head.
- Indigestion: digestion weak with cramping, pressing pains and rumbling.
- Insomnia: disturbed sleep with anxious dreams.

APIS MELLIFICA (*Apis.*)
Honey bee

Emotional state
Apathetic. Fearful: of being alone; of death. *Irritable. Jealous. Restless. Tearful.*

Emotional stress: jealousy.

These types are sensitive to emotional shock, especially jealousy, quickly becoming irritable if they feel displaced. The arrival of a new baby can cause an older child to feel jealous, to become difficult and mildly hyperactive (busy rather than manic). They don't want to be alone and they become demanding and whiney, also crying without knowing why.

Older people who feel displaced (whatever the reason) may slip into apathy, becoming absent-minded and clumsy. This apathy is accompanied by a restlessness. They flit from one thing to another, without achieving much.

General state
Clumsy: drops things. *Face:* puffy; red. *Lips* swollen. *Pains:* burning; stinging. *Swelling* of affected parts. *Symptoms:* right-sided; move from the right side to the left. *Thirstless. Tongue* fiery red.
Better for cold (anything); cool air.
Worse 3.00–5.00 p.m.; heat (hot anything); pressure; for stuffy heat; touch.

Physical stress: bites.

Those needing *Apis* have burning, stinging pains that may also itch, that are better for cold and worse for heat. With a fever or any localized inflammation, the surface of the body or the affected part itself (throat, eyes, insect bites, etc.) are generally swollen, sore, shiny red and sensitive, especially to touch and pressure. These are warm-blooded people who can become ill if over-heated. But despite being generally hot they are thirstless, even with a fever.

Typical physical complaints as a result of stress include:
- Conjunctivitis: with swollen eyelids; eyes raw red and burning.
- Cough: worse at night and for lying down.
- Cystitis: constant urge to urinate; scanty urine.
- Diarrhoea: painless.
- Earache: with sore throat; pains worse when swallowing.
- Exhaustion: with restlessness, fidgeting and twitching.
- Fever: dry, burning heat; better for uncovering.
- Headache: head feels hot, scalp feels tight and sore.
- Hives: angry red swellings.
- Hot flushes.
- Joint pains: joints are red and shiny and painful.
- Sore throat: mouth dry; throat/tongue are red; throat swollen; stings; tonsils ulcerated.

ARGENTUM NITRICUM (*Arg-n.*)
Silver nitrate

Emotional state
Anxious: before an exam/interview, etc.; about the future; about health. *Dull/confused. Excitable. Fearful:* of being alone; claustrophobic; of failure; of heights; of being late; of heights; of public speaking. *Hurried:* while walking/speaking/waiting. *Impatient. Impulsive. Panic. Restless. Stubborn.*
Worse for mental exertion/thinking.

Emotional stresses: failure; fear; mental strain; uncertainty; worry.

These are lively, extrovert types who express their feelings openly. They are generally hurried, highly strung and speedy – verging on manic at times. They move and speak fast, they are impatient and impulsive. They tend to live in the future rather than in the present and this can add to their anxiety.

Punctuality is important to them – they get into a real state about being on time for appointments (however unimportant). They also expect others to be punctual, becoming anxious if they are late.

They worry about their health and their future and this can

quickly get out of hand, developing into more deep-seated fears. It is then that they are prone to panic attacks, typically becoming claustrophobic. Their fears and anxieties are worse when they are on their own and better for company.

They can be superstitious, from mild forms such as always doing things in a certain way (putting the left shoe on first), to more obsessive behaviour like not walking on the cracks in the pavement.

These are headstrong, stubborn types who dislike feeling helpless, who have a need to feel in control because of their inner turmoil.

They dread ordeals (from exams to public speaking), trembling with nervous excitement and suffering from frequent urination, diarrhoea, wind or palpitations. They may even lose their voice before an important event. Anxious and impulsive thoughts and vivid pictures torment them, typically about failing or about terrible things happening like having an accident.

Those needing *Argentum nitricum* become fidgety and walk hurriedly around (especially in circles) to calm themselves, to try and gather their thoughts, because the physical exertion actually eases the anxiety. Time seems to pass inexorably slowly. They can become obsessive and make endless lists to try and control the inner chaos that is threatening to overwhelm them. They can forget everything when the time comes to perform because the intensity of their feelings overshadows their mental processes.

They know this about themselves and because of it have a fear of failure. They can get to the point where they won't even try because they know there isn't any point. This is a useful remedy for school children who won't revise, who lack perseverence, who say that they are going to fail anyway so why bother?

Afterwards the stress of it all gets on top of them and they become dull, confused and unable to concentrate or think or remember anything. They can then become silently depressed – not wanting to talk about how they feel. There is, in fact, a lot going on emotionally and they will still feel nervous and anxious inside, but it may not show.

General state
Appetite: likes chocolate; salty foods; sugar/sweets; sweet foods. *Desires* fresh air. *Pains:* needle-like; splinter; stitching. *Symptoms:* left-sided. *Taste in mouth* sour. *Thirsty. Tongue* red-tipped.

Better for cold; fresh air; for a walk in the fresh air.
Worse for heat; sugar/sweets; at night; tight clothing.

Physical stresses: sugar/sweets; strain/overexertion – of voice.

These people are warm-blooded types who are generally worse for heat, who suffer in hot, stuffy rooms and feel better for fresh air. They love salty and strong-tasting foods but these do not affect them badly the way sweet things do. They crave sugar (they can eat it straight from the sugar bowl) and sweets, more so when they are under stress, but these make them feel ill, typically with diarrhoea and/or indigestion which is accompanied by flatulence and belching. This is worse for tight clothing and is difficult to expel and noisy, even explosive when it does come out, usually providing relief from the bloating and discomfort, but not always. The diarrhoea is a common symptom with the anxiety state and the panic attacks.

Their nervous exhaustion is often accompanied by anxiety and trembling and may follow a period of intense mental work or study where the whole system feels worn out.

Typical physical complaints as a result of stress include:

- Diarrhoea: stools green, smelly, watery; worse immediately after drinking.
- Exhaustion: with trembling.
- Eye inflammation: eyes sticky, red; sensitive to light; with stitching pains; better for cold and cold compresses.
- Flatulence: painful bloating; worse after eating.
- Headache: better for pressure of a scarf or headband and for cold bathing.
- Hoarseness: from over-using voice (singers, public speakers); may lose voice altogether.
- Hot flushes: with sweating; breaks out into anxious sweat.
- Indigestion: bloating with loud belching, worse after eating.
- Palpitations: felt throughout body; worse thinking about them; worse lying on the right side.
- Sore throat: pains splinter-like; throat red, raw.

ARNICA MONTANA (*Arn.*)
Leopard's bane

Emotional state
Denial: of illness/of suffering. *Dislikes* being touched/examined. *Fearful:* generally; of being touched. *Forgetful* following injury. *Irritable. Memory* loss after head injury.

Emotional stress: shock.

Arnica is for physical or emotional injury, for those suffering from delayed shock, i.e. for shock after an injury which isn't expressed. People needing *Arnica* deny that they are ill and say they are well when they aren't. They can moan and complain about their pains, but more usually the sicker they are, the finer they insist they are feeling.

This is a remedy for those who don't want to be touched after an injury because their bodies are still in shock. They become irritable, not letting anyone near and refusing treatment, saying they want to manage things on their own. At the scene of an accident they will say they are all right and insist on going home – in spite of quite nasty looking injuries.

On coming round after a concussion they are apathetic and can have difficulty with their memory, forgetting words whilst they are speaking.

General state
Breath smells. *Pains:* sore, bruised. *Taste in mouth* of rotten eggs.
Worse for jarring movement; for lying on the injured part; for moving the affected part; for touch.

Physical stresses: altitude; injury – to bones, bruises to head, to muscles; sprain with swelling; general physical strain/from travel; shock after injury.

Arnica promotes healing by controlling bleeding, reducing swelling and preventing pus forming. It is therefore a very important remedy for physical stresses but especially stresses from injury. It is the first remedy to think of for any bruising to the muscular (or soft) tissues of the body or any injury that involves bruising, i.e. accidents, surgery, dental treatment, childbirth, etc.

The pains are sore and bruised, and sensitive to being touched or jarred, so that sufferers will avoid crowded places in case they get inadvertently jostled. Even lying down can aggravate, making people feel that their bed is too hard, causing them to appear restless as they try to find a pain-free position.

Overexertion (physical strain) with muscular aching, will also respond to *Arnica*, if the characteristic sensitivities are also present, whether the exertion is due to childbirth, gardening, jet lag or mountain climbing!

Typical physical complaints as a result of stress include:

- Bleeding gums: after dental treatment (including extraction).
- Blood blister: from a blow or injury.
- Bruises: with swelling, without discoloration – to any part of the body.
- Eye inflammation: from injury to the eye; eye is red.
- Injuries: with sore, bruised pains and swelling – to any part of the body.
- Jetlag: feels achy, sore and bruised and worse for movement.
- Muscle strain: pains sore, bruised after overexertion.
- Nosebleed: from injury or overexertion (strain).
- Swelling: from injury; feels sore, bruised (first stage sprain, first stage fractures/broken bones).
- Toothache: after head injury or dental work.

ARSENICUM ALBUM (*Ars.*)
Arsenic trioxide

Emotional state
Anxious: when alone; with fear; during a fever; at night; about others; on waking. *Bites fingernails. Blames* others. *Busy. Complaining. Critical. Depressed. Desires:* to be carried (fast); company. *Despair:* with the pain. *Fearful:* generally; or being alone; of burglars; of death; of illness; of losing control; at night. *Fussy. Insecure. Irritable. Restless. Selfish. Tidy.*

Emotional stresses: fear; guilt; resentment; transition; uncertainty; worry.

These are generally anxious, tense, restless types. The anxiety is always worse at night (typically around 3 a.m.), is overwhelming and often felt physically in the pit of the stomach.

This state can arise out of a period of insecurity – often financial, although it may be emotional. In attempting to right this imbalance they seek order and perfection in their external life – in their environment at home and at work. At their worst they become obsessively neat and tidy in an attempt to feel secure and in control.

They have a reputation for being selfish and stingy, compulsively hoarding things like paper bags and rubber bands – tidily of course!

They set impossible standards and goals for themselves, and can easily become guilt-ridden when they fail to achieve them. They also expect a lot from others and don't hesitate to say so! They can become picky, and critical – more so when under stress.

Once ill they become frightened of being alone. They fear for their own safety at night and can become obsessed with being robbed – to the point of looking under the bed just in case. They also fear death (however minor the illness) and want desperately to be looked after. They become quickly depressed and despair of getting well again.

They are demanding, difficult patients who find fault and make a fuss. In spite of being too weak to get out of bed to make a cup of tea they may clear up for visitors or the doctor because of their obsession with tidiness.

Children needing this remedy are also fussy – wanting their food on certain plates, disliking getting their hands dirty and ordering their parents around. Babies and infants want to be carried around when they are ill but prefer to be carried fast.

It is possible to fall into a temporary *Arsenicum* state under stress, either emotional or physical. You will then see the characteristic anxiety and irritability, which, if left unchecked, can lead to depression.

General state
Appetite poor/lost: likes hot food/drinks. **Breath** smells. *Discharges* burning; smelly; thin; watery. *Dryness* generally. *Expression*

anxious/haggard; suffering. *Eyes* sensitive to bright light. *Face* pale. *Lips:* cracked; dry; pale; licks them. *Mouth* dry. *Pains* burning – better for heat. *Senses* acute. *Symptoms* right-sided. *Taste in mouth* bitter. *Thirsty* for sips. *Tongue:* red-edged; red-tipped; white coated. **Better** for bathing (a hot bath); heat; for hot drinks; for lying down; for warmth of bed.

Worse after midnight, at 1.00 a.m.; for change of temperature; for cold; for cold wet weather; for damp; for physical exertion; at night; on waking.

Physical stresses: burns and scalds; chemicals; cold; food poisoning; ice-cold food/drink; swimming in the sea; wet weather.

A person who needs *Arsenicum* looks pale and anxious, even haggard. When ill they quickly become weak and exhausted, sometimes to the point of collapse in an acute complaint like food poisoning, often out of proportion to the severity of the illness. The tiredness comes on suddenly, especially after physical exertion, or even a short walk.

They are generally better for lying down, although many of the physical symptoms are worse for this, for example the cough, and this causes their general restlessness.

They are extremely sensitive to cold and to getting chilled *and* they need fresh air so their ideal is to have the heating on and a window open! Because of their sensitivity to cold they can become ill (typically with a cough or a cold) after swimming in cold water, especially cold seawater.

When ill they become dried out, with dry lips and mouth. Their pains are characteristically burning and, except for the headaches, are better for heat (a useful, unusual symptom) and for warm drinks, food or compresses. Cold drinks and food aggravate, especially with digestive problems. They lose their appetites when ill – the sight or smell of food will make this worse. Their worst time of day is between midnight and 2 a.m., usually around 1 a.m., when their symptoms, including the anxiety, are worse.

Typical physical complaints as a result of stress include:

• Anaemia: exhaustion with a pale face.

- Common cold: with burning, watery nasal catarrh; dry, sore eyes; frequent sneezing.
- Cough: dry; painful; tickling; better for hot drinks.
- Cystitis: burning pains, better for heat.
- Diarrhoea: stools are smelly, watery; worse for cold drinks; burning pains after stool.
- Exhaustion: extreme, sudden, with faint feeling and restlessness; with trembling and anxiety.
- Fever: dry, burning heat; worse at night.
- Flu: with fever and restlessness, anxiety, etc.
- Food poisoning: severe, with vomiting and diarrhoea.
- Headache: pains burning, throbbing; better for fresh air.
- Indigestion: with heartburn, better for hot drinks.
- Insomnia: with anxious dreams, nightmares and restless sleep.
- Palpitations: worse lying down at night.
- Piles: pains burning, better for hot compresses/water.
- Sore throat: with ulcers in the throat, burning pains, better for hot drinks, worse swallowing.
- Stomach ache: burning pains, better for hot drinks.
- Vomiting: with diarrhoea.

AURUM METALLICUM (*Aur.*)
Gold

Emotional state
Angry: with difficulty expressing anger. *Blames* self. *Depressed. Despair. Gloomy. Lacks self-confidence. Lonely. Prays. Quarrelsome. Sensitive* to music.

Emotional stresses: betrayal; depression; failure; guilt; loneliness; loss; shame.

Those who need this remedy are sensitive and take life seriously. They have integrity and a strong sense of duty – especially with regard to their family – and can take on too much. They then can become irritable (typically reacting badly to contradiction), guilt-ridden and, ultimately, full of regret.

This remedy is needed for someone who has set themselves a high goal, and failed to achieve it. It can be a personal goal, or a work goal – and could be materially based, i.e. including the gain of money (gold!), and may have become all consuming.

Children who may also need *Aurum*, are typically mature, responsible children who want to be top of the class. They become withdrawn and melancholy after a lost dream, a lost goal, a failed exam or even a disappointment such as a rejection from a loved one – for example, after their parents divorce. They feel as if they have fallen from a great height. They also feel increasingly lonely and abandoned as they keep their emotions (especially their anger) inside. If the anger isn't expressed they can spiral down into a depression full of feelings of hopelessness, despair and worthlessness.

These types become sensitive to rejection, to possible failure and to criticism. They are conscientious types with a tendency to workaholism who feel they have tried hard to do the right thing and take criticism to heart, reacting with thoughts of death because they feel others have lost confidence in them and they don't feel useful any more.

The depression is a deep, dark, quiet despair which is worse in the evening, when they re-evaluate their lives and where they are going, and may well seek solace in prayer or meditation – reconnecting with their neglected spiritual side. They find music soothing in a melancholy sort of way rather than uplifting.

Once depressed they find it difficult to think and don't want to talk about how they feel. They may become so gloomy that the present *and* the future look black.

General state
Desires fresh air. *Pains* in the bones; boring; tearing. *Symptoms:* right-sided.
Better in the evening; for movement; walking slowly in the fresh air.
Worse for cold; lying down; at night; for rest; in the winter.

There is a general sensitivity to the cold, sometimes with a feeling of heat in the face, but their desire for fresh air over-rides this. They are sensitive to pain.

They may feel generally better in the evening but emotionally they feel worse then, more depressed and their pains are often worse at night.

Typical physical complaints as a result of stress include:

- Cough: takes deep breaths because of a feeling that they can't get enough air into their lungs.
- Headache: pains tearing; in bones; worse for mental exertion; worse when blowing nose; for cold air; with dizziness.
- Insomnia: restless sleep; with frightful, vivid dreams.
- Palpitations: heart seems to stop, then starts again with a thump.
- Ulcers: in mouth and/or nose; painful.

BARYTA CARBONICA (*Bar-c.*)
Barium carbonate

Emotional state

Bites fingernails. Childish. Concentration difficult/poor. *Dull/ confused. Easily embarrassed. Fearful* of strangers. *Forgetful. Indecisive. Lacks self-confidence. Shy. Slow. Sluggish mentally.*

Emotional stresses: boredom; bullying; embarrassment; transition.

These types are shy and nervous, especially with people they don't know, finding social situations difficult because of their insecurity. They prefer to be at home but don't want to be on their own. Small children hide behind their mothers or the furniture when strangers are around, whilst older children slink around the edges of gatherings, feeling embarrassed and out of place.

They lack self-confidence and are either emotionally immature (at any age) or find it difficult to grow up into their next phase of life, and especially to make the transition from childhood to adulthood. They are naive and can behave childishly in a way that is delightful when they are strong in themselves (they love to play the clown) and irritating when they become sluggish (they whine, and can regress into babytalk).

Elderly people may seem to go through a second childhood and appear to those around them to be surprisingly scatty – forgetful and indecisive – and sluggish, physically as well as emotionally and mentally.

They can get stuck in boredom and become spaced-out, sitting around doing nothing much – and not wanting to do anything anyway. There may even be nothing going on inside – not even a pleasant little daydream! – and they need a little help to get them going again.

Their own particular blend of personal characteristics plus a dislike of being teased will tend to attract the unwelcome attention of the school (or office) bully. They very quickly think that others are laughing at them, or criticizing them – even when they aren't. This can set up a vicious cycle of being bullied or even harassed which is hard to break. They become emotionally withdrawn if this continues.

They are self-conscious about their bodies (because of their lack of confidence) and compare themselves to others in a childish attempt to look 'right'. They are cautious, especially with regard to making decisions and can take ages to make up their minds on trivial issues, like what to wear.

They are studious but have difficulty remembering and are easily distracted, which makes studying, especially for exams, a struggle. Children may lag behind or be unable to concentrate or take in new concepts (this includes bright children who have come up against a learning block).

This remedy is useful for those who are generally slow and shy and lacking in self-confidence as well as for those who have become so temporarily. It is especially useful for children who are stuck and not living up to their own potential – either mentally, emotionally or physically.

General state
Eyes sensitive to bright light. *Glands* sensitive; swollen. *Slowness* (of children) to grow; to learn. *Sweaty* feet (smelly).
Worse for cold.

Physical stresses: cold, damp weather; getting wet.

These types are sensitive to cold, damp weather and need to wrap up warmly due to a tendency to catch colds and coughs, which usually come with swollen glands – they can have huge tonsils and glands like peas at the back of their necks.

They are usually sensitive to the heat – wilting in the hot weather and in stuffy rooms, getting hot and sweaty in bed at night and poking bits of their bodies out or kicking the covers off altogether. Their eyes are sensitive to bright light, especially sunlight – babies will cry if their eyes aren't shaded in the car or pushchair.

They can also come down with a cold, cough or sore throat if their feet get wet. They have sweaty feet which causes rawness between the toes and if this sweat is suppressed (with sprays or powders) they can actually become ill – with a sore throat or a cough.

Babies that need *Baryta carbonica* are slow to develop, to walk and talk. They have an old look about them, an old expression. They don't lose their 'toddler's tummies' when the other children do but they aren't necessarily fat either. Adults needing *Baryta carbonica* may also have trouble losing weight from around their middles.

In spite of having a generally dry mouth they may dribble into their pillows at night. If they become nervous and insecure they will bite their nails and suffer from nightmares.

Typical physical complaints as a result of stress include:
- Colds: with swollen glands and a congested nose; with cough.
- Cough: dry and/or rattling; worse for cold air/drinks, at night.
- Exhaustion: worse after eating.
- Headache: with dizziness.
- Indigestion: after eating, food lies like a stone in the stomach.
- Sore throat: throat raw; tonsils swollen; worse for swallowing food (liquids are fine); worse at night.

BELLADONNA (*Bell.*)
Deadly nightshade

Emotional state
Cheerful alternating with sadness. *Delirious* with hallucinations. *Dislikes* being touched or examined. *Dull/confused. Excitable. Fear*

of animals; of dogs. *Jumpy. Rage/tantrums:* with desire to bite or hit. *Screaming* or moaning with pain. *Sensitive:* generally: to light; to noise. *Tearful* with a fever.

Emotional stress: shock.

These are happy, easygoing, lively types who become wild and unmanageable under stress. They may be generally scared of animals, especially dogs, and this can be acute when they are ill. They may also be fascinated with fire – something to watch out for in young children!

When ill they become hypersensitive to light and noise. With a fever they become delirious, seeing and talking to imaginary beings. They become agitated and restless – and will jump out of bed at night to try and 'escape'.

They look terrified but may also be angry at what has happened. They can have violent rages when unwell or in pain. They cry, scream and even hit and bite. They talk, scream and/or kick in their sleep or start as if frightened when falling asleep as well as during sleep.

General state
Appetite: likes lemonade. *Dryness. Expression* fierce. *Eyes* shining. *Face* red (flushed); red in spots. *Glands* sensitive; swollen. *Onset* of pain/complaint – sudden. *Pains* appear and disappear suddenly; shooting; throbbing. *Pupils* dilated. *Sensation* of constriction. *Senses* acute. *Sweat* absent during fever; on covered parts. *Swelling* of affected parts. *Symptoms* right-sided. *Thirstless. Tongue* red or white-coated; strawberry.
Better for lying down; for pressure; for rest.
Worse for draughts; for jarring movement; at 3.00 p.m.

Physical stresses: getting head wet; sunstroke.

A *Belladonna* illness comes on suddenly and strongly. Pains (headache, teething, earache, etc.) come and go suddenly. A cold may start if the head is chilled, especially if the head/hair is wet (after a swim or haircut or getting wet in the rain).

Generally symptoms are worse at 3.00 p.m. although 3.00 a.m. may also be a bad time. Lying in a quiet, darkened room helps, although some symptoms are better for standing.

They have a fierce look because of the flushed face, shiny eyes and dilated pupils. The tongue is red, coated with white dots (strawberry) or it has a white coating. In spite of a dry mouth they can be thirstless, although with a fever they may crave lemonade.

Any part of the body can become inflamed or infected, going red and throbbing painfully, radiating heat. With a fever the artery in the neck may throb visibly, and they can tremble and twitch with the heat. Violent throbbing pains are intensified by movement or being moved, touched or jarred (for example, during a car journey). Whilst they can have a hot face and head, typically their hands and feet are cold.

In women many problems may occur around menstruation and during the menopause when the periods can become very heavy.

Typical physical complaints as a result of stress include:

- Common cold: with fever and headache.
- Convulsions: in teething babies.
- Cough: dry, barking, tickling, tormenting; with hoarse voice; worse at night, for deep breathing.
- Cramps: in hands or feet; in muscles (anywhere in the body).
- Cystitis: pains in bladder pressing, sore; worse for jarring motion.
- Diarrhoea: after getting chilled in hot weather; in teething infants; after a haircut.
- Earache: pains stitching, tearing, throbbing; spread down into the neck; face aches; worse at night, on the right side.
- Eye inflammation: eyes bloodshot, burning, dry, watering, sensitive to light; with a cold; worse for light, for heat.
- Fever: heat alternating with chills; dry, burning; with delirium; with hoarse voice; without sweating.
- Headache: pains bursting, hammering, pulsating, throbbing, violent; migraines: better for rest, lying down, for pressure; worse for bending down, for light, for walking.
- Hot flushes: at the menopause.
- Insomnia: with grinding of teeth; with sleepiness; anxious dreams.
- Joint pains: joints are hot and swollen.

- Nosebleeds: blood is hot, bright or dark red with or without dark clots.
- Piles: very painful; with backache; worse for touch.
- Period problems: periods very heavy; painful; blood is hot, bright red with dark clots.
- Sore throats: throat constricted, irritated, raw; pains severe, stitching; worse for swallowing liquids.
- Sunstroke: with fever and headache.
- Teething: painful in babies; with restless sleep.

BORAX VENATA (*Bor.*)
Sodium biborate

Emotional state
Anxious. Fearful: generally; of downward motion; of sudden noises. *Irritable. Jumpy.*

Emotional stresses: fear; shock.

An emotional shock in childhood or the shock of a difficult or fast childbirth can upset the nervous system.

This remedy is useful for nervous children who haven't recovered from a particular shock, who become easily startled by sudden noises – someone sneezing unexpectedly can make them jump and set them off crying. They wake up screaming with the slightest noise, or they may scream in their sleep without waking up.

Babies and children are irritable leading up to passing a stool and change to being cheerful directly afterwards. Babies dislike downward motion and will cry on being rocked or being put down in their cots. They don't like being thrown in the air as do many babies and small children (because of the coming down part!)

Adults needing this remedy are phobic about lifts – feeling scared going down rather than generally claustrophobic.

General state
Expression anxious. *Pains* sharp. *Sensitive* to downward motion. *Symptoms* right-sided.

Better after passing a stool.
Worse at 10.00 a.m.; before a stool.

Physical stress: travel.

The sensitivity to downward motion is physical as well as emotional and this is therefore a useful remedy for travel sickness where the nausea and vomiting are worse for downward movement, i.e. when the car goes downhill, the ship dips or the aeroplane lands everything in the stomach comes up!

Typical physical complaints as a result of stress include:
- Cough: dry, painful; stitching pains worse for deep breathing.
- Diarrhoea: painless; with mucus; in teething infants.
- Dizziness: with downward motion (including walking downstairs).
- Headache: worse at 10.00 a.m.
- Hiccoughs: in nervous babies.
- Insomnia: sleep disturbed; difficulty sleeping if too hot.
- Teething: difficult in sensitive babies.
- Thrush (genital): burns; discharge like egg white.
- Thrush (oral): of the tongue and mouth; bleeding; hot; painful.

CALCAREA CARBONICA (*Calc-c.*)
Calcium carbonate

Emotional state
Affected by hearing of tragic events/sad stories. *Anxious:* about the future; during the evening; about health. *Depressed.. Despair* of getting well. *Dull/confused. Fearful:* of death; of dogs; of heights; of illness; of insects; worse in the evening. *Forgetful. Melancholic. Self-pitying. Slow. Sluggish. Stubborn. Tearful.*
Worse for mental exertion/thinking.

Emotional stresses: fear; uncertainty; worry.

When well, these are robust, happy, contented types. But under the stress of a shock or even overwork they can become deeply anxious. They then have a tendency to worry about all sorts of things, but especially about their own health. They can become hypochondriacs and read endless medical books. This can get them down and can get out of hand so that, for example, they become anxious about their future, about something bad happening to them and frightened of catching an infection or becoming seriously ill.

They also have a fear of heights that is accompanied by dizziness – even watching someone else on a high place can be excruciating. They may be phobic about flying (because of their fear of heights), animals (especially dogs), birds and insects. They are also scared of the dark and can become claustrophobic. These fears, if unchecked, can be the stress or stresses that cause them to become ill.

When depressed they have a tendency to self-pity or melancholy. Naturally slow types (plodders), under stress they become sluggish mentally and physically as well as dull and confused. This, combined with the depression, a despair of ever being well again and their general state of anxiety can make them feel as if they are going crazy.

They have a strong imagination and hate hearing of horrible things happening to others. They can't bear to read newspapers or watch the news on television because they retain the images in their minds. They have strong wills (stubborn!), are hard workers who see things through and take life and their responsibilities seriously. They are dependable, reliable types who can become workaholics (reacting with irritability when they don't have anything to do). When their stress load becomes too much and their anxieties surface, they can plod on and on, gradually becoming more and more fearful and exhausted. They become especially worried about losing their job (and becoming poverty stricken). They become concerned about what others think of them, not wanting to appear foolish and confused, which adds to their already untenable stress load.

General state
Appetite good: digestion poor/slow; dislikes coffee, meat; likes boiled eggs, indigestible things (coal/earth/sand, etc.). *Clumsy.* *Cracks* in skin. *Discharges* sour; thick. *Face* pale. *Glands* swollen. *Pains* cramping; stitching. *Sense* of smell lost. *Slowness:* of children to teethe; to walk. *Sweat:* on head; from mental exertion; from

slightest physical exertion; profuse; during sleep; sour. *Symptoms* right-sided. *Taste in mouth:* bad; sour. *Tongue* white-coated.
Better for heat; for lying down; for massage; for touch.
Worse for cold; for damp; for darkness; draughts; for mental or physical exertion; for fasting; for fresh air; for milk; full moon; for wet weather.

Physical stresses: damp weather; food sensitivities – milk; medication (aspirin); moon (full); joints, wrist, strain/over exertion of ankles, of hips/back – from lifting; digestion sluggish; teething; slow metabolism; getting wet.

People needing this remedy vary in their general state depending on how stressed they are. They can be resilient, strong and robust, only falling ill with occasional unhealthy stress.

Under continued stress they become sluggish, moving slowly, looking white and pasty. They may become so worn out that they have a spineless and flabby look about them, and slump in the chair when sitting down. At this stage exertion of any sort (physical *or* mental) leaves them weak, trembly, sweaty and breathless and they feel better for lying down and for loosening their clothes. They feel a need to take deep breaths.

Children are typically fast to grow physically but slow to learn to walk and produce teeth, and their fontanelles are slow to close. They tend to have large heads and bellies and put on weight easily. They may also be slow learners at school, although they will manage by sheer hard work.

People who need this remedy feel worse for cold and damp although they can over-heat easily and then be subject to hot flushes. Their feet and hands are always cold and often clammy, even in bed. (Typically they have a clammy, limp handshake). They sweat on their heads and at the back of the neck, especially whilst asleep when they may leave wet patches on their sheets or pillows. They sweat when they exert themselves. Their sweat smells sour, as do their other discharges (stools and urine, etc.) They have a sour taste in their mouths.

They have a slow metabolism and they put on weight easily. They can sprain their ankles (and back easily) because of the extra weight, and these are slow to mend. They may have difficulty assimilating their food, especially milk which turns sour in the stomach, causing nausea. They may also want to eat strange, indigestible things (mainly children and pregnant women!) like chalk or pencils. They love sweet things and eggs – especially boiled eggs.

They dislike draughts and can catch cold easily after swimming or getting wet. Warmth relieves their symptoms. Their fears and anxieties are worse at dusk. Their faces become lined from worry with lots of fine lines rather than deep creases.

Typical physical complaints as a result of stress are:

- Anaemia: with exhaustion.
- Backache: lower back aches, feels weak and sprained; worse getting up from sitting.
- Common cold: nose blocked; catarrh yellow.
- Constipation: stools hard at first, large, pale; no urging; then sour-smelling diarrhoea.
- Cough: dry at night, loose in the morning; difficulty coughing up yellow sour-smelling mucus.
- Cramps: calf, hand, sole, toes; worse when stretching in bed.
- Diarrhoea: stools sour, watery with undigested food.
- Earache: pains throbbing; with noises in ear.
- Exhaustion: with breathlessness and dizziness.
- Eye inflammation: eyes gritty, glued together, watery, sensitive to light; with a common cold.
- Headache: pains bursting, maddening; worse for light with dizziness (worse on turning head quickly).
- Indigestion: painful bloating worse for tight clothing; sour belches; with flatulence.
- Insomnia: anxious dreams; sleepless before midnight or waking at 3.00 a.m. with inability to get back to sleep.
- Joint pain: pains cramping; worse in wet weather.
- Palpitations: at night; worse after eating.
- Periods: heavy; breasts swollen and painful before period.
- Sore throat: throat dry; painless hoarseness.
- Stiff neck: pains sprained.
- Toothache: pains gnawing; worse for drawing cold air in between teeth.
- Vomiting: vomits curdled milk, smells sour.

CALCAREA PHOSPHORICA (*Calc-p.*)
Phosphate of lime

Emotional state
Anxious. Complaining. Desire to travel. *Discontented. Dull/confused. Fear* of thunderstorms. *Restless. Sighing. Sluggish* mentally. *Stubborn.*
Worse for mental exertion/thinking.

Emotional stresses: disappointment; mental strain; shock; transition.

These are lively, sympathetic types whose genuine concern for others can tip over into anxiety if stressed by overwork, shock or a disappointment in love, etc. Then they become fearful, discontented and negative – even depressed.

They are generally restless types who like to have new experiences, especially to travel, but under stress they become aimlessly restless – wanting to go somewhere, only to want to return home once they reach their destination. This can be especially infuriating in children. The travelling acts as a distraction from thinking about their problems and reflects an inner desire to escape or get away from their troubles.

Under stress they lose interest *and* complain about it – they know there's something wrong but can't pinpoint what. Trying to work out what is wrong only makes them feel worse.

They can become mentally worn out from too much studying, turning dull and sluggish and finding it hard to concentrate. Children find schoolwork difficult and complain of boredom – along with the typical head or stomach aches. They are peevish and have no 'go' in them.

General state
Appetite: likes smoked foods. *Face* pale. *Glands* swollen. *Slowness* of children to grow; learn; to teethe; to walk. *Thin.*
Worse for cold; for cold, wet weather; for damp; for draughts; after eating; for fresh air.

Physical stresses: drafts; growth spurt; convalescing from illness; injury – to bones; insomnia from tension/nervous strain; soft drinks; teething; wet weather.

Calcarea phosphorica is for skinny types whose food is assimilated poorly as a result of a fast metabolism. This remedy helps with calcium absorption, with the health and strength of teeth and bones. Fractures (in a person of any age) are slow to mend because of poor food assimilation and the bones of elderly people are brittle because of a poor diet.

Babies have difficulty teething, with diarrhoea, coughs and colds. Their teeth are slow to come through and they decay easily. Children are slow learning to walk and have weak ankles. They can be slow to grow and to gain weight – or find growing difficult, becoming tired and anaemic after each growth spurt. At puberty, the menstrual periods are late to start.

This is a wonderful tonic to give to children who have had a growth spurt and have become pale and exhausted as a result. It is also useful for growing pains in children. These are more usually felt in the muscles or the joints, although it can be in the bones.

Those who are weak and tired while convalescing from an illness will likewise benefit from this remedy – typically they look pale and thin or just generally flabby.

Those needing this remedy are generally sensitive to the cold, the damp, draughts and suffer with cold hands and feet (melting snow can bring on joint pains and a general aggravation of symptoms). They have a love of strong-tasting foods, especially smoked meats (salami, ham and bacon), fish and salty foods like olives. Their illnesses are often accompanied by swollen glands.

Typical complaints as a result of stress include:

- Anaemia: with exhaustion.
- Backache: worse for cold and draughts.
- Common cold: recurring, catches colds easily; worse for cold.
- Cough: with yellow mucus.
- Cramp: calves; worse when walking.
- Diarrhoea: with green stools.
- Exhaustion: with heaviness and weakness in limbs.
- Growing pains: in bones or muscles; after a growth spurt.

- Headache: from mental exertion; in schoolchildren; better for cold compresses.
- Insomnia: sleepless before midnight; wakes late with difficulty.
- Joint pain: in hips or feet with cramping and aching numbness.
- Nosebleeds: from blowing nose.
- Stiff neck: and shoulders; worse for draughts.
- Sore throat: with hoarse voice and swollen tonsils.
- Stomach ache: in children; with loud belches; better for eating.
- Teething: slow, difficult; teeth decay easily.

CAPSICUM (*Caps.*)
Cayenne pepper

Emotional state
Depressed. Excitable. Irritable. Sensitive.

Emotional stress: homesickness.

This is a small remedy for stubborn, sensitive, excitable types who find it difficult to be away from home, who suffer from insomnia and melancholy when homesick, who may become almost paralysed with unhappiness if, for example, they are sent away to boarding school.

General state
Appetite: desires alcohol; coffee; pepper; spicy foods. *Face* red. *Lips* burning, cracked, swollen. *Mouth* dry. *Pains* burning. *Symptoms* left-sided. *Tongue* burning.
Worse for cold; slightest draught.

If homesick they lose their vitality and can then start putting on a lot of weight in a short space of time, becoming clumsy and awkward.

Although generally chilly they become flushed easily and quickly, without necessarily feeling hot. They may crave stimulants to keep going, especially alcohol, coffee and spicy foods with lots of pepper!

Burning pains accompany most of their complaints, which, under stress, include the following:

- Cough: nervous; spasmodic (coughing fits).
- Eye inflammation: painful; eyes water.
- Headache: bursting, throbbing.
- Indigestion: acid burning in stomach.
- Insomnia: with homesickness or cough.
- Piles: burning; with flatulence.
- Sore throat: burning; with swollen tonsils and hoarseness.

CARBO VEGETABILIS (*Carb-v.*)
Wood charcoal

Emotional state
Anxious: in bed; worse during the evening. *Apathetic* about everything. *Dull/confused. Irritable. Sluggish* mentally.

Emotional stress: shock.

This is a remedy for people who become inactive and so sluggish that they find it difficult to rouse themselves to do anything. They may become indifferent to the point that they do not care if they live or die because they don't feel they are going to get better.

Alongside this apathy is a surprising irritability that surfaces mainly with those close to them, when they rouse themselves to make cutting, nasty comments.

They suffer from anxiety which is worse in the late afternoon and the evening and intensifies when they go to bed and shut their eyes.

General state
Appetite: dislikes fatty foods; likes salty foods; salty and sour foods; sweet foods. *Breath* smells. *Desires:* to be fanned; fresh air. *Discharges* smelly. *Face:* cold; pale; sallow. *Lips:* chapped, cracked. *Pains:* burning; pressing. *Sweat:* cold; profuse. *Taste in mouth* bitter.
Better for being fanned.
Worse for physical exertion; after eating rich/fatty foods; for humidity.

Physical stresses: digestion sluggish; food poisoning; car or gas/ coal/charcoal fumes; heat; humidity; convalescing from illness; loss of fluids; overeating; fatty, rich food; travel.

Carbo vegetabilis is for those who are debilitated, sluggish and low in vitality. This may have been caused by an emotional shock but it is commonly caused by a physical stress such as food poisoning (typically from bad eggs or vegetables) or carbon dioxide poisoning (from car exhausts or gas, coal or charcoal fumes) or an illness. The lack of oxygen on a long distance flight is stressful for some. The other main stress calling for this remedy is a loss of body fluids, i.e. after diarrhoea or a haemorrhage or even while breastfeeding.

People of any age struggling to recover from an illness (glandular fever or chest infections, including children recovering from childhood illnesses such as measles or whooping cough) can need this remedy if the whole picture fits.

They feel generally chilly, their legs are cold to the touch, but they don't want to be covered. They want to be fanned and feel much better out in the cool, fresh air, especially if there is a breeze. Indoors they want the electric fan (or the air conditioning) on and when travelling they want the windows open so they can feel the breeze. Becoming overheated makes them feel worse as does humidity. They sweat easily, especially whilst eating, and their perspiration feels cold to the touch.

They want to lie down and sleep but may feel worse lying down, in spite of feeling too weak and heavy to do otherwise. The arm or leg that is lain on goes to sleep. Mornings and evenings are their worst times of day. The slightest exertion exhausts them, making them feel faint and weak – they have to force themselves to get going.

The digestion is easily upset, especially by eating fatty, rich foods, although it can accompany any of the physical stresses. The stomach feels full and bloated after eating. Belching relieves the bloating for a while and then the gas builds up quite quickly again. They can be thin or they can put on weight easily.

Typical physical symptoms as a result of stress include:
- Breathlessness: with wind or after over-eating; worse lying down; better for belching.

- Common cold: frequent, difficult sneezing; nose blocked; voice hoarse.
- Cough: racking, painful, in fits; breathing fast, wheezing.
- Diarrhoea: smelly stools; with bloating and flatulence.
- Exhaustion: with cold sweat; worse for any exertion.
- Fainting: worse on getting up from sitting, on waking.
- Flatulence: worse at night; better for passing wind.
- Gums bleeding: gums are sore, recede and bleed easily.
- Hair falls out: in pregnancy; after childbirth.
- Headache: dull, heavy pains; worse for pressure, for lying flat, for over-heating; with nausea, burping and dizziness.
- Hoarseness: painless; voice deep; worse talking, in the evening.
- Indigestion: with bloating and stomach pains; with heartburn; better for belching; worse after eating.
- Insomnia: sleepy but can't sleep before midnight; with vivid, unpleasant dreams.
- Jetlag: with exhaustion and indigestion.
- Nosebleeds: worse at night; with dark blood.
- Sore throat: larynx sore and irritated; with hoarseness.
- Voice lost: worse in the evening.

CAUSTICUM (*Caust.*)
Potassium hydrate

Emotional state
Absent-minded. Anxious about others. *Concentration* poor. *Defiant. Depressed. Fearful:* worse in the evening; that something bad will happen. *Forgetful memory* weak. *Sensitive:* to injustice. *Sympathetic. Tearful.*

Emotional stresses: conflict; loss; uncertainty.

These are sensitive souls who suffer when others, especially those close to them, are hurting – either emotionally or physically or both. They care about injustice in any shape or form, and can become actively rebellious (because of their defiant streak), joining organizations and actually fighting for justice. They care so much *for* others that they are vulnerable to misfortune and sensitive to loss, both personally and on others' behalf.

Being pessimistic by nature, they tend to look on the dark side of things and become gloomy, negative and full of anxious forebodings, suffering from (sometimes irrational) fears that something bad will happen.

They cry easily, especially if they see a sad news item in the paper or something touching on television. Children also cry easily and are frightened of the dark, of ghosts, of going to bed on their own. They don't want to be alone, especially in the evening when all their fears and worries are at their worst.

They are naturally anxious and cautious but their worrying can get out of hand under stress, and it is then that they are vulnerable to becoming depressed and emotionally paralysed.

Under stress they can stammer. Their memory is affected and they have difficulty concentrating. They can have an uneasy feeling that they have forgotten something. On leaving their home they will go back to check they have locked the front or back door and turned off the gas, and will even get out of bed at night for the same reason. Only a short time later they may question again whether they have done it.

General state
Appetite: dislikes sweets; likes smoked foods (salami, ham, bacon). *Clumsy,* trips easily while walking. *Discharges:* burning; watery. *Eyelids* heavy. *Pains* burning. *Slowness* (of children) learning to walk. *Thirsty. Tongue:* painful blister/pimple on tip; red stripe down centre (white edges).
Better for cold drinks (especially water); for heat; for warmth of bed; in wet weather.
Worse for changes in weather to dry; for coffee; for cold; for draughts; during the evening; for walking in the fresh air.

Physical stresses: burns; change in weather to dry; dry weather; lead.

These are chilly people who are affected by draughts, by changes in the weather, and especially by clear, dry, cold weather. They can feel unusually well in the damp or even wet weather. Mild, wet weather makes them feel emotionally and physically better, especially their joints and their chests.

Their acute complaints, like the cough and even the stomach pains, are better for cold drinks, especially cold water. Typically, there is a marked dislike of sweets and sweet foods, even in children. Whilst they feel generally worse in the evenings, they can also feel bad on waking in the morning.

Children needing this remedy are sensitive and late learning to walk. Their coordination is poor and they trip easily when walking.

Once run-down, painful blisters on the tongue, typically the tip of the tongue, often accompany or precede a physical complaint.

Typical physical complaints as a result of stress include:

- Backache: back sore, stiff; worse getting up from sitting.
- Common cold: nose blocked without discharge; with sneezing and itching.
- Constipation: with piles; burning pain after stool and ineffectual urging.
- Cough: hacking, constant, distressing, painful; worse lying down; difficulty coughing up phlegm.
- Cramp: feet, toes, sole of foot – worse at night.
- Cystitis: painful, burning during urination with constant, ineffectual desire to urinate; with involuntary urination.
- Exhaustion: overwhelming; feels faint; legs feel weak and trembly; worse in the evening, in the morning on waking.
- Headache: tearing pains from cold, dry air.
- Hoarseness: with a cold; with a cough; from over-using the voice; worse in the morning.
- Indigestion: empty belching and cramping pains.
- Insomnia: sleep unrefreshing; sleepy but can't sleep.
- Joint pain: pains tearing, with stiffness and weakness; joints crack.
- Restless legs: in the evening, in the night in bed, in sleep.
- Rheumatism: worse for cold.
- Sore throat: pains burning, irritating, dry, raw; constant desire to swallow; worse for talking; may lose voice.
- Stomach ache: worse after eating bread.
- Stress incontinence: from coughing or sneezing or getting chilled.
- Voice loss: in singers; from over-using voice; sudden.

CHAMOMILLA (*Cham.*)
German chamomile

Emotional state
Abusive. Angry. Capricious. Contrary. Depressed. Desires: to be carried. *Despair* with the pain. *Dislikes* being touched/examined. *Excitable. Impatient. Quarrelsome. Rage/tantrums. Screaming* with pain. *Sensitive:* to pain; to touch. *Stubborn. Tearful.*

Emotional stress: conflict.

This remedy is indicated for anyone who has been in a highly emotional state (typically angry) for some time, becoming over-sensitive as a result, either mentally or physically or both – with severe pains that cause more anger.

They become impatient and excitable and sensitive to pain, seeming to take it personally and becoming enraged by it. They are difficult to help because they don't want to be questioned or touched (children can become hysterical if examined).

Children are demanding but they don't know what they want. They ask for things which they then reject, which may even be hurled across the room (drinks, toys, etc.) or they cry and scream if they can't have what they want. Babies and children cannot be comforted; they demand to be carried but are quiet only for a short time, as long as they are being rocked vigorously. A bumpy car drive can help. They can get into such a state they hit out at those who are trying to help.

They are quarrelsome (to the point of being abusive) and difficult when sick, with their anger erupting in explosive outbursts (tantrums). It is very hard to be sympathetic towards a child or friend or relative who needs *Chamomilla!*

General state
Appetite: doesn't want breakfast; likes cold drinks. *Breath* smells. *Dislikes* fresh air. *Face:* feels hot; red -- one-sided, in spots. *Pains* unbearable. *Sweat* clammy; hot; better for uncovering. *Thirsty:* extreme, with the pains.

Better for fasting; for uncovering.
Worse for coffee; in the evening; for heat; whilst sweating; for touch; for warmth of bed; for wet compresses; for wind.

Physical stresses: caffeine/coffee; pain; teething; wind.

The keynote of this remedy is unbearable pain – with teething, earache, colic, childbirth, etc. They are also sensitive to coffee – suffering from stomach ache and becoming even more irritable if they drink too much of it.

There may be sweating with the pains, especially on the scalp and face, along with a fever. The face feels hot and flushed and sweaty after eating or drinking. They generally feel worse whilst sweating but better afterwards. They become hot with the pains or a fever and don't like it, kicking off the covers or sticking their burning, hot feet out of bed, but they don't want fresh air either.

Teething is difficult and painful (at any age!), babies dribble and are beside themselves with the pains. The cheek on the side of the erupting tooth is red or has a red patch on it.

They are sensitive to getting chilled by the wind (to the point of being frightened by it) suffering from earache or a cough after being out in it.

Typical physical complaints as a result of stress include:

- Colic: with flatulence; abdomen/stomach feels bloated.
- Conjunctivitis: eyes feel hot, swollen and painful.
- Cough: dry; irritating; tickling; worse at night; chest feels tight
- Diarrhoea: stools are green, hot, painful, smell of bad eggs; in teething children.
- Earache: pains aching, pressing, stitching, tearing; worse bending down; worse for touch.
- Fever: heat burning, one-sided; with shivering; heat alternating with chills.
- Headache: pressing pain; worse for thinking about it.
- Insomnia: restless with sleepiness and vivid dreams.
- Joint pain: with numbness; worse in bed at night; must get up and walk about.
- Periods: cramping pains; flow is dark and clotted; period comes on early.

- Stomach ache: after anger, excitement or coffee; dull pains with painful belching and painful bloating.
- Sore throat: with swollen tonsils; throat feels constricted; larynx feels raw, irritated; voice hoarse.
- Teething: painful/difficult in children; worse for pressure, for any warmth.
- Toothache: pains unbearable; worse for any warmth (including hot drinks); for pressure.
- Vomiting: easy; of bile; after anger.

COCCULUS INDICUS (*Cocc.*)
Indian cockle

Emotional state
Anxious. Dazed. Dull/confused. Forgetful/memory weak. Introspective. Mild (gentle). *Sensitive* to noise; to pain. *Time* passes too quickly. *Uncommunicative.*

Emotional stress: mental strain.

Usually easy-going. If they are overstressed – from worry, mental strain or sometimes from the loss of a loved one, *and* loss of sleep – they become introspective, uncommunicative and closed off from the world, appearing sad, dazed and passive to those close to them. Everything slows down. They feel that time passes quickly, especially at night when they try to sleep but can't because of their worrying. Their anxieties centre around the health of those close to them (more than their own health). They worry for others, especially those close to them and are especially upset by rudeness *to* others.

They become tired, anxious and confused and begin to forget things. They may become trembly if they have difficult emotional situations to deal with.

General state
Appetite: lost. *Dislikes* fresh air. *Senses* acute. *Sweat* on single parts of the body; cold; from slightest physical exertion. *Taste in mouth* metallic. *Trembling.*

Better for lying down.
Worse for movement; for physical exertion; for touch; for walking in the fresh air.

Physical stresses: altitude; loss of sleep; strain from travel.

This remedy is useful in situations where there is a loss of sleep and worry, after nursing a sick person or with travelling, for instance. There is complete (paralytic) exhaustion – they tremble with tiredness, are dizzy and feel worse for fresh air and physical exertion. There is a feeling of numbness, with parts of the body (an arm or a leg) going to sleep easily.

They want to lie quietly in bed and sleep, but this is difficult because the habit of sleeping is lost, which creates a dreadful vicious circle of exhaustion.

Typical physical complaints as a result of stress include:

- Diarrhoea: with travel sickness.
- Dizziness: with nausea; has to lie down; worse on getting up from lying down; as if drunk.
- Exhaustion: with trembling (legs whilst walking; hands/arms when lifting them, i.e. for eating); feels stiff and dizzy; legs feel heavy, numb, feet go to sleep easily.
- Headache: pains in back of head, at nape of neck, in forehead; with nausea.
- Hot flushes: with exhaustion.
- Insomnia: from anxiety; restless sleep; with anxious dreams and/ or nightmares.
- Jetlag: with exhaustion and dizziness.
- Nausea: appetite lost; empty, faint feeling in stomach; worse after eating/drinking, for smell or thought of food.
- Nosebleeds: in pregnancy.
- Period: cramping pains, worse with every breath; periods are heavy and come on early.
- Stomach ache: cramps or dull aching, worse for motion; with bloating and wind.
- Travel sickness: with dizziness, headache and nausea; worse for fresh air, for sitting up, for looking out of the window; better for lying down.

• Vomiting: with diarrhoea and dizziness; better for lying down; worse for fresh air, after eating/drinking; for sitting up.

COFFEA CRUDA (*Coff.*)
Unroasted coffee

Emotional state
Cheerful. Despairs with pain. *Excitable. Lively. Restless. Screaming* with pain. *Sensitive:* to noise, to pain. *Thoughts* active.

Emotional stresses: excitement; mental strain.

This is a remedy for excessive excitability – those who have been overstressed by a pleasant or happy surprise or excitement. They feel cheerful and well in themselves but they can become over-stimulated. The mind then races with ideas and thoughts that whir around uncontrollably, preventing sleep and winding up the nervous system. At this stage they can appear euphoric with excitement.

Their cheerfulness (laughing and joking) can alternate with crying once they are seriously overstressed. The slightest pain induces despair: they make a fuss (screaming and crying) over minor aches and pains.

General state
Dislikes fresh air. *Pains* unbearable. *Senses* acute. *Thirst* at night.
Worse for fresh air; for heat; at night; for wine.

Physical stresses: caffeine/coffee; soft drinks; difficulty sleeping – from over-excitement.

Coffea affects the nerves, causing overexcitement and oversensitivity, agitation and restlessness. All the senses become acute. Pains (headache, toothache, etc.) are severe and are worse for touch or heat.

Soft drinks with caffeine (colas) can affect some people (including children) who become 'wound up', excitable and unable to sleep, as can any drug/medication which has caffeine in it. Both coffee as a drink and *Coffea* can counteract the effect of some homeopathic remedies.

Typical physical complaints as a result of stress include:

- Exhaustion: nervous agitation with insomnia.
- Fever: with chilliness and headache.
- Headache: stabbing pains worse for noise (especially music).
- Insomnia: sleep light and restless; can't get to sleep; with sweating, racing thoughts and vivid dreams.
- Palpitations: with trembling; after excitement.
- Sore throat: pains are worse for swallowing.
- Toothache: shooting pains; better for cold drinks; worse for hot drinks and food.

COLOCYNTHIS (*Coloc.*)
Bitter cucumber

Emotional state
Despairs of getting well. *Indignant. Moaning* with pain. *Restless. Sensitive.*

Emotional stresses: conflict; humiliation.

This remedy is for those who have had a difficult, humiliating situation to deal with, involving feelings of anger combined with indignation. Physical symptoms develop after feeling exposed and insulted – the nervous system is directly affected with cramping or shooting (neuralgic) pains in response to the emotional stress.

The pain causes intense anguish, restlessness and irritability.

General state
Pains cramping; in the muscles; neuralgic; stitching. *Symptoms* right-sided. *Taste in mouth* bitter.
Better for hard pressure; for lying doubled up.
Worse for eating/drinking; for fruit.

Neuralgic or stitching pains or cramps anywhere in the body after feeling angry or humiliated. These pains are worse after eating (especially fruit) or drinking, and are relieved by pressure, for example the abdominal pains are better for bending double.

Typical physical complaints as a result of stress include:

- Backache: worse lying on the back, for breathing in.
- Colic: pains aching, cramping, violent, in waves; with bloating; with nausea, diarrhoea, vomiting.
- Cramps: in thigh, leg, calf.
- Diarrhoea: stools green, pasty; with colic and flatulence.
- Headache: pains tearing, on left side of face, spreading to the ear.
- Insomnia: from anger or humiliation.
- Periods: stop – from anger or humiliation.
- Period pains: cramping pains better for hard pressure; worse after eating/drinking.
- Sciatica: pains tearing, in right leg; with numbness; worse for lying on the painful side, motion, touch, walking.
- Stomach ache: with colic.

CONIUM MACULATUM (*Con.*)
Common hemlock

Emotional state
Anxious. Apathetic. Depressed. Dull/confused. Forgetful/memory weak. Sensitive to light; to noise. *Slow.*

Emotional stress: mental strain.

These are down-to-earth types who become melancholic after a period of mental strain.

People who need this remedy become generally anxious and jumpy, easily startled by noise and also sensitive to light. The mind slows down and they can end up sitting looking (and feeling) vacant, unable even to read. There is no interest in working and they feel quickly tired if they try.

Conium is useful for elderly people who become apathetic and forgetful if the stresses and the symptoms fit.

General state

Glands: hard; lumpy; sensitive; swollen. *Pains* sharp. *Sweat* on closing eyes; during sleep; hot; worse at night. *Symptoms* right-sided.

Better for fasting.

Worse for alcohol; for eating; for physical exertion; for frosty/snowy weather; at night.

Physical stress: injury – to breasts/testicles, to glands; snow.

Conium is useful for injuries to glands (including the testes/testicles and the breasts) where there is continued soreness or a lump or hardness remaining.

Under stress, especially with mental strain as well as with many of the physical complaints below, sweating may be profuse and occurs strangely on closing the eyes as well as during sleep.

Frosty, snowy weather can bring on many complaints or aggravate existing complaints, as can alcohol. Those needing this remedy may feel better when sitting letting the limbs hang down, i.e. not cross-legged, or with folded arms.

Typical physical complaints as a result of stress are:

- Backache: stitching pains in the lower back; worse standing.
- Breasts: are sore, itchy and lumpy; stitching pains; worse before a menstrual period.
- Constipation: painful, ineffectual urging; with straining; with weakness and trembling after.
- Cough: dry, hacking, tickling, exhausting; worse lying down; has to sit up to cough.
- Dizziness: worse lying or turning head (especially quickly); everything whirls around.
- Exhaustion: with trembling, heaviness and numbness; better for fresh air; worse for slight exertion.
- Headache: pains bursting, shooting; worse stepping heavily, when coughing.
- Hot flushes: with sweating.
- Insomnia: sleepless before midnight; with lots of bad dreams; with sweating.
- Palpitations: after passing a stool.

- Sore throat: dryness and tickling in the larynx and bronchi (air passages).

GELSEMIUM SEMPERVIRENS (*Gels.*)
Yellow jasmine

Emotional state
Anxious: before an exam/interview, etc. *Apathetic:* during a fever; when stressed. *Depressed* but cannot cry. *Desires* to be alone. *Dull/ confused. Fearful:* agoraphobic; of failing an exam or test; of losing control; of public speaking. *Shy. Sluggish* mentally.

Emotional stresses: fear; loss; shock; uncertainty; worry.

Gelsemium is for those paralysed with anxiety and fear, mentally and physically, before an important event – an exam, interview, test or performance – and any ordeal, including going to the dentist or into hospital for an operation. They are shy about appearing in public and will suffer from shaking legs, frequent urination and diarrhoea. They look, as well as feel stupid. They may even forget their lines or fluff their driving test because they tremble and stutter and can't collect their thoughts.

These are dull, sluggish types who want to be left alone, to be quiet. They become apathetic and physically exhausted when stressed. They find it difficult to cry if depressed, typically after a loss or after receiving a piece of bad news, when they can become paralysed with grief.

A *Gelsemium* state can also come on from overexcitement.

General state
Eyelids heavy. *Heavy* feeling. *Onset of pain/complaint* – slow. *Pains* bruised, sore. *Sweat* absent during fever; from fright. *Thirstless. Trembling.*
Better for rest; for sweating; for urinating.
Worse for heat; for physical exertion.

Physical stresses: convalescing from illness; strain from travel.

Those needing this remedy feel drowsy, listless and intensely weary. There is a general feeling of heaviness: the body feels heavy (arms and legs feel as if weighted down with lead); keeping the eyes open is difficult because the eyelids feel heavy; talking is difficult because the tongue feels stiff and heavy.

They tremble with exhaustion and are worse for heat, especially the heat of the sun in the summer months, and for any additional physical exertion, peculiarly only feeling better temporarily after urination. They pass a lot of clear (colourless) urine.

Acute *Gelsemium* complaints (for example, flu) take days to develop, coming on when the weather changes to warm after the cold of winter, for those who spend their lives in over-heated houses. Their complaints are accompanied by thirstlessness and a reluctance to move for heaviness and weariness.

Typical physical complaints as a result of stress include:

- Backache: with exhaustion.
- Diarrhoea: from anxiety, shock or excitement; on going into battle.
- Dizziness: with staggering; feel they will fall; with blurred vision.
- Exhaustion: paralytic; with trembling and a feeling of heaviness.
- Fever: burning heat without sweating, with shivering; heat alternating with chills; chills run up and down back.
- Flu: pains in muscles, eyeballs ache, with exhaustion; heaviness; numbness; shivering/chills in back.
- Headache: pains aching, sore, bruised; head feels very heavy; with frequent urination.
- Jetlag: with exhaustion and head or backache.

IGNATIA AMARA (*Ign.*)
St Ignatius' bean

Emotional state

Brooding. Conscientious. Depressed from unexpressed grief. *Desires* to be alone. *Despair. Dislikes:* consolation; contradiction. *Idealistic. Introspective. Moody. Sensitive:* generally; to pain. *Sentimental. Sighing. Tearful:* cries on own; with involuntary weeping.

Emotional stresses: criticism; disappointment; guilt; homesickness; humiliation; loneliness; loss; reprimand; shame; shock.

These are gentle, idealistic, sentimental types who lose themselves in poetry and country walks and daydreams. They are refined and sensitive, especially to emotional stress because they find it difficult to express their feelings.

Ignatia is needed typically after emotional stress, be it grief (a loss or bereavement), or shock, or anger where anxiety is also present, or from being told off, punished or contradicted. These types become broody and resentful, tormenting themselves with recollections of the offence or emotional injury they have received. They suffer inwardly, feeling numb and becoming introspective, secretive and moody. When feeling guilty or humiliated, they blame themselves.

They can have hysterical outbursts of anger or even laughter once the emotional pressures have built up to a certain level. They tend to be conscientious in everything they do and can snap, becoming irritable or even angry if contradicted.

They appear sad but don't express it publicly because they can't, but once they are alone thoughts of their loss or loneliness etc., crowd in. They hold their tears back and this causes a feeling of constriction in their chest or even a lump in their throat. They are using so much tension in their chests to hold in their feelings they take the odd deep breath, or sigh and yawn in an (unconscious) attempt to get some oxygen, and of course, this makes them feel a bit better.

They become anti-social, not wanting company or sympathy (although they will not be openly resentful of sympathy). They want to be alone to cry but if they do break down in front of others they will sob convulsively and feel embarrassed so they may laugh at the same time.

Ignatia is valuable at all stages in life, for sensitive children who have developed sore throats or a stomach ache or insomnia after being punished or severely frightened, or are homesick; for teenagers who brood and pine after a disappointment in love (and they fall in love easily); for men and women of all ages and in all walks of life who have suffered inwardly and become introspective and depressed; for older people, who, after losing a partner or beloved pet, or close friend or relative, grieve silently whilst struggling on and appearing to be coping but suffer from ill health as a result.

General state
Appetite: dislikes fruit; milk. *Dislikes* fresh air. *Pains* constricting; neuralgic. *Sweat* hot; on single parts of the body. *Symptoms* contradictory.
Better for eating; for heat.
Worse after drinking coffee; for tobacco.

Physical stresses: caffeine/coffee; smoke.

Contradictory symptoms are a strong indication for this remedy. For example, an empty feeling in the stomach that is *not* relieved by eating, a sore throat that is worse when *not* swallowing, constricting pains that are *better* for pressure. The sensation of a lump in the throat is often associated with a suppressed desire to cry or express some upset.

The emotional suppression is expressed in the body with feelings of constriction and emptiness as well as neuralgic pains, spasms and twitches.

They sweat on single parts of their body when feverish and at other times may sweat easily on the face, especially when eating.

They are generally sensitive to coffee, which brings on shakiness, and smoke, especially tobacco smoke, which causes a headache. They feel generally worse for fresh air which quickly chills them, and better for warmth, especially during a fever.

Typical physical complaints as a result of stress include:

- Backache: muscles go into spasm.
- Cough: dry, hacking, irritating, painful; larynx/bronchi are irritated; worse for coughing; in the evening in bed.
- Fainting: feels faint in a crowded room.
- Fever: thirsty when chilly (not when hot and feverish).
- Exhaustion: nervous.
- Headache: crushing, stabbing pains (like a nail in the side of the head).
- Indigestion: sour belching – stomach feels weak and empty (no better after eating).

- Insomnia: from emotional stress; with busy dreams.
- Menstrual periods: stop after emotional stress.
- Palpitations: from emotional stress.
- Piles: shooting pains; worse after a stool; better for walking.
- Sore throat: constricting, stitching pains and a feeling of a lump; better for swallowing (worse when not swallowing).
- Stomach ache: cramps with bloating.

KALI PHOSPHORICUM (*Kali-p.*)
Potassium phosphate

Emotional state
Anxious. Depressed. Forgetful/memory weak. Jumpy. Sensitive. Sluggish mentally.

Emotional stresses: depression; excitement; mental strain; worry.

This remedy is for those who are exhausted following a heavy work or study period, a period of anxiety, or over-excitement, and whose nerves are worn out. The physical and mental exhaustion is combined with a feeling of nervousness. They are sensitive to noise and to light, and easily startled.

They can't work because they can't concentrate even if they try, and they lose confidence in themselves because of this, becoming anxious and depressed.

General state
Breath smells. *Pains* sharp. *Sweat:* profuse; after the slightest physical exertion; when tired. *Symptoms* one-sided.
Better for heat; for rest.
Worse for cold; for excitement; for mental or physical exertion.

Physical stress: convalescing from illness; insomnia from tension.

This remedy is indicated in cases of nervous exhaustion where there is anaemia, nervous headaches and/or insomnia. It is useful in the convalescent stage of an acute illness (especially after flu) where there is muscular weakness and nervous exhaustion. The tiredness is accompanied by sweating from even the gentlest exertion.

There is a great sensitivity to cold air and cold in general and the physical complaints are worse for cold. People who need this remedy feel better for – and desperately need – warmth and rest, and a healthy diet to build themselves up again.

The physical complaints responding to *Kali phosphoricum* are mostly caused by or accompany nervous exhaustion, and include:

● Anaemia: with exhaustion.
● Backache: spine feels sore/bruised; better for movement.
● Exhaustion: nervous; muscular.
● Gums: spongy; receding.
● Headache: nervous headaches; one-sided; pains stitching; worse for thinking.
● Heaviness: of limbs; with coldness.
● Indigestion: nervous indigestion, stomach feels empty.
● Insomnia: with empty feeling in the pit of the stomach.

LACHESIS (*Lach.*)
Bushmaster snake

Emotional state
Abusive. Anxious. Blames others. *Cheerful. Concentration* difficult. *Depressed. Eccentric. Excitable. Jealous. Lively. Sensitive* to touch. *Sluggish* mentally. *Suspicious. Talkative. Tearful. Thoughts* active. *Vindictive.*
Worse on waking.

Emotional stresses: depression; jealousy.

These are lively, excitable eccentrics who are so talkative it is hard to get a word in edgeways. They can even talk in their sleep. They are exuberant characters who live life to the full, who work and play hard. They experience strong emotions which are generally expressed freely. It is the suppression of these feelings that can cause ill-health.

Typically, those needing *Lachesis* will feel deeply jealous (or envious) of something or someone, or will be trying to suppress these feelings. Children feeling displaced by the birth of a new baby can become wild with jealousy or depressed, deceitful and spiteful if they try to hold their aggression in.

Any suppression of feelings quickly causes an inner turmoil that must have an outlet, like being able to have a good cry (which does help), otherwise the pressure will build up and cause physical symptoms to develop.

Under stress these types become difficult – critical, sarcastic, suspicious and aggressive. Thoughts and ideas whir around uncontrollably in their minds and come out in a jumble as they jump from one subject to another. If this goes on, they can become exhausted and generally sluggish, finding it difficult to remember what they have read, and finding it particularly hard to get going in the morning.

In fact, all their symptoms, emotional and physical, are worse on waking – the depression, the sluggishness and the anxiety. They may be reluctant to go to sleep because they know that they will feel dreadful when they wake up.

General state

Appetite: desires alcohol, starchy foods. *Desires* fresh air. *Face* red (flushed). *Pains:* pressing; sharp. *Sweat:* from mental exertion; from pain. *Symptoms* left-sided or start on the left and move to the right. **Better** for fresh air; during a menstrual period.
Worse for alcohol; before a menstrual period; for heat; for pressure; after sleep; for tight clothes; on waking.

Physical stresses: heat; humidity.

Generally, *Lachesis* types are affected by heat, by humidity and the heat of the sun – suffering from hot flushes, headaches and exhaustion. They feel better for fresh air and generally better during the winter months. All their symptoms are worse on waking, and are typically on the left side of the body or will move from the left to the right. Their complaints can recur on a fortnightly cycle.

Acutely sensitive to touch, they cannot bear the pressure of tight

clothes anywhere on their bodies but especially around the neck.
They may not even want to be touched around their neck. They
have a love for alcohol which has a bad effect if they over-indulge,
causing hot flushes and headaches. If run down, their gums can
become spongy and bleed easily and their breath smells.

They can become unwell if any of their natural discharges are
suppressed (stopped) – for example, nasal catarrh with decongestants or menstrual periods with the contraceptive pill or even
during pregnancy or menopause. Pre-menstrual tension is a strong
symptom of *Lachesis* with pains, depression and/or irritability all
clearing up once the flow of the period starts. Young girls can
develop a *Lachesis* state before the onset of their first period.

Typical physical complaints as a result of stress are:

- Backache: lower back is stiff and sore.
- Constipation: with ineffectual urging and straining.
- Cough: dry, hacking, suffocative, tickling; worse at night (wakes
  coughing on falling asleep).
- Dizziness: worse on closing eyes and on waking.
- Earache: severe pains worse for swallowing.
- Exhaustion: worse for slightest exertion (physical or mental), on
  getting up in the morning.
- Fainting: with nausea and palpitations.
- Gums inflamed: spongy, bleeding easily; with smelly breath.
- Hair falls out: in pregnancy.
- Headache: pains bursting, throbbing, violent; head feels heavy.
- Hot flushes: with or without sweating.
- Insomnia: light sleep; wakes with a start and can't get back to
  sleep; sleeps on the right side; extraordinary dreams.
- Menstrual periods: painful; flow is dark, clotted and scanty; pains
  occur before the period starts and cease once bleeding starts.
- Nosebleeds: on blowing the nose; the blood is dark.
- Palpitations: in the morning on waking; worse for exertion and
  when lying on the left side.
- Sciatica: pains go down the leg; worse for touch, after a sleep.
- Sore throat: pains spread to ears; choking or lump sensation in
  throat is worse for swallowing liquids or saliva and better for
  solid food – returning after swallowing; with swollen glands;
  tickling and irritation in larynx.

- Sunstroke: with bursting headache.
- Toothache: teeth sensitive to cold water, heat and touch.

LYCOPODIUM (*Lyc.*)
Club moss

Emotional state
Angry with difficulty expressing anger. *Anxious* before an exam/interview, etc. *Bites* fingernails. *Concentration* poor. *Desires* to be alone. *Dictatorial*. *Dislikes:* being alone; being contradicted. *Easily* embarrassed; offended. *Fearful:* claustrophobic; of failure; of failing an exam/test; of getting lost; of public speaking. *Forgetful/memory weak. Impatient. Indecisive. Intellectual. Irritable. Lack* of self-confidence. *Moody. Rude. Sensitive. Shy. Sluggish mentally. Tearful.*

Emotional stresses: bullying; fear; humiliation; transitions; worry.

Lycopodium individuals are bookish intellectuals who don't like sports, who work hard and do well (in spite of their nerves) and because of this attract a fair amount of bullying as children. They are anxious and worry about many things because they feel inferior and lack self-confidence. They dislike responsibility and will naturally shy away from marriage and a family life.

They dread taking on new things, but in anticipation of an event prepare meticulously and usually shine. They are loners who have many fears, but they feel especially threatened by people. They can cry easily, especially if reprimanded or if they feel others don't appreciate them, but also if people are especially nice to them.

They can be moody because they find it difficult to express their feelings, especially their anger, which tends to come out in impatient, irritable bursts. They are easily offended and will fly into a rage over the smallest thing. They are irritable after a sleep – *Lycopodium* infants kick and scream after a nap or on waking in the mornings and can be generally difficult to live with.

These types are easily offended, in spite of not being especially sensitive to others' feelings, and can be rude and domineering to

those close to them. This behaviour is a compensation for their low
self-confidence. They become bullies as their way of dealing with
the world but will make sure they pick on those weaker then
themselves. They don't like to be alone, but dislike company; their
ideal is to know that there is someone else in the house – in another
room! When tired and overstressed, they become forgetful and find
it difficult to concentrate.

General state
Appetite: feels quickly full up (after eating only a little); digestion is
slow/poor; dislikes onions; likes chocolate, hot food/drinks, starchy
foods, sugar/sweets, sweet foods. *Discharges* yellow. *Expression*
confused. *Face* pale and drawn. *Glands* swollen. *Pains* tearing.
Slowness of children to learn. *Sweat* clammy; cold; on feet; profuse;
smelly; sour; better for uncovering. *Symptoms* right-sided; start on
the right side and move to the left. *Taste in mouth* sour.
Better for fresh air; for warmth of bed.
Worse around 4.00–8.00 p.m.; during the afternoon and/or the
evening; for fasting; for flatulent food (beans, cabbage, etc.); for
onions; for pressure; in stuffy rooms; for tight clothes; for wind.

Physical stresses: aluminium; chocolate; food sensitivities – flatulent food (beans, cabbage, etc.); sluggish digestion; sugar/sweets;
food poisoning (from sea food, especially oysters).

These types have trouble with food: either feeling full up and
bloated after eating very little or having no appetite at all until they
start eating, and then becoming ravenous. They can have an empty
sensation in the stomach which is no better for eating. They can
wake hungry at night. They are big sweet-cravers, often eating
several bars of chocolate a day. The stomach feels heavy after eating
and they may also feel sleepy. They are worse for fasting or missing
meals, becoming tired and nauseous. They digest their food poorly
and become bloated with gas, especially after eating beans, onions
or brassicas (cabbage, sprouts, etc.), with acidity and sourness, and
can't then tolerate tight clothes around their waist.

Lycopodium symptoms are predominantly right-sided, or they
may start on the right and move to the left. The symptoms are worse

between 4 and 8 p.m. Despite feeling generally chilly and hating draughts, these people feel worse in stuffy rooms and generally better for fresh air and many of their complaints (i.e. headaches and back pain) are better for a walk outside. They have sweaty, smelly feet that may be different temperatures, i.e. one colder than the other.

Lycopodium children, in spite of being bright, can, under stress, go through phases where they can't seem to learn anything.

Adults look anxious, may even have a lined forehead and their hair can go grey prematurely, either all over or in patches.

Typical physical complaints as a result of stress include:

- Backache: lower back pain; better for urinating (may have strained/pulled back).
- Blisters: burning, on tip of tongue.
- Common cold: nose and sinuses blocked, worse in bed at night; catarrh is yellow.
- Conjunctivitis: eyes are sticky, sore and sensitive to light.
- Constipation: with straining; stools knotty, hard at first then loose.
- Cough: dry, irritating, painful, better for hot drinks.
- Cramps: in calf at night.
- Cystitis: frequent, painful urging to urinate; can only pass a little at a time; urine is cloudy.
- Dizziness: in the morning on getting out of bed.
- Earache: ears feel blocked up; smelly discharge from ear.
- Exhaustion: worse for mental or physical exertion.
- Fever: one-sided; chills with shaking alternating with burning heat.
- Flatulence: belly bloated with loud rumbling after eating; better passing wind.
- Hair loss: after childbirth.
- Headache: pains pressing, tearing, in forehead/temples; worse for mental exertion.
- Indigestion: heartburn with sour belches; better for belching.
- Insomnia: sleepless until midnight; wakes with a start from vivid, anxious dreams or nightmares.
- Joint pain: pains tearing, better for walking and warmth.
- Mouth ulcers: under the tongue.

- Palpitations: after over-eating; in the evening in bed.
- Sciatica: better for walking and for warmth.
- Sore throat: throat dry, raw, sore; with swollen glands; with tickling in larynx/bronchi; better for hot drinks.
- Stomach ache: aching or cramping pains which radiate to the back.

NATRUM CARBONICUM (*Nat-c.*)
Sodium carbonate

Emotional state
Anxious. Cheerful. Conscientious. Depressed. Dull/confused. Fearful. Forgetful/memory weak. Gloomy. Jumpy. Lively. Sensitive: in general; to music. *Shy. Sluggish mentally.*
Worse for mental exertion.

Emotional stress: mental strain.

These are shy, sensitive, gentle types who prefer a quiet life. They are especially sensitive to emotional hurts which they harbour quietly inside, although without bitterness. They put on a brave face and avoid conflict by appearing cheerful, but this masks a feeling of being cut off, and they can then become depressed, lonely and anxious with persistent sad thoughts. Listening to music increases their sense of melancholy in a comforting but negative way.

They look after the needs of others before their own. Whilst they dislike being on their own they aren't happy in company either, partly because they can take against certain people. They can be mentally weakened as a result of emotional pressure, becoming jumpy and finding it difficult to think and impossible to work.

General state
Ankles weak. *Appetite:* digestion is slow/poor; dislikes milk. *Dislikes* fresh air. *Face* pale. *Sweat:* from pain; from slightest physical exertion. *Taste in mouth:* metallic; sour.
Better after eating; for massage.

Worse before eating; for fresh air; mid-morning; for physical exertion; for sun; during a storm.

Physical stresses: extremes of temperature; food sensitivities – milk; heat; sluggish digestion; sun/sunstroke; thunderstorms.

Natrum carbonicum types have pale faces with dark circles under the eyes and their eyelids may be puffy. They are aggravated generally by excessive summer heat and exposure to the sun (especially the head), but there is also an aversion to fresh air.

Once run down, any exercise will aggravate their general condition. They are extremely sensitive to thunderstorms and can sense them coming, often getting a headache and feeling anxious during the build-up to a storm as well.

They have difficulty assimilating their food, especially dairy products, suffering from digestive problems and suspecting other food allergies as well. They feel better generally after eating.

This is a useful remedy for nervous types who cannot tolerate milk or sunshine and who suffer from weak ankles (who trip easily on uneven surfaces).

Typical physical complaints as a result of stress include:

- Common cold: nose blocked; catarrh is thick and drips down the back of the throat, has to hawk it up to spit it out.
- Constipation: with an unfinished feeling.
- Cystitis: burning pains during and after urinating.
- Diarrhoea: with wind; after drinking milk.
- Dizziness: worse in a stuffy room and for thinking.
- Exhaustion: nervous; legs weak and heavy; arms and legs feel cold; worse for mental or physical exhaustion.
- Fever: burning heat with sweating.
- Headache: head feels heavy; pains pressing; with sweating on the head; worse after eating, for thinking.
- Indigestion: with stomach ache, bloating, nausea and sour belches.
- Insomnia: anxious dreams; wakes early and can't get back to sleep.

NATRUM MURIATICUM (*Nat-m.*)
Sodium chloride or common table salt

Emotional state
Anxious: before an exam/interview, etc. *Bites fingernails. Depressed:* and cannot cry; from suppressed grief. *Desires* to be alone. *Dislikes* consolation. *Dull/confused. Dwells* on unpleasant events. *Easily* embarrassed; offended. *Fearful* of being late. *Irritable. Private. Resentful. Sensitive:* in general; to rudeness. *Tearful:* with difficulty crying; cries on own. *Unforgiving.*

Emotional stresses: betrayal; depression; disappointment; humiliation; loss; resentment; transition; worry.

These are sensitive, intensely private people who can appear cool and prickly because of their reluctance to express their emotions. They are sensitive to other people's feelings and other people seem to instinctively know that they won't gossip, that they can be confided in without getting too involved.

They dislike small talk or having to make polite conversation, neither are they willing to talk about themselves, and so they avoid parties or social gatherings. They can become especially insular when depressed, preferring to stay at home alone. They actually like to be on their own, and need and feel better for some time to themselves on a regular basis.

Even when sad they don't want others to see they are in pain. They find it difficult to cry and will only cry on their own, if at all. It is rare to see them crying in front of others but their feelings can burst out under certain conditions, especially to a sensitive, sympathetic ear, when they may cry in spite of themselves. This makes them feel exposed and they respond by getting cross. They don't want comforting and will get irritated with anyone who tries to console them.

Unfortunately, they do expect others to be sensitive to their feelings. But they don't show them! This makes them easy to hurt or offend and then, of course, they do not show they have been upset, but harbour criticisms, insults and grudges inside, becoming very bitter. They find it difficult to forget or forgive and will dwell on past grievances, tormented by revengeful thoughts.

They close themselves off more and more to avoid being further hurt, suppressing more feelings, not wanting anyone to help them, and becoming more and more unhappy.

With emotional stress the suppression of their feelings – of sadness and anger especially – builds up inside and eventually affects their health.

They have an anxious side, worrying about their health, about exams and interviews, etc., and about meetings that involve other people. They can hide these feelings too – the only evidence being their lack of fingernails, which they bite in private. They can be scared at night, specifically of burglars, and may even dream of being robbed – this also because their privacy is so important to them.

Children are serious and sensitive and tend to dislike too much physical contact. They hate to be teased and are often best ignored if they get upset, leaving them to come round in their own time. They may be slow to learn to talk – not speaking until their second or even third year – and can also be slow learning to walk.

In women, the depression and irritability can be worse pre-menstrually, when nothing pleases them.

General state
Appetite: poor; dislikes bread, chicken, slimy foods (oysters, okra, undercooked egg white, etc.); likes salt/salty foods, salty and sour foods; starchy foods. *Discharges:* like egg white; white. *Dryness* generally. *Eyes* sensitive to bright light. *Face* sallow. *Lips:* chapped; cracked. *Mouth* dry. *Pains:* pressing; tearing. *Slowness:* of children to talk; to walk. *Taste in mouth:* bitter; salty. *Thirsty:* extremely; for large quantities; with the pains.
Better for fasting; for lying down; rest; for sea air; for sweating.
Worse after eating; for heat; for hot baths; mid-morning (10.00–11.00 a.m.); for physical exertion; for sea air; for sun.

Physical stresses: food sensitivities – salt, bread; heat; medication (quinine); sea air; sun.

Dryness and an intense thirst (usually for cold drinks) are characteristic, especially with a fever or a headache. Lips dry up and become chapped and cracked (either at the corners of the mouth or a single crack in the middle of the lower lip). The skin can be generally dry with the hands being dry and cracked and the skin around the nails prone to hangnails.

Discharges are generally profuse and watery, often like egg white, or thick and white. They sweat profusely when ill, especially with a fever, and feel better for doing so.

People needing this remedy dislike hot weather and hot, stuffy rooms. They are sensitive to the direct heat of the sun, commonly suffering from headaches if they are out in it for even a short period of time. They may feel cold in their bodies, their hands and feet may feel cold to touch but this doesn't bother them.

They have a love for both salt (or a combination of sour and salt i.e. pickles) and pastry, both of which can cause them health problems under stress. They also have an affinity with the seaside, often feeling better for salty, sea air but there are times when it can make them feel worse. They dislike slimy foods and can go off bread at times.

They feel better for fasting and can lose their appetites under stress, only feeling hungry in the middle of the morning. Children tend to be skinny and don't gain weight in spite of eating a lot.

An unusual symptom is that they find it difficult to pass urine in the presence of others – they need privacy to do so and will therefore avoid public toilets or situations where they can't be completely alone.

They feel generally worse mid-morning around 10 or 11 a.m., and any physical symptoms will be aggravated at that time.

Typical physical complaints as a result of stress include:
- Anaemia: with exhaustion.
- Backache: weakness and aching in lower back; better for lying on a hard surface; worse for prolonged bending down.
- Blisters: on tip of tongue.
- Cold sores: on lips; around mouth.
- Common cold: copious nasal discharge alternates with blocked nose; with sneezing; can't smell or taste anything.

- Conjunctivitis: eyes burn and water, feel gritty and are sensitive to light.
- Constipation: ineffectual straining; stools like sheep dung; with unfinished feeling.
- Cough: dry, hacking; with watery eyes; with tickling in larynx/bronchi (air passages).
- Cystitis: burning or cutting pains after urination; urine clear.
- Dandruff: thick white flakes; with dryness of scalp.
- Diarrhoea: daytime only; painless, smelly and watery.
- Dizziness: in the morning on getting up; whilst walking or looking out of the window; with nausea; worse for tea/coffee/tobacco/alcohol; with loss of balance.
- Exhaustion: with heaviness; worse during the evening.
- Fever: burning heat with nausea, better for uncovering.
- Gums bleeding: easily, inflamed and swollen; with smelly breath.
- Hair falling: after childbirth.
- Hay fever: with cold sores and symptoms of a common cold.
- Headache: pains pressing, splitting, throbbing; better for firm pressure; with watery eyes and visual disturbances; worse for close work (reading/sewing) or thinking.
- Indigestion: cramping pains; sour belches; violent hiccoughs; with bloating; worse after eating.
- Insomnia: wakes and can't get back to sleep; with anxious, vivid dreams/nightmares.
- Menstrual periods: late to start in young women.
- Palpitations: with anxiety; worse lying on the left side.
- Prickly heat: skin itches when overheated.
- Retention of urine: can't pass urine in front of strangers.
- Sore throat: burning, dry; with lump sensation and hoarse voice; with tickling in larynx/bronchi.
- Thrush (genital): with exhaustion; discharge like egg white.
- Thrush (oral): on the gums; burning.
- Toothache: teeth sensitive to cold air, cold drinks and to touch.
- Stress incontinence: when walking or coughing.

NITRICUM ACIDUM (*Nit-ac.*)
Nitric acid

Emotional state
Angry. Anxious about their health. *Compassionate. Complaining. Depressed. Forgetful/memory weak. Irritable. Sensitive:* generally; to noise; to pain. *Unforgiving. Vindictive.*

Emotional stresses: conflict; resentment.

These are cheerful, compassionate, determined types who hold strong opinions and are profoundly affected by the sufferings of others. They are generally impatient and don't suffer fools gladly. They have an irritable streak which is worse in the mornings, when they will snap if spoken to.

They are very sensitive to conflict – to quarrels and arguments – reacting in a particular way by quickly becoming angry and even verbally abusive. Then, in the aftermath, they complain and blame others for what has happened, feeling vindictive towards those they have quarrelled with, or those who have offended them. They may use the word 'hate' when describing the object of their derision. They are (in this unforgiving state) not interested in apologies and carry this hatred around with them, plotting and scheming revenge or fantasizing about how they will get back at the 'enemy'. In this state their anger can explode in unpleasant outbursts of rage where they shout and swear freely. Afterwards they tremble and carry on feeling angry. This eats away at them like an acid, and they become negative and depressed.

They have a lot of anxiety about their health and may well consult doctor after doctor in order to find out what is wrong, not believing the diagnoses, particularly if they are told they are not seriously ill. They believe they have something seriously wrong with them, are frightened of death, and get cross with doctors who try and reassure them.

Under stress they may throw themselves into their work and then become irritable and mentally worn out and swing to the opposite extreme of not wanting to work at all. In this state they become oversensitive to noise, especially shrill noises (which make them jump) and forgetful – they can't collect their thoughts and their minds go blank when they try.

General state
Appetite: dislikes cheese; likes fat/fatty foods, salty foods. *Breath* smells. *Cracking* joints. *Cracks* in skin. *Discharges:* like ammonia; burning; smelly; thin; yellow-green. *Pains:* appear and disappear suddenly; in bones; flying around; needle-like/splinter-like. *Sensation* of constriction. *Sweat:* on single parts of the body; smelly; sour; from slightest physical exertion. *Tongue:* cracked; sore.
Better for lying down.
Worse for cold; for fresh air; for jarring movement; at night; for touch; on waking; for walking.

Physical stresses: chemicals; cold; getting chilled; loss of sleep; medication (drugs in general); mercury.

These are chilly types – worse for cold in any form, including draughts. They are sensitive to being touched or jarred and to pain, which is typically splinter- or needle-like and which comes and goes suddenly. Whilst they are worse for jarring, they can feel better when going out for a ride in a car.

Their urine smells strong (like a horse's); and their sweat also smells. They can have smelly, sweaty feet. They crave fatty, fried foods and adore the fat on meat. They suffer from nervous exhaustion caused by too little sleep or broken nights and they always feel better for lying down.

Once run-down, they suffer from cracks: in the corners of the mouth, in the fingers and hands, in the anus. These can be deep and painful and bleed easily. The tongue is also cracked – with a crack down the centre or lots of cracks all over. They can also have cracking joints: the ankles crack whilst walking (and are generally weak), and the jaw cracks whilst they eat. They can find themselves biting their inner cheek whilst eating or talking.

Ulcers are another strong guiding symptom and these are painful (with stitching pains) and sensitive to touch. They are found in the mouth, on the lips and even in the nostrils. They can have injuries (especially punctured wounds) which are slow to heal – usually accompanied by anger towards the cause of the injury.

Typical physical complaints as a result of stress include:

- Anaemia: with exhaustion.
- Backache: sharp pains between shoulder blades; with stiff neck.
- Common cold: nasal catarrh burns and is thin and watery.
- Conjunctivitis: eyes water and eyelids are swollen.
- Constipation: with painful straining and an unfinished feeling; stools are dry and hard; alternating with diarrhoea.
- Cystitis: painful whilst urinating; with scanty, smelly urine.
- Earache: splinter-like pains on swallowing; crackling in ears when chewing; with sore throat.
- Exhaustion: muscular or nervous; with dizziness and sleepiness; worse from exertion, after passing a stool.
- Flatulence: smelly wind that is difficult to expel.
- Gums: gums are swollen and bleed easily; breath smells.
- Hair loss: after childbirth.
- Headache: pains pressing, sore/bruised, in bones; head feels constricted; worse for noise, pressure, jarring.
- Indigestion: with nausea, bloating and wind; from drinking milk.
- Insomnia: wakes between midnight and 2 a.m., can't get back to sleep, many anxious dreams; sleep is unrefreshing.
- Joint pain: pains in bones; splinter-like, stitching.
- Mouth ulcers: ulcers on edges of tongue; painful.
- Nosebleed: blood is thin and dark red.
- Piles: painful, large, bleeding; pains are splinter-like and last for hours after passing a stool.
- Sore throat: throat sore, raw; with swollen glands; pains are sharp, like splinters or needles, they radiate to the ear, and are worse for swallowing even a small amount of fluids.
- Thrush (genital): discharge burns, smells and itches.

NUX VOMICA (*Nux-v.*)
Poison nut

Emotional state
Abusive. Affectionate. Angry over little things. *Anxious. Concentration poor. Depressed. Easily* offended. *Excitable. Impatient. Impulsive. Irritable. Mischievous. Quarrelsome. Sensitive:* generally; to rudeness; to light; to music; to noise; to pain; to smells; to touch. *Sentimental. Sluggish mentally. Spiteful. Stubborn. Tidy.*

Emotional stresses: boredom; conflict; criticism; failure; humiliation; mental strain; shame; worry.

These are intense types: excitable and enthusiastic, sentimental and affectionate, they embrace life (and especially work) with a passion. Bright and capable, they are ambitious high-achievers with creative minds. Full of ideas, they are also hard-working, capable of seeing things through, of 'delivering the goods' so to speak.

But their enthusiasm can get out of hand if they do not manage the stresses in their lives carefully. They can become driven workaholics who worry more and more, usually about their work, and become worn out. Their mental efficiency is affected (but they don't admit to this initially): they can't concentrate, they find reading as well as writing difficult and their memory is also affected.

They are impulsive, impatient individuals who know what they want and who want it now! They like to be in charge and move at a fast pace in everything they do, becoming irritated by others who can't keep up with them, or worse, who get in their way or keep them waiting. They will be first to beep their horn in traffic queues or overtake, and hate supermarket queues or slow shopkeepers.

They are critical, fussy and exacting, easily frustrated by any limitations. They are tidy but not obsessively so, more out of a desire for efficiency, and will get angry if things aren't in their 'right' place.

They are irritable and argumentative, taking things out on those closest to them, both at work and at home. They dislike being disturbed or contradicted. Their irritability must have an outlet and it usually does – they will shout or scream and swear at those who have offended them. Which is easy to do. Relatively small things going wrong will set them biting off other people's heads.

Seeing nothing wrong in their own rudeness, they are paradoxically sensitive to rudeness in others. When humiliated, they become angry and take an aggressive position – although they may not express it. If they do suppress their anger they feel awful and quickly develop physical symptoms. They tend not to keep their anger in but it can escalate into physical violence if they don't find other ways to deal with their feelings.

They seek help to keep them going in the form of caffeine at work and alcohol or even drugs to sleep at night. The nervous system becomes overstimulated and they become oversensitive to any extra stimulation like bright lights, noise, smells, etc.

Once their physical health is affected they are prone to sinking into a depressed and worried state where they fear they will lose the goodwill of those close to them. With good reason!

Nux vomica children are mischievous and full of contradictions. They can be spiteful, stubborn, irritable and headstrong on the one hand, and extremely sensitive, affectionate, jealous and easily offended on the other. As they grow up they become difficult, getting cross if things are not going their way.

Anyone can fall into a *Nux vomica* state given the right combination of stresses including a heavy workload, a few too many late nights and too much alcohol.

General state
Appetite: poor in the morning; doesn't want breakfast; digestion is slow/poor; dislikes water: likes alcohol, coffee, meat, spicy foods. *Breath* smells. *Dislikes* fresh air. *Pains* cramping. *Sensation* of constriction and tension. *Senses* acute. *Sweat:* hot; one-sided; smelly. *Symptoms* right-sided. *Taste in mouth* bitter or sour in the morning. *Tense feeling*.
Better for heat; for hot drinks; for lying down; for rest; for sitting down; for warmth of bed.
Worse for alcohol; for coffee; for cold food and drinks; cold wind; after eating; for tight clothes; for tobacco; getting feet wet.

Physical stresses: alcohol; caffeine/coffee; getting chilled; cold in general; cold, dry weather; cold wind; complaints from a sedentary lifestyle; drafts; drugs in general; insomnia from tension; overeating; junk/processed food; sluggish digestion; soft drinks; spicy foods; tea.

Those needing this remedy have become run down from overwork and living on stimulants (tea, coffee, alcohol, cigarettes and/or medication) without eating well or getting enough rest or exercise. They overdo everything: they work too hard, stay out too late, take no exercise, eat too much rich food, drink too much alcohol, become too wound up to sleep and then consume vast quantities of coffee in order to get going the next day. They become tense, physically as well as emotionally, and prone to cramps and because of this can't stand constriction from tight clothes, jewellery, watches etc.

They are extremely chilly individuals who hate the cold in any shape or form; they catch cold easily, especially if exposed to draughts or after becoming chilled, and they hate dry, windy weather. They are always better for warmth and if sick will not want any part of their bodies to be uncovered; they become so sensitive to cold that the slightest draught under the bedclothes will upset them. All they want to do when sick is to sit or lie down and keep warm.

Nux vomica is useful for all sorts of disturbances that follow overindulgence in food, alcohol, coffee or tobacco. Once sick, any further indulgences will make them worse, but they find it hard to stop and will often carry on drinking and smoking in spite of feeling ghastly. Children become irritable after too much junk food.

Mornings are their worst time of day, especially after a disturbed night, which is not unusual. Worrying about work keeps them from getting to sleep, carries on in their dreams and they wake in the middle of the night to worry some more, only falling back to sleep around dawn. In the mornings they are at their most irritable and their physical complaints are worse then. Their mouths taste terrible, they feel bilious, liverish and hungover, especially if they have drunk too much the night before.

They don't want to eat breakfast and because they feel generally worse after eating anyway, they will drink coffee and get to work, thereby perpetuating their vicious circle. Their illnesses can return in monthly (or four-weekly) cycles.

Typical physical complaints as a result of stress include:

- Backache: lower back is stiff and achy; must sit up in bed to turn over; worse in the morning in bed.
- Colic: cramps after 'indulgence'; better for passing wind/stool and hot drinks; worse for tight clothing.
- Common cold: with sneezing and watery eyes, catarrh runs in the daytime and blocks up at night (on the side lain on).
- Constipation: alternating with diarrhoea; stools small (or large) and hard; with ineffectual urging and straining.
- Cough: dry, painful, racking; worse after midnight and in the morning in bed; with tickling in the larynx/bronchi.
- Cramps: in legs and feet.
- Cystitis: burning, pressing pains during urination; constant urge to urinate; only passes small amounts.
- Diarrhoea: watery stools; urging to pass stool when urinating; feels faint after.
- Dizziness: worse on getting up in the morning; with staggering.
- Earache: stitching pains; worse for swallowing; with itching in the Eustachian tubes.
- Exhaustion: nervous; with trembling; feels heavy and weary; worse on waking in the morning.
- Fainting: feels faint with digestive complaints (after vomiting, diarrhoea, etc.) and pains (menstrual/stomach cramps).
- Fever: with shivering and sweating (which doesn't help); heat alternating with chills; worse for slightest uncovering.
- Flatulence: bloated stomach worse for eating and tight clothing, rumbling; better for passing wind.
- Flu: with exhaustion, pains in joints and great chilliness.
- Gastric flu: with nausea and vomiting and flu symptoms.
- Headache: head feels heavy; brain feels loose; with dizziness; typical 'hangover' headache with sore eyes; worse moving eyes or head or for thinking; accompanies a cold or gastric upset.
- Heartburn: after eating; in the morning before breakfast.
- Indigestion: with wind and sour belches; stomach feels heavy and bloated after eating; better for passing wind.
- Insomnia: with anxious thoughts about work; sleepy daytime

(especially after dinner); can't get to sleep easily then wakes around 3 a.m.; with anxious dreams about business or conflict situations.
- Menstrual periods: heavy; painful cramps with urging to pass stool; feels faint during pains.
- Nausea: constant; accompanies gastric flu/travel sickness, etc.
- Palpitations: from coffee; worse after dinner, on lying down.
- Piles: large; painful after passing a stool.
- Sore throat: throat feels raw; stitching pains spread to ears on swallowing.
- Stomach ache: cramping pains; with nausea; worse in the morning, after eating; better for warmth, after passing a stool.
- Toothache: after a filling or a tooth extraction; better for wrapping up head, for external warmth.
- Travel sickness: with nausea and feeling of faintness, better for lying down; aggravated by tobacco smoke.
- Vomiting: biliousness after overeating/indulging in rich food especially when travelling; vomit is sour or bitter.

OPIUM (*Op.*)
White poppy

Emotional state
Apathetic: and doesn't complain; during a fever. *Depressed.*
Dreamy. Drowsy. Dull/confused. Indecisive. Sensitive to noise.
Stupor.

Emotional stresses: excitement; reprimand; shame; shock.

Normally bright and lively hardworkers, in an acute illness like fever or after an emotional stress such as a shock, *Opium* types become dull, confused and apathetic to the point of stupor. They don't complain, don't ask for anything and are overwhelmingly sleepy. They may look spaced-out or simply serenely peaceful and dreamy. Before reaching this state they may go through an excitable, delirious stage.

They suffer from fear with apathy after a telling off or a bad shock such as witnessing a serious accident or after an operation. Images or pictures of the situation that caused the shock come into their minds during their waking hours and every time they think about what happened the same feelings rush in all over again.

Whilst they are emotionally dull and unresponsive, their senses are acute – with a special sensitivity to noise, especially when they are trying to get to sleep.

General state

Expression sleepy. *Eyes* glassy. *Face* flushed, red. *Pains* absent. *Pupils* contracted. *Senses* dull. *Sweat:* from fright; hot; profuse; on single parts of the body.

Worse during sleep; for warmth of bed.

Physical stresses: alcohol; anaesthetics (general); fumes (gas, coal or charcoal); shock after injury.

Those needing *Opium* look drunk, glassy-eyed with eyelids half-open. The face is flushed dark red or drawn. There can be a lack of pain in complaints that are normally painful, for example, the constipation, although with this complaint there may be abdominal cramps. Generally, there is profuse sweating with scanty urination, and with a fever *Opium* types don't find any relief from sweating. They become hot in bed, feel worse for the heat and will kick off the covers.

The shock that can follow alcohol poisoning can be helped with this remedy, if the symptoms agree, but this is only useful in an unusual, mistaken accident and not for habitual drinkers. After a poisoning with alcohol or gas or coal fumes it is important that you seek urgent medical advice as well as (or even instead of) taking a homeopathic remedy.

They may be able to sleep soundly once they drop off but they find it difficult to get to sleep after an emotional stress. They sleep very heavily, with their eyes and mouth half open – and have difficulty waking up. They can have all sorts of problems breathing in their sleep, from loud snoring (again common with a fever), to breathing that slows down and even stops from time to time.

Typical physical complaints as a result of stress include:
- Bed-wetting: in children after a shock or reprimand.
- Constipation: stools like sheep-droppings or black balls; no desire to pass a stool; difficulty passing stools.
- Cough: breathing difficult, slow, snoring/laboured.
- Diarrhoea: from sudden excitement; stools watery.
- Exhaustion: feels faint and trembly and sleepy.
- Fainting: after a shock/excitement.
- Fever: heat burning; with thirst, sweating and deep sleep.
- Insomnia: with overpowering sleepiness; difficulty getting to sleep; vivid dreams.
- Retention of urine: in adults or children after shock or reprimand; tries to pass urine but only passes a small amount.
- Trembling: arms and legs tremble with fear (after shock).

PHOSPHORIC ACID (*Pho-ac.*)
Phosphoric acid

Emotional state
Apathetic: about everything; during a fever. *Brooding. Concentration* difficult. *Depressed. Forgetful/memory weak. Slow:* in thinking; in speaking. *Sluggish mentally. Uncommunicative.*

Emotional stresses: betrayal; disappointment; homesickness; mental strain.

After an emotional trauma such as a disappointment in love, a betrayal, homesickness, or during a fever, these types sink into an apathetic state. This apathy is worse on a mental level – they do not want to talk, to think or to answer questions because they cannot concentrate, and they may even forget words while they are speaking. They speak slowly and answer questions monosyllabically.
They may be able to summon up the energy to do physical things but there is a great stillness mentally and emotionally. If depressed, they will grieve silently and may not even be able to summon up the energy to cry. There is a tranquillity about them, a very still depressiveness.

General state

Appetite: likes fizzy drinks, fruit, refreshing things. *Expression* vacant. *Face* pale. *Pains* in bones. *Sweat:* clammy; profuse. *Symptoms* one-sided. *Thirstless.*
Better after a good sleep.
Worse for cold; in the evening; in the morning; for sweating.

Physical stresses: growth spurt; convalescing from illness; loss of fluids.

This remedy benefits those who are weak and tired from studying too much or from a significant 'fluid loss', for example during breastfeeding, after an attack of diarrhoea, a heavy period, bleeding or vomiting. It is also for those who are convalescing from an acute illness. Those with diarrhoea do not become as debilitated by it as expected.

They look pale and sickly; with dark rings around their eyes and they sweat a lot. Their appetite isn't very good and they tend to want refreshing food to eat, such as fruit and vegetables (to replace the liquid), but may not be especially thirsty – and they often feel tired after eating. They are generally worse for cold and better for a sleep, even a short nap.

This remedy benefits young people with pains in the bones of their legs who have recently had a growth spurt, anyone convalescing from an acute illness, especially where they have lost a lot of their own fluids (even sweat), and those (especially schoolchildren) who are suffering from headaches as a result of eye or brain strain (before, say, an exam).

Typical physical complaints as a result of stress include:
- Backache: soreness in upper or lower back; back feels weak.
- Cough: dry, tickling, violent; worse for talking.
- Diarrhoea: painless; stools profuse, thin, watery with rumbling; worse after eating solid/dry food.
- Exhaustion: nervous, paralytic; worse after eating, in the morning after getting up, for the slightest exertion, after eating.
- Fainting: feels faint after a loss of fluids.
- Growing pains: pains in the bones, in the legs.
- Hair loss: of head and beard; after loss or grief.

- Headache: head feels heavy, pains top or back of head; one-sided, pressing; worse getting up from lying down.
- Indigestion: with stomach cramps, loud rumbling and bloating.
- Insomnia: wakes frequently, can't sleep after midnight; sleep is unrefreshing.
- Palpitations: with anxiety; worse after eating (evening meal).

PHOSPHORUS (*Phos.*)
White phosphorous

Emotional state
Affected by hearing of tragic events/sad stories. *Affectionate.* *Anxious* when alone. *Apathetic. Concentration* difficult. *Depressed. Desires* company. *Easily* consoled. *Excitable. Fearful:* of being alone; of the dark; of illness; at night; during a thunderstorm. *Irritable. Jumpy. Lively. Sensitive. Slow. Sympathetic. Uncommunicative.*

Emotional stresses: conflict; fear; uncertainty.

In health these are lively, affectionate, gregarious, open and excitable individuals – although they may also have the classic *Phosphorus* fears. They don't like to be alone, especially in the dark at night when their vivid imaginations conjure up all sorts of ghosts and monsters creeping out of the shadows. They are scared of thunderstorms and jump with each thunderclap, but as they grow older they may find the lightning exciting.

These are people who want company, who feel things strongly, are sensitive, and, being highly strung, are easily startled. They are especially sensitive *and* sympathetic to the feelings of others, picking up on anyone who is upset and wanting to help them. These are people who will stop at the scene of an accident and give comfort to those that need it.

But it is as if they have no emotional skin for protection and because of this they can become overstressed with worrying about and helping others. And then they become anxious, irritable, mentally sluggish and apathetic, and may even lose interest in those close to them. They slow down and don't want to think, talk or work. They can become anxious about their health when unwell, or suffer from an anxiety that something bad is going to happen and need (and ask for) lots of reassurance. Despite being fearful and irritable they are easily comforted and reassured.

General state
Appetite: good; doesn't want breakfast; dislikes hot food/drinks; likes chocolate, cold drinks and food, fizzy drinks, ice (in drinks, etc.), ice-cream, milk (cold), salt and sour foods, salty foods, spicy foods, water. *Discharges* blood-streaked. *Expression* frightened. *Face* flushed red in spots. *Glands* sensitive. *Pains:* burning; pressing. *Senses* acute. *Sweat:* clammy; on single parts of the body; from slightest physical exertion. *Taste in mouth* sour. *Thirsty* for large quantities.
Better for bathing (a hot bath); for cold drinks; for massage; after a good sleep.
Worse for cold; for any change of weather; in the evening; for fasting; in the morning (especially on waking); at twilight; for wind.

Physical stresses: anaesthetics (general); change of temperature or weather; cloudy weather; electricity; fast metabolism; growth spurt; salt; soft drinks; thunderstorms.

These types have fast metabolisms; they burn up their food quickly and therefore need to eat often. They usually have a good appetite, and may even get up at night for a snack! They don't like hot food (they wait for a cooked meal to cool down before eating) as it makes them feel uncomfortable and can give them hot flushes. Under stress they may skimp on breakfast – a big mistake as they will end up running on adrenaline. They like salty and sour foods (salt pickles) and spicy foods, but they don't agree with them when they are unwell, especially with a gastric complaint.

They are very thirsty with a liking for cold or iced drinks, usually water although they may want milk and/or fizzy drinks instead or as well!

They tend not to look ill, i.e. they will often have sparkly eyes and flushed cheeks (even with anaemia), although if you look closely there is a hectic quality about their red cheeks *and* their eyes.

They bleed easily and profusely, suffering from heavy periods and nosebleeds of bright-red blood. They are prone to anaemia and hair loss because of this.

These are chilly individuals who are sensitive to the weather, feel worse for getting cold, and hate the wind. Changes of weather may bring on colds which have a tendency to go onto their chests. Their chest and throat complaints are then worse for cold (and better for heat) whereas their headaches and stomach complaints are better for cold (and worse for heat).

They have lots of energy which flares up in bursts, and is followed by a slump. When stressed, they can still summon up bursts of nervous energy but the slumps become more severe and increasingly difficult to climb out of. They are then prone to feeling heavy and cold; their feet and hands become icy, especially in bed and after mental strain. Their legs fall asleep easily.

They also grow in spurts and can become debilitated as a result – especially in adolescence, when those who are self-conscious of their height can become stooped.

Once exhausted, they feel better after a sleep, however brief. They prefer to sleep on their right side, finding it difficult (or impossible) to sleep on their left. Many of their symptoms are worse when they lie on their backs or left sides. They are sensitive to touch and feel better for being rubbed or massaged.

They are sensitive to smells and when sick, usually with a headache or digestive problems, they find strong smells and especially the smell of flowers hard to tolerate. Their eyes are sensitive to bright light (the sun or electric light) and they are also generally sensitive to pain, not dealing with it stoically.

Their worst times of day are the morning and the evening between twilight and midnight and they are also sensitive to the moon's phases.

Typical physical complaints as a result of stress include:

- Anaemia: with exhaustion.
- Backache: of lower back, between shoulder blades; pains burning or as if broken; better for massage; worse on getting up from sitting.
- Common cold: catarrh blood-streaked, one-sided; sense of taste/ smell lost; nose blocked; with hoarseness or a sore throat.

- Cough: dry, croupy, irritating, hacking, painful; chest feels tight; has to sit up to cough; with copious mucus; worse for cold air, laughing, talking, lying on left side.
- Diarrhoea: painless, profuse, watery, blood-streaked; worse during the morning.
- Exhaustion: nervous, extreme; body feels heavy; with anaemia, diarrhoea, fever, etc.; worse for slightest exertion.
- Fever: heat burning; with sweating; with increased appetite and great thirst.
- Gums bleeding: easily; with anaemia; after dental work.
- Hair loss: hair falls out in handfuls or in spots.
- Headache: pains burning, throbbing; nervous; better for cold compresses, fresh air, massage, sleep; worse before a storm.
- Hoarseness: painful; after over-using voice; with a cold.
- Indigestion: pressing or burning pains after eating; stomach gurgles and rumbles; with bloating and belching.
- Insomnia: with sleepiness and anxious dreams; sleeps on right side, can't sleep on left.
- Menstrual period: is very heavy; comes on early.
- Nausea: empty feeling in stomach not relieved by eating; with belching.
- Nosebleeds: copious, persistent; worse for blowing nose.
- Palpitations: with anxiety or excitement; worse lying on left side, for motion, on getting up, sitting or lying down.
- Sore throat: larynx raw, sore; tickling in bronchi/air passages; tonsils swollen; worse breathing in (especially cold air), coughing, talking.
- Ulcers: of gums, when run down.
- Voice lost: painless; in singers; with a cold.
- Vomiting: of even a little food or drink as soon as it is warm in the stomach (after a little while); stomach feels sore or burns; vomits bile.

PICRIC ACID (*Pic-ac.*)

Emotional state
Dull/confused. Forgetful/memory weak. Sluggish mentally. *Thinking* difficult.

Emotional stress: mental strain.

This is a small remedy for mental exhaustion after a heavy work or study period for people whose minds become worn out without their feelings being much affected. After a period of mental strain there is an intellectual weariness – with difficulty concentrating however much they try, and becoming quickly confused if they do try. Can't think or work and doesn't want to. The sluggishness is on a mental level, with a loss of mental willpower and an inability to get anything done or to take on anything new.

General state
Appetite poor. *Heavy feeling.*
Better for lying down; for rest.
Worse for physical or mental exertion.

There is also a physical tiredness with burning and prickling sensations in the back and legs. Physical symptoms (backache, headache, tiredness and even diarrhoea) are all worse for mental or physical exertion. They feel better for lying down and having a good rest or a sleep.
Typical physical complaints as a result of stress include:
- Backache: burning pains in back; lower back feels heavy and tired.
- Diarrhoea: with flatulence (after stool); stools thin, watery.
- Exhaustion: nervous, muscular; legs ache and feel heavy and tired; staggers and stumbles when walking; worse for slightest exertion, after stool.
- Headache: head feels heavy, pains pressing; in back of head, nape of neck, forehead; worse for mental exertion.
- Indigestion: with heavy feeling in stomach, empty belching.
- Insomnia: with sleepiness; worse before midnight, then wakes early.

PULSATILLA NIGRICANS (*Puls.*)
Pasque flower

Emotional state

Affected by hearing of tragic events/sad stories. *Affectionate.*
Anxious. Changeable. Clingy. Depressed. Desires: to be carried
(slowly); company. *Easily* consoled. *Excitable. Fearful:* claustropho-
bic; of dogs. *Introspective. Irritable. Lonely. Mild* (gentle). *Moody.*
Self-pitying. Sensitive. Shy. Sluggish mentally. *Sympathetic.*
Tearful. Whiney.

Emotional stresses: betrayal; conflict; depression; embarrassment;
humiliation; jealousy; loneliness; loss; transitions.

These are gentle, yielding, mild individuals, easily moved to
laughter or tears. They are shy with people they don't know, but
only for a little while, quickly making friends and usually having
lots of them.

They are affectionate creatures who are deeply compassionate
about others, who love animals (although they can be scared of
dogs, especially big black dogs) and cannot bear to see them (or
anybody else) hurt. They crave affection and reassurance especially,
when they are feeling low or unwell, and this will make them feel
better.

They are big softies who are easily influenced by others and who
easily become dependent on others. Because of this, they can be
picked on, especially when they are young. They are particularly
clingy and dependent when sick, when they also become irritable
and whiney (moaning and groaning) and feeling hard done by.
Babies and small children are literally clingy – wanting to be carried
around (gently and slowly) – older children and adults are more
subtle about it.

Their dependence on others makes them vulnerable to envy
and jealousy, and to loneliness and loss. There is a whiney,
child-like quality to their reaction, with them feeling that 'It isn't
fair'.

They are easily hurt but may suppress it, becoming introspective, moody, even irritable. If they feel humiliated and exposed, they tend to blame themselves for what happened.

Most of their complaints, including the emotional ones such as depression and worry, are better for fresh air and worse during the evening and in warm, stuffy rooms.

They are highly emotional with surprising mood swings, weeping one moment, irritable the next and then full of anxiety. Because of their dependency the opinions of others are terribly important to them and they worry about this. There is a tendency to claustrophobia which makes them anxious indoors, and this is worse at night (especially on airless hot nights).

They cry easily, and especially over hurts that they or others have suffered, or when talking about their stresses and/or complaints. They always feel better for a good cry, especially if they are also offered some sympathy or consolation at the same time.

General state

Appetite: changeable; dislikes bread, egg yolk, fatty meat, fatty/rich foods, fruit, hot food/drinks; likes cold food/drinks. *Breath* smells. *Desires* fresh air. *Discharges:* bland; thick; yellow; yellow-green. *Glands* swollen. *Lips* and mouth dry. *Pains:* on parts lain on; wandering. *Sweat:* one-sided; on single parts of the body; smelly; worse at night. *Symptoms:* changeable; right-sided. *Taste in the mouth* bad or bitter in the morning. *Thirstless. Tongue* coated; white; yellow.

Better for bathing; for fresh air; for movement; for pressure; for walking in fresh air.

Worse for sun; for rich fatty food; for getting wet – especially feet or head; for heat; before or during a menstrual period; at night; in stuffy rooms; at twilight; for wet weather; for wind.

Physical stresses: food sensitivities – fatty/rich foods, ice cream; food poisoning (rotten meat); heat; convalescing from illness; medication (the contraceptive pill/HRT); sun (feet or head).

These types have dry mouths and lips and an absence of thirst, even with a fever. They may be chilly, with cold hands and feet, but dislike heat (including hot baths, hot food and drinks, getting hot in bed, stuffy rooms and the heat of the sun), becoming quickly flushed and headachy. They will wait for hot foods and drinks to cool down before eating or drinking them. Their feet get hot in bed at night so they stick them out of the covers, when they quickly cool down and need covering up again. Small children kick the covers off and then wake their parents up crying when they become cold.

They love the seaside for the cool breezes and also like swimming in cool or even cold water. They always feel better in the fresh air, where their moods lift and their symptoms (especially coughs) improve. They are sensitive to getting wet or being exposed to wet, windy weather, when they can go down with a cough, a cold, an earache or can even miss a period. Twilight can be their worst time of day.

Their discharges (from nose, eyes, etc.) are typically thick and yellow in colour but they aren't irritating. Their glands become swollen with many complaints. Their complaints, especially the chests and joints, are worse for rest and better for moving about, especially in the fresh air.

They don't like rich, fatty foods, which give them indigestion and nausea, but they may have a liking for butter and sometimes even cream.

Many complaints (including feelings of depression and moodiness) coincide with the menstrual cycle in women – coming on before or during a period. This remedy is useful during puberty, pregnancy or menopause or if the periods have ceased for a while with the Pill or after, say, a loss.

Typical complaints as a result of stress include:

- Anaemia: feels faint and dizzy.
- Backache: in small of back, aching, dragging down; better for gentle exercise; worse on beginning to move, before a period.
- Common cold: catarrh yellow or yellow/green, thick; watery in fresh air; nose blocked up in a stuffy room; sense of smell/taste lost; with sneezing.
- Cough: dry at night, loose in the morning; racking; worse at night, for lying down and after meals; disturbs sleep; mucus difficult to cough up; chest feels tight.
- Cystitis: frequent, painful, ineffectual urging; pains after urinating.

- Diarrhoea: stools changeable; worse at night (from rich food/ fruit).
- Dizziness: has to lie down; worse bending down, getting up from lying down.
- Earache: aching, pressing, throbbing; external ear is red; ear feels blocked with noises, deafness and/or itching; with yellow discharge.
- Exhaustion: nervous; worse for heat, mental exertion, in the morning in bed; may be caused by loss of sleep (broken nights).
- Eye inflammation: eyes ache, burn, itch and water; eyelids glued together in the morning; discharge is thick and yellow; better for bathing with cold water.
- Fainting: in a warm or stuffy room.
- Fever: heat burning, with chilliness; better for uncovering; worse at night in bed.
- Flatulence: stomach bloated, rumbles; wind difficult to expel.
- Food poisoning: with vomiting and diarrhoea; from 'off' meat (including sausages) or fish.
- Headache: nervous, pains pressing, throbbing; with vomiting; better for pressure; worse after eating, on bending down, for exertion.
- Indigestion: stomach feels empty; heartburn (pains pressing); belches bitter, empty, tasting of food; worse at night.
- Insomnia: with sleepiness; restless sleep with frequent waking; anxious dreams; worse for heat; sleeps on back.
- Joint pain: pains sore, wandering; better for cold, including cold compresses; worse on beginning to move, for heat.
- Menstrual periods: scanty, irregular, late; flow is changeable, clotted, only in the day time; pains aching (beforehand), dragging down (during) or pressing.
- Nausea: with vomiting in pregnancy; worse after hot drinks, eating (especially rich foods).
- Nosebleeds: especially when the menstrual periods are suppressed.
- Palpitations: with anxiety; worse after eating, at night in bed.
- Sinuses: blocked, painful.
- Snuffles: in babies, especially teething babies.

- Sore throat: throat dry, irritated, raw – as if there's dust in it; tickling in larynx/air passages; chokes on food.
- Stomach ache: colic from rich or hot foods; dull aching with flatulence; has to bend double.
- Styes: upper eyelids.
- Thrush: discharge creamy; worse in pregnancy.
- Toothache: better for cold air/drinks/food; worse for hot things.
- Vomiting: bilious; vomits food or sour stuff; from rich, fatty foods or food poisoning.

SEPIA (*Sep.*)
Cuttlefish ink

Emotional state
Anxious. Apathetic. Depressed. Desires: to be alone. *Dislikes:* consolation; contradiction. *Dull/confused. Forgetful/memory weak. Indifferent:* to own children; to family; to loved ones; to work. *Irritable. Sluggish* mentally. *Tearful.*

Emotional stresses: depression; transitions.

When well, these individuals are energetic, productive, lively hardworkers. Once overstressed, they are prone to dreadful emotional troughs where they become apathetic, sluggish, irritable, weepy *and* depressed. This remedy is useful for those who have become worn out, who are struggling without enough support, for example, single parents, women who are worn down by worries and/or too many children with not enough time between them for their bodies to recover. Women (and men and sometimes children also) may be worn out from having too much to do and not enough resources to see them through.

When stressed they sag mentally and physically; they grind to a halt, sitting silently, feeling empty and enjoying nothing. They are indifferent to things that formerly gave them enjoyment, including partners, children and their work.

They find it hard to rouse themselves to do anything, including think, *but* they feel much better if they do drag themselves out of their torpor to do something physically strenuous, such as exercise, dancing, running, swimming or even spring cleaning.

They respond to sympathy with irritability, preferring to be quiet and alone to avoid any further stress. They may cry when talking about their problems and this makes them feel worse. They can be surprisingly sharp-tongued, especially in response to the concern of others – this helps to keep others away!

In this state their irritability can erupt in angry outbursts with shouting, screaming or nagging and sarcasm – if contradicted, or if others make demands on them, especially the demands of children on parents. They can turn to religion for comfort at this time.

This remedy is useful for women who are affected by their menstrual cycle – their symptoms are worse before a period, especially the depression and/or the irritability, and during menopause.

General state

Appetite: poor; dislikes milk, meat; likes lemonade, sour foods, vinegar, pickles. *Discharges* yellow. *Face:* pale; pasty. *Heavy feeling*. *Lips* cracked. *Pains:* pressing; stitching; tearing. *Sweat:* cold; hot; profuse; smelly; sour; from slightest physical exertion; from mental exertion; from pain; on single parts of the body. *Symptoms* left-sided.

Better after eating; for rest; for running; for vigorous exercise; for walking fast.

Worse before/during/after menstrual period; at night; for cold; for mental/physical exertion; for fasting; for frosty air; for sea air; for sweating; for touch; for walking in the wind.

Physical stresses: cold; frost; medication (the contraceptive pill/ HRT); sea air; snow; getting wet.

Sepia has a profound effect on the female hormones and is therefore often needed for many problems associated with the menstrual period from puberty onwards, during and after pregnancy, when breast-feeding, to help after a miscarriage or an abortion, and around the time of the menopause.

These are tense, chilly types, with cold hands and feet, extremely sensitive to cold in almost any shape or form. They sweat easily and profusely, with any exertion of the body or mind or when experiencing strong emotions. Coughing can also make them sweat. The sweat smells sour and can aggravate their complaints and/or make them feel generally worse.

They feel exhausted and run down, lose their muscle tone, feel and look physically saggy. They can feel as though something heavy is dragging down inside of them.

The typical *Sepia* face is yellow, earthy and pale, with dark rings under the eyes. There may be yellow or brown marks over the nose which appear typically in pregnancy or whilst taking the Pill and usually disappear afterwards.

Their exhaustion can be caused by a loss of body fluids, i.e. whilst breast-feeding or after a bout of diarrhoea, but there will usually be other emotional stresses contributing to a general feeling of ill-being.

Despite their general aggravation from mental and/or physical exertion *and* their state of exhaustion, they are usually better for exercising vigorously – this energizes them, even if they are feeling unwell or exhausted. They tend to feel weary in the morning on waking, especially after a bad night's sleep. Many of their complaints (backache, period pains, etc.) are worse for having to stand and better sitting with their legs crossed as this eases the dragging down sensations.

They will have a dry mouth and lips, especially with a fever, and the lower lip will become cracked.

Eating helps temporarily (they are much worse for missing meals), although some complaints (the vomiting) are worse for eating and the emptiness in the stomach isn't any better after food. They do not want to be touched or massaged.

Typical complaints as a result of stress include:
- Backache: lower back stiff and achy; pains dragging down; better for pressure; worse bending down, when sitting.
- Common cold: catarrh green or yellow-green, in sinuses, drips down back of throat; sense of smell lost.
- Conjunctivitis: eyes burning, gritty; lids swollen, glued together; worse during the evening, in a cold wind.
- Constipation: stomach feels full; stools large, hard; with straining.

- Cough: dry, exhausting, hacking, tickling, violent; worse lying down; better sitting up; lots of yellow mucus.
- Cystitis: constant, painful urging; dragging-down, pressing pains; urine cloudy, scanty, smelly.
- Exhaustion: nervous, sudden; worse for sweating, exertion, on getting up in the morning.
- Faintness: with a feeling of emptiness; during a period or with a fever; worse on exertion, in a stuffy room.
- Fever: with anxiety and sweating; worse for sweating.
- Hair loss: after childbirth.
- Headache: pains bursting, throbbing; in temples, forehead or back of head; extremities icy-cold; worse bending down.
- Hot flushes: flush of heat moves up the body; as if warm water were poured over; exhausted after; worse afternoon/night.
- Indigestion: gnawing pains after eating; with burping after fatty foods.
- Insomnia: with sleepiness; can't get to sleep before midnight; wakes around 3.00 a.m. and can't sleep; wakes frequently.
- Nausea: intermittent; empty feeling in stomach; with vomiting and gnawing pains; worse in the morning before breakfast; only temporarily better for eating; worse for smell of food.
- Palpitations: from irritability.
- Period problems: periods late, scanty, delayed (absent); pains dull/aching, dragging down, pressing; better sitting; worse standing, before and/or during a menstrual period.
- Prolapse: with constipation and bearing-down sensation; better for sitting with legs crossed.
- Thrush: discharge lumpy (cottage cheese), smelly; itches.
- Toothache: pains tearing, throbbing, radiate to ear; in pregnancy or during a menstrual period; worse for biting teeth together, for cold.
- Travel sickness: with biliousness, headache and nausea.
- Vomiting: vomits bile; worse after eating, mornings.

SILICA (*Sil.*)
Pure flint

Emotional state

Anxious: before an exam/interview, etc. *Concentration* poor. *Conscientious. Dislikes* consolation. *Dull/confused. Fearful* of public speaking. *Irritable. Jumpy. Lacks self-confidence. Mild* (gentle). *Sensitive* to noise. *Shy. Sluggish* mentally.

Emotional stresses: boredom; bullying; criticism; failure; mental strain; worry.

These are sensitive, self-contained types who are incredibly resilient emotionally. They take life seriously and, whilst they will typically give way if pushed, they will often quietly do what they wanted to do in the first place when no one is looking.

They can be delicate and lacking in stamina – usually physically, but also mentally. They can appear to lack grit (flintiness), becoming worn out from too much work (usually mental, for example, studying). Alternatively they can be gritty, hard-working and conscientious under pressure, able to sustain seemingly superhuman feats of endurance, collapsing only once the job in hand is completed. Under stress they may become obsessed with minutiae, wasting their time on small tasks and putting off tackling the big ones.

They are naturally shy, and anxious about appearing in public because of a fear of failure and can suffer horribly with exam or interview nerves. Unassertive, lacking in confidence, they give way rather than take a position and fight for it, although deep down they won't change their mind – rather they will keep their own opinions to themselves.

Once overstressed they can become restless, nervous inside and jumpy. In this state they are sensitive to noise, especially small noises which make them start and increase their feelings of anxiety. Once worn out, they can't concentrate and find reading and studying as well as any kind of thinking, difficult. They don't want to talk or make decisions. They become irritable if consoled or sympathized with when feeling low.

General state
Ankles weak. *Appetite:* poor: digestion slow/poor: dislikes meat;
likes raw foods, indigestible things like coal, sand, chalk, pencils,
etc. *Dislikes* fresh air. *Glands* swollen. *Pains* stitching. *Sensation* of
a hair on the tongue. *Slowness* (of children) to teethe. *Sweat:* acidic;
on the feet; on the head; worse at night, during sleep; profuse;
smelly; sour. *Thin. Thirsty.*
Better for heat; for wrapping up head.
Worse for change of weather; for cold; for damp; for draughts; for
fasting; for fresh air; for getting feet wet; for touch; for being
uncovered; for wet weather; wind.

Physical stresses: change of temperature from hot to cold;
chemicals; getting chilled; cold; cold wind; drafts; dust; injury – to
bones, incisions; splinters; teething; vaccination; wet weather;
getting feet wet.

Silica types feel the cold intensely and have icy-cold hands and feet.
They are sensitive to cold air, to draughts and wind, and changes of
weather, and are always better for warmth and being wrapped up
well, especially the head. They may even want to wear a hat or scarf
in mild weather. They are easily chilled: if they go out into the cold
air after swimming, or if they become wet and chilled in the rain
they become sick, with a cold or a cough. They are also vulnerable if
just their feet get wet. They are susceptible to colds (also with
teething or after vaccination) which have a tendency to go onto the
chest and are generally accompanied by swollen glands.

They sweat at night, particularly on the back of the head and
neck. Their sweat smells sour and their feet are cold, with smelly
and acidic sweat which may even eat holes in their socks! The feet
may be smelly without sweating. They can get all sorts of feet
complaints from bunions and corns, to cracks between the toes
(usually associated with athletes' foot) and toenails which become
thick and distorted.

They tend to be skinny, have trouble assimilating their food and
the bones in these children may not form as well or as quickly as in
others. Children have weak ankles and can be slow in learning to
walk. Their teeth are slow to come through and decay easily. Adults

can have difficulties with wisdom teeth taking a long time to come through.

There may be white spots on the nails, and the nails themselves can be brittle, splitting easily. They have a peculiar sensation that there is hair on the back of the tongue (when there isn't).

Cuts and injuries take a long time to heal – the scar becomes red or keeps reopening or becomes lumpy on healing. This particular remedy is always indicated for wounds where there is a suspicion that there is something (a tiny piece of dirt or a splinter) left in the body, i.e. under the skin or in the eye, etc., even after your doctor has prounounced it clean.

Typical physical complaints as a result of stress include:

- Abscesses: at roots of teeth – better for wrapping up head; of glands.
- Athletes' foot: cracks between toes; with sweaty, smelly feet.
- Backache: sore, stiff back; feels lame, weak; worse sitting, getting up from sitting, at night, for pressure.
- Broken bones: slow to mend.
- Common cold: catarrh smelly, thick; sinuses painful; sense of smell/taste lost; wants to sneeze but can't.
- Conjunctivitis: eyes sore with yellow discharge; worse for cold air.
- Constipation: strains (without success) to pass a large, hard stool which keeps slipping back; unfinished feeling; burns after passing stool.
- Cough: irritating, tickling with thick, yellow mucus; better for hot drinks; worse on waking, for becoming cold, for cold drinks.
- Diarrhoea: with smelly flatulence; especially in teething babies.
- Earache: tearing pains behind ear; ear feels blocked, itches inside; hearing may be affected; discharge from ear is thick and smelly.
- Exhaustion: nervous; wants to lie down; from overwork, diarrhoea or breast-feeding, etc.
- Fever: worse for movement, for uncovering, evenings/night; with characteristic sweat – feels icy cold and shivery.
- Flatulence: wind difficult to expel, smelly; stomach rumbles.
- Gumboil: gums are sore and inflamed.
- Headache: pains tearing, pressing, throbbing; in forehead, back

of head spreading over to eye (especially the right eye), in sinuses; with dizziness; better for lying in a dark room with eyes closed, for wrapping up head; worse for jarring movement.

- Ingrowing toenails: with smelly and/or sweaty feet.
- Injuries: cuts/wounds are slow to heal, become inflamed, painful, with pus/dirt inside; scars are painful, lumpy, break open.
- Insomnia: wakes after midnight and can't get back to sleep; restless sleep with vivid dreams/nightmares.
- Joint pains: worse for cold; better for heat.
- Sore throat: throat dry, stitching pains; glands swollen; worse swallowing, uncovering throat.
- Stomach ache: with constipation; with blocked wind (flatulence).
- Thrush: vaginal; acrid, burning, itching, profuse.
- Toothache: worse in the winter; better for wrapping up the head.
- Vomiting: babies vomit (or posit) milk (bottle or breast).

STAPHYSAGRIA (*Staph.*)
Palmated larkspur

Emotional state
Affected by hearing of tragic events/sad stories. *Angry:* with difficulty expressing anger; with trembling. *Apathetic* about everything. *Capricious. Conscientious. Depressed. Destructive. Dislikes* contradiction. *Dwells* on unpleasant events. *Easily* offended. *Indignant. Irritable. Lacks* self-confidence. *Mild* (gentle). *Resentful. Sensitive:* to pain; to rudeness.

Emotional stresses: betrayal; bullying; conflict; criticism; disappointment; humiliation; loss; reprimand; resentment; shame.

These are romantic, sentimental people who are deeply affected by hearing sad or terrible stories. They tend to be inhibited emotionally and whilst they may feel things strongly, they don't show their feelings, or at least don't show the depth of them. They have a tendency to blame others.
They are sensitive and touchy and easily offended – especially by

rudeness in others, in spite of being sharp-tongued themselves at times. If offended, they suppress their feelings (smiling sweetly all the while), but will then tremble afterwards, feeling angrily indignant. It is anger in particular that isn't expressed.

These are compliant people who are conscientious and hard-working. They find it hard to say 'no', they take on too much and allow pressure to build up inside. They are vulnerable to feeling exposed or humiliated because they are generally sensitive, suffer from low self-esteem *and* are unable to express their own needs.

They avoid confrontation at any cost, not letting their feelings show, biting back an angry reaction and ending up feeling resentful. They may re-live the event, when alone, often late at night, and may walk around talking to themselves as they do so. After a disappointment, a conflict or any difficult situation they will literally shake with anger (although they may be able to hide this too). They may cry instead of getting angry, and this makes them feel even more humiliated.

The more anger they hold in, the more difficult they find it to speak. This emotional suppression can turn into an active resentment, spilling out into all areas of their lives. Work becomes more difficult and they have trouble sleeping, lying awake at night replaying the event or situation and imagining what they wish they'd said or done and feeling furious. They wake in the morning feeling irritable and it is then that they can snap at those around them, especially if contradicted.

They may be so effective at hiding their feelings that they are unaware of the depth of them themselves, and it is only in the telling of what happened that a note of indignation in the voice gives the game away.

Children (or adults) may become ill after having been told off, or after being bullied or humiliated, even though they appear to have taken it well. Adults who have suffered at the hands of an angry boss or partner, or are in any situation where they feel abused and seethe inside, become ill if they don't find a way of dealing with their feelings.

The anger will either come out at some point, in a violent outburst when they may throw things but not *at* people, or be kept inside when they will either become physically ill or become depressed – or both. The depression isn't generally overwhelming, it is more of an apathy, and in the same way that they can pretend to be okay when they are feeling angry inside, they are also able to do the same when they feel depressed.

General state
Appetite: dislikes milk, water; likes meat, sweet foods. *Pains* stitching. *Sweat* worse for mental exertion.
Worse for physical exertion; for fasting; after an afternoon nap; for tobacco; for touch.

Physical stresses: injury – incisions; tobacco.

These individuals are extremely sensitive, physically and emotionally, and suffer pain acutely. Wounds and cuts are unusually painful, especially if they feel they have been assaulted. The pains are typically stitching or shooting and worse for touch. They feel generally worse for exercise, smoky rooms and missing meals. They feel worse for a daytime sleep, being irritable, anxious and thirsty on waking.
Typical complaints as a result of stress include:
- Anaemia: with exhaustion.
- Colic: pains cramping; worse for drinking.
- Cough: nervous; tickling; air passages feel irritated.
- Cystitis: frequent urging to urinate; scanty urine; caused by unaccustomed sexual intercourse.
- Exhaustion: nervous, with trembling.
- Gums: inflamed; pale; bleed when brushing teeth.
- Headache: pains pulling, pressing, in back of head or forehead.
- Injuries: punctured wounds; very sensitive to touch; pains tearing; stinging; injuries to nerve-rich parts, to the eye.
- Insomnia: sleep unrefreshing; sleepy during the day, sleepless at night; body aches all over.
- Piles: excruciatingly sensitive to touch.
- Stomach ache: after anger or surgery/injury, etc.; stomach feels heavy; pains aching, cramping; with flatulence; better for passing wind; worse after eating or drinking.
- Styes: sensitive to touch; on eyelids; eyes may water.

- Toothache: pains tearing, spread to ears, in decayed teeth; worse after eating, for cold drinks; teeth decay easily.

STRAMONIUM (Stram.)
Thorn-apple

Emotional state

Anxious at night. *Apathetic* and doesn't complain. *Clingy. Destructive. Dull/confused* (sense of unreality). *Fearful:* claustrophobic; of the dark; of dogs; of glittering surfaces; of water. *Hyperactive. Lonely. Mischievous. Rage/tantrums. Talkative.*

Emotional stresses: fear; shock.

This remedy is for shock with fear. The shock may date back to childbirth (for mother *or* baby) or an accident or injury (especially bad burns), surgery or a natural disaster, i.e. any situation that was a 'nightmare'.

The fears are many and include: fear of the dark (babies and children, especially, are terrified of the dark and wake with nightmares, knowing no one); fear of water and glittering surfaces such as mirrors – children don't want to learn to swim and dislike having their hair washed, especially having water poured over their heads; of death and/or of all things dark and black; of animals, especially dogs and especially black dogs; of violence, of being hurt; of being closed in (claustrophobia).

In the early stages of shock they may become hysterical, laughing loudly, being talkative and cheerful. Apathy and confusion are common, either after the hysterical stage or instead of it – there's a feeling that nothing is real, as if it is all a dream. Adults may turn to prayer for solace.

Children (and sometimes adults) needing this remedy may be prone to anger after a shock – to tantrums, to impulsive, explosive, destructive outbursts of violence where they shout and scream and kick and may even hit out and bite those close to them. There is a particular restlessness – they wander around aimlessly achieving nothing, and children may be labelled hyperactive.

General state
Appetite: dislikes water. *Expression* frightened. *Pain* absent. *Pupils* dilated. *Sensation* of constriction. *Thirsty*.
Better for light.
Worse for dark.

Physical stress: shock after injury.

After a shock, including surgery or injury of any sort, someone needing this remedy will *look* frightened – their pupils may be dilated, they tremble, and they may even have trouble speaking, stuttering and stammering.

They don't experience as much (or even any) pain with complaints that are normally painful, although they may have feelings of constriction.

They feel emotionally and physically worse at night when it gets dark, and correspondingly better with the light. They are thirsty, especially with a fever but have a dread of cold water and may have difficulty swallowing if the feeling of constriction affects the throat.

Typical complaints as a result of stress include:
• Convulsions: with rage from overexcitement or shock.
• Cough: barking, deep; croupy.
• Diarrhoea: from shock; in children.
• Fever: burning heat with sweating; worse for uncovering.
• Headache: in back of head; severe; worse for exposure to the sun.
• Insomnia: in a dark room; with night terrors – wakes knowing no one.
• Sore throat: throat dry; feeling of constriction; swallowing difficult.

SULPHUR (*Sul.*)
Flowers of sulphur

Emotional state
Anxious: about others. *Bites* fingernails. *Critical. Depressed. Despair. Discontented. Dull/confused. Eccentric. Fearful* of heights; for others; claustrophobic. *Hurried. Impatient. Intellectual.*

Irritable. Lazy. Quarrelsome. Restless. Selfish. Sluggish mentally. Stubborn. Untidy.

Emotional stresses: boredom; embarrassment; fear; transitions.

These are enthusiastic, ambitious, self-confident, generous extroverts who have lots of energy and make many plans. They may be pure intellectuals (academics) or lean to being more practical types. Either way they start many things and do not finish them. Their dreams, likewise, may never materialize because they tend to be lazy and are happiest talking about what they are going to do!

They are also self-centred, stubborn, impatient and irritable, critical of others and how they run their lives, with lots of ideas about how they could do it better themselves.

Mess doesn't bother them, although they may get periodical cravings for a limited external order (their cupboards and drawers are still chaotic). They don't take any trouble over their personal appearance and tend to always look untidy and/or unwashed, no matter what they do. They are often eccentric in their dress sense (as well as the rest of their lives!) and don't care how they look, not noticing the odd socks, the hem coming down, the collar escaping from inside a jumper. They can also be hoarders, not wanting to throw anything away.

Under stress they become introverted, sloppy and disorganized; they feel constantly rushed and hurried, putting off what they know they have to do – preferring not to do it at all! They can become anxious nail-biters, suffering from worries which plague them in the evening and stop them sleeping at night. They worry about their health (about 'catching' things), and about those closest to them, especially if they are late home from work or school. They become depressed, sluggish and despairing when ill.

Sulphur children are restless, boisterous, impatient, always on the go and intensely curious – always asking the question 'Why?' Children of all ages dislike being washed or bathed. When ill, they become quarrelsome and sluggish but never lose their restlessness.

General state
Appetite: good; dislikes bread, eggs, meat; likes alcohol, fatty foods,

raw foods, spicy foods, sweet foods, sweet and sour foods, water. *Breath* smells. *Desires* fresh air. *Discharges:* smelly, sour, watery. *Eyes* sensitive to bright light. *Face:* red (flushed); sallow; red in spots. *Glands* swollen. *Lips:* chapped; cracked; dry; red. *Mouth* dry. *Pains* burning. *Sweat:* on feet; profuse; during sleep; smelly; sour; from slightest physical exertion. *Symptoms* left-sided. *Taste in mouth:* bitter; bad. *Thirsty* for large quantities. *Tongue:* white-coated; red-edged; red-tipped.
Better for cold; for fresh air.
Worse around 10.00–11.00 a.m.; for alcohol; bathing; for change of weather; for physical exertion; for fasting; for heat; for milk; for standing; in stuffy rooms; for warmth of bed.

Physical stresses: alcohol; change of temperature – cold to hot; heat; drugs in general; tension from sedentary lifestyle; fast metabolism; sun/sunstroke; vaccination.

These are warm-blooded types who feel the heat, who have hot feet which they poke out of bed at night, who can wear sandals all the year round. Their complaints can be caused by heat and hot weather (especially by the change of weather to warm) *or* they can be aggravated by heat. Whilst they are always worse for being in a stuffy room, and better for fresh air, they may also be sensitive to the cold, especially cold draughts.

They are lazy about washing, often feeling worse for it, especially for hot baths. They slump when sitting and stoop when walking, and are always worse for having to stand up for long – ending up with a backache and sore feet.

They become flushed and red when hot, and when ill their lips become red, dry and cracked. The tongue is white-coated with red edges and tip. They are thirsty types, consuming large quantities of water whether sick or well, and have huge appetites. Their discharges are usually hot, smelly and burning. They sweat profusely and easily but feel worse while sweating.

Their complaints under stress may have a weekly cycle, often coming back at the weekend, typically on Sunday or on their day off.

They have a characteristic aggravation mid-morning, usually

around 11.00 a.m. when they become suddenly hungry and then headachy and faint if they don't have something to eat. They have fast metabolisms and need to eat regularly, although if they aren't careful they do have a tendency to put on weight. They have a soft spot for beer (and also whisky) but it can give them indigestion, flatulence and diarrhoea.

There can be many problems around menstruation with backache and painful periods as well as periods that are short and scanty. The menopause can also be difficult, with hot flushes and headaches, etc.

NB This remedy is hailed for its effect on eczema and skin rashes, but I strongly advise you not to prescribe for these complaints without consulting a professional homeopath, as the aggravations can be severe and need to be monitored carefully.

Typical physical complaints as a result of stress include:

- Anaemia: with exhaustion and fainting.
- Backache: in lower back; back aches, feels weak/tired/stiff; worse for long sitting, standing, bending down.
- Common cold: catarrh smelly, yellow; nose dry, itching; with frequent sneezing.
- Conjunctivitis: eyes burning, gritty, sensitive to light, watering; eyelids itching, burning and red; worse for washing eyes.
- Constipation: with itching, burning, redness around anus; stools large, hard, knotting; with straining and/or an unfinished feeling.
- Cough: dry evening/night, loose day/morning; painful, irritating disturbs sleep; worse lying down; with green mucus.
- Cradle cap: dry, itchy scalp which may smell.
- Cramps: in thighs, legs, calves, soles of feet; worse at night in bed.
- Cystitis: frequent, urgent desire to urinate; pains burning; worse when urinating, at night; urine smelly, brown.
- Dandruff: dry, itchy scalp – especially at the back of the head.
- Diarrhoea: slimy, smelly, sour, watery; morning only – drives sufferer out of bed; painless; with smelly flatulence; worse at 5.00 a.m.
- Dizziness: worse getting up from sitting or lying, on bending down.
- Earache: pains stitching, tearing; with painful noises in ear; worse in left ear, for noise; external parts of ear itch.

- Exhaustion: from hunger; worse during the afternoon, in the hot weather.
- Fainting: feels hot, flushed and faint; worse for digestive upsets.
- Fever: heat alternating with chills; with sweating and shivering; worse at night, for sweating (feels worse when hot and sweating).
- Flatulence: stomach bloated, gurgling, rumbling; with smelly wind (smells of rotten eggs); better for passing wind.
- Hair loss: after childbirth.
- Headache: head feels hot/constricted; pains burning, bursting, in top of head; better for cold; worse after eating, bending, sneezing, coughing, blowing nose.
- Hot flushes: with faint feeling and exhaustion; worse mid-morning.
- Indigestion: stomach bloated, feels empty around 11.00 a.m.; empty, sour belches; with flatulence; pains burning; worse after eating, after milk.
- Insomnia: sleep unrefreshing, restless; wakes frequently, late in the morning; with unpleasant dreams; worse after 3.00, 4.00 or 5.00 a.m.; better for a daytime nap.
- Joint pain: pains burning, tearing; worse for walking, for warmth of bed.
- Nappy rash: skin is red, itchy, burns – becomes red raw and may bleed; better for uncovering; worse for heat, for washing.
- Menstrual periods: come on later, are scanty and painful; with backache during a period.
- Piles: painful, bleeding, burning, itching; with constipation; worse for touch, for standing, when walking.
- Prickly heat: skin itches, worse for heat.
- Restless legs: worse for heat.
- Sore throat: throat dry, raw, burns; choking sensation; worse for coughing, for swallowing; glands swollen; voice hoarse.
- Sunstroke: hot, thirsty, feverish; with profuse sweating, dizziness, headache; skin sore, itchy; worse for washing and heat.
- Thrush (genital): yellow discharge, burns and itches.

TARENTULA HISPANIA (*Tarent.*)
Spanish spider

Emotional state
Angry. Contrary. Destructive. Disobedient. Hurried. Hyperactive. Mischievous. Quarrelsome. Restless. Sensitive to music. Stubborn.

Emotional stress: reprimand.

This remedy is for excitable, restless, highly-strung types who are particularly sensitive to reprimand. After being told off, children become hysterical, hyperactive, naughty and destructive. They can have massive tantrums when they turn their anger on to things rather than people.

These are generally impatient, speedy types who want everyone to move at their pace, who have a natural tendency to workaholism. Under pressure they become stubborn and contrary.

They are particularly sensitive to music and to dancing. These make them feel better – the louder and wilder the music, the better!

General state
Thirsty.
Worse for cold; for touch.

The nervous system is like a tightly coiled spring which wants to be continually on the go. These types are restless day and night. They sleep badly, twitching in their sleep and tossing and turning all night. Their restlessness is better for exercise, especially dancing! They are very thirsty, and feel the cold. They are generally sensitive to touch and their pains are worse for touch.

Typical physical complaints as a result of stress include:
- Constipation: with ineffectual straining and anxiety.
- Cough: dry; in fits.
- Exhaustion: nervous; with sweating.
- Headache: pains pressing, severe; worse for light, on waking in the morning.
- Indigestion: digestion is slow; with empty burping and flatulence.

- Restless legs: in bed at night; with itching.
- Sore throat: air passages feel raw, burning; worse on coughing or swallowing.
- Vomiting: in the morning; worse after eating, on coughing.

VERATRUM ALBUM (*Verat.*)
White hellebore

Emotional state
Anxious. Arrogant. Bites fingernails. Blames others. Brooding. Busy. Critical. Depressed. Despair. Forgetful/memory weak. Hyperactive. Lively. Prays. Rude. Sluggish mentally. Uncommunicative.

Emotional stresses: failure; loss.

These are bright, critical people who like to be occupied, who are always busy with something, who worry about their social position, about their place in their family, in their community, etc.

The loss of that position (after a bankruptcy or even a house move) is incredibly stressful and can lead to depression and illness. Under stress they become rude and blaming and even busier than usual. They worry about their losses and become sluggish and forgetful. They are arrogant and sullen and don't want to talk.

When depressed, they brood on what they have lost and turn to prayer for comfort, praying in a compulsive but despairing way. Normally lively children become hyperactive, precociously rude and difficult to control.

General state
Appetite: increased; likes cold drinks/food, fruit, ice (in drinks, etc.), lemon, refreshing foods, salt/salty foods; salty and sour foods, sour foods. *Expression* anxious. *Face:* cold; drawn; pale. *Mouth* dry. *Onset of pain/complaint* – sudden. *Pains* pressing. *Sweat* clammy, cold. *Thirsty.*
Worse for cold; for fruit.

Physical stresses: food poisoning; fruit.

Coldness runs through this remedy. They feel cold and feel worse for cold; even their breath may be cold and they can complain of ice-cold hands and feet. They feel worse in the winter and especially when it first changes to cold. The sweat is cold – especially on the forehead and face, particularly the sweat that accompanies a physical complaint. Sweating doesn't give a relief of symptoms.

In spite of their physical coldness, there is a desire for cold (even ice-cold) drinks. They want refreshing things to eat and drink – tangy (sour) and salty foods – and may even eat lemons. They eat a lot and burp afterwards but the empty feeling in the stomach isn't relieved by food.

Physical complaints come on suddenly and in some instances violently, for example, the vomiting or the headache.

Typical physical complaints as a result of stress include:

- Cough: deep, hollow; coughing fits with feeling of tightness in chest.
- Diarrhoea: profuse, exhausting; with vomiting; passes stool with flatus; stools watery, explosive; with exhaustion; worse for fruit, for movement.
- Exhaustion: sudden, extreme (to the point of collapse).
- Headache: severe, nervous; waves of pain; top of head feels cold; with vomiting; worse cold; better for pressure.
- Palpitations: with anxiety.
- Period pains: severe; with vomiting and diarrhoea.
- Stomach ache: pains aching, cramping; with burping; with flatulence; worse after eating, after fruit.
- Vomiting: violent, frothy; vomits food, bile; hiccoughs during or after vomiting; with diarrhoea (at the same time); with fainting; worse for fruit.

ZINCUM METALLICUM (*Zinc.*)
Zinc

Emotional state
Depressed. Dull/confused. Irritable. Sensitive to noise. *Sluggish mentally. Uncommunicative.*

Emotional stress: mental strain.

This remedy is useful for those who are suffering from nervous exhaustion caused by mental strain. They become depressed, irritable, sensitive to noise and generally worn out. They have difficulty in thinking and, whilst they may not want to talk much (because conversation is too noisy!), they may go on and on whining about their complaints. Their thoughts wander, they are slow to answer (they can irritatingly repeat all questions before answering them) and they forget what they are saying halfway through a sentence.

General state
Appetite: doesn't want breakfast. *Face* pale. *Pains* pressing. *Sweat:* clammy; profuse; sour. *Taste in mouth* metallic. *Twitchy. White* spots on fingernails.
Worse after eating; for fasting; during the evening; at night; for wine.

Physical stresses: difficulty sleeping/from tension; repetitive strain injury.

For people of any age who are weary and run-down from overwork, especially if it is accompanied by a loss of sleep. The nervous system becomes run-down, causing them to tremble, twitch and jerk. They suffer from restless legs when exhausted which is worse in bed; their legs will carry on twitching even during their sleep.
    Their symptoms tend to be worse at night, from drinking wine and after eating, although they may feel better whilst they eat. Like *Sulphur* types, they have an empty feeling in the stomach around 11 a.m.
    Typical physical complaints as a result of stress include:
• Backache: sore, aching, burning; in spine, coccyx, neck; with weak feeling in back; worse for sitting.
• Conjunctivitis: eyes sore, gritty, burning; worse during evening, at night.
• Constipation: stools dry and hard.
• Cough: dry; worse eating sweet things, before a menstrual period.

- Diarrhoea: after drinking wine.
- Exhaustion: with restless legs.
- Gums: pale, bleeding easily.
- Headache: nervous; pains bursting, tearing; better for fresh air.
- Indigestion: worse after eating.
- Insomnia: with restless legs; sleep light and unrefreshing.
- Restless legs: worse in bed at night.
- Stomach ache: worse after eating; with nausea after drinking wine.

List of remedies and abbreviations

Entries in bold are covered in detail in the 'Homeopathic Remedies' section on pages 251–349.

Ac-sul.	*Acid sulphurosum*	*Chin.*	*China officinalis*
Aco.	**Aconitum napellus**	*Chlorum*	*Chlorum*
Adren.	*Adrenalin*	*Choc.*	*Chocolate*
Agar.	*Agaricus muscarius*	**Cocc.**	**Cocculus indicus**
Alu.	*Alumina*	**Coff.**	**Coffea cruda**
Ambr.	**Ambra grisea**	**Coloc.**	**Colocynthis**
Anac.	**Anacardium orientale**	**Con.**	**Conium maculatum**
Ant-c.	*Antimonium crudum*	*Cort.*	*Cortisone*
Apis	**Apis mellifica**	*Elect.*	*Electricitas*
Arg-n.	**Argentum nitricum**	**Gels.**	**Gelsemium**
Arn.	**Arnica montana**		**sempervirens**
Ars.	**Arsenicum album**	*Glon.*	*Glonoine*
Aur.	**Aurum metallicum**	*Hep-s.*	*Hepar sulphuris*
Bar-c.	**Baryta carbonica**		*calcareum*
Bell.	**Belladonna**	*Hyp.*	*Hypericum perfoliatum*
Bell-p.	*Bellis perennis*	**Ign.**	**Ignatia amara**
Bor.	**Borax venata**	*Kali-bi*	*Kali bichromicum*
Brom.	*Bromium*	**Kali-p.**	**Kali phosphoricum**
Bry.	*Bryonia alba*	*Kali-s.*	*Kali sulphuricum*
Cad-s.	*Cadmium sulphuratum*	**Lach.**	**Lachesis**
Calad.	*Caladium*	*Led.*	*Ledum palustre*
Calc-c.	**Calcarea carbonica**	**Lyc.**	**Lycopodium**
Calc-p.	**Calcarea phosphorica**	*Mag-c.*	*Magnesia carbonica*
Calend.	*Calendula officinalis*	*Mag-m.*	*Magnesia muriatica*
Canth.	*Cantharis vesiticatoria*	*Mag-p.*	*Magnesia phosphorica*
Caps.	**Capsicum**	*Merc-s.*	*Mercurius solubis*
Carb-an.	*Carbo animalis*	**Nat-c.**	**Natrum carbonicum**
Carbn-s.	*Carboneum sulphuratum*	**Nat-m.**	**Natrum muriaticum**
Carb-v.	**Carbo vegetabilis**	*Nat-s.*	*Natrum sulphuricum*
Caust.	**Causticum**	*Nicc.*	*Niccolum*
Cham.	**Chamomilla**	**Nit-ac.**	**Nitricum acidum**

Nux-v.	**Nux vomica**	**Sil.**	**Silica**
Op.	**Opium**	*Spig.*	*Spigelia*
Petr.	*Petroleum*	**Staph.**	**Staphysagria**
Pho-ac.	**Phosphoric acid**	**Stram.**	**Stramonium**
Phos.	**Phosphorus**	*Stront-c.*	*Strontium carbonicum*
Pic-ac.	**Picric acid**	**Sul.**	**Sulphur**
Plb.	*Plumbum*	*Sul-ac.*	*Sulphuric acid*
Puls.	**Pulsatilla nigricans**	*Symph.*	*Symphytum*
Rad-br.	*Radium bromatum*	*Tabac.*	*Tabacum*
Ran-b.	*Ranunculus bulbosis*	**Tarent.**	**Tarentula hispania**
Rhod.	*Rhododenron*	*Thea*	*Thea*
Rhus-t.	*Rhus toxicodendron*	*Thu.*	*Thuja occidentalis*
Ruta	*Ruta graveolens*	**Verat.**	**Veratrum album**
Sep.	**Sepia**	**Zinc.**	**Zincum metallicum**

INDEXES OF
STRESSES

Index of Emotional State

Absent-minded *Caust.*

Abusive (see also Angry, Irritable, Rage) *Cham., Lach., Nux-v.*

Affected by hearing of tragic events/sad stories (see also Compassionate, Sensitive, Sympathetic) *Calc-c., Phos., Puls., Staph.*

Affectionate *Nux-v., Phos., Puls.*

Angry *Anac., Aur., Cham., Lyc., Nit-ac., Nux-v., Staph., Tarent.*

with difficulty expressing anger *Aur., Lyc., Staph.*

with trembling *Staph.*

over little things *Nux-v.*

Anxious *Aco., Ambr., Anac., Arg-n., Ars., Bor., Calc-c., Calc-p., Carb-v., Cocc., Con., Gels., Kali-p., Lach., Lyc., Nat-c., Nat-m., Nux-v., Phos., Puls., Sep., Sil., Stram., Sul., Verat.*

when alone *Ars., Phos.*

in bed *Carb-v.*

before a test, exam, interview, performance or any ordeal i.e. a visit to the dentist, hospital etc. *Aco., Ambr., Anac., Arg-n., Gels., Lyc., Nat-m., Sil.*

during the evening *Calc-c., Carb-v.*

with fear *Aco., Anac., Ars.*

during a fever *Ars.*

about the future *Arg-n., Calc-c.*

about their health *Arg-n., Calc-c., Nit-ac.*

at night *Ars., Stram.*

about others *Ars., Caust., Sul.*

on waking *Ars.*

Apathetic *Ap., Carb-v., Con., Gels., Op., Pho-ac., Phos., Sep., Staph., Stram.*

and doesn't complain *Op., Stram.*

about everything *Carb-v., Pho-ac., Staph.*

during a fever *Gels., Op., Pho-ac.*

Arrogant *Verat.*

Bites fingernails *Ars., Bar-c., Lyc., Nat-m., Sul., Verat.*

Blames

others *Ars., Lach., Verat.*

self *Aur.*

Brooding *Ign., Pho-ac., Verat.*

Busy *Ars., Verat.*

Capricious *Cham., Staph.*

Changeable *Puls.*

Cheerful *Coff., Lach., Nat-c.*

alternating with sadness *Bell.*

Childish *Bar-c.*

Clingy *Puls., Stram.*

Compassionate *Nit-ac.*

Complaining *Ars., Calc-p., Nit-ac.*

Concentration difficult/poor *Anac., Bar-c., Caust., Lach., Lyc., Nux-v., Pho-ac., Phos., Sil.*

Confused – see **Dull/confused**
Conscientious *Ign., Nat-c., Sil., Staph.*
Contrary *Cham., Tarent.*
Critical *Ars., Sul., Verat.*
Dazed *Cocc.*
Defiant *Caust.*
Delirious with hallucinations *Bell.*
Denial of illness/of suffering *Arn.*
Depressed *Ambr., Ars., Aur., Calc-c.,*
     Caps., Caust., Cham., Con.,
     Gels., Ign., Kali-p., Lach.,
     Nat-c., Nat-m., Nit-ac., Nux-v.,
     Op., Pho-ac., Phos., Puls., Sep.,
     Staph., Sul., Verat., Zinc.
     but cannot cry *Gels., Nat-m.*
     from unexpressed grief *Ign.,*
          Nat-m.
Desires
     to be alone *Gels., Ign., Lyc.,*
          Nat-m., Sep.
     to be carried (infants/children)
          Ars., Cham., Puls.
     fast *Ars., Cham.*
     slowly *Puls.*
     company *Ars., Phos., Puls.*
     to travel *Calc-p.*
Despair *Ars., Aur., Ign., Sul., Verat.*
     of getting well *Calc-c., Coloc.*
     with pain *Ars., Cham., Coff.*
Destructive *Staph., Stram., Tarent.*
Dictatorial *Lyc.*
Discontented *Calc-p., Sul.*
Dislikes
     being alone *Lyc.*
     being touched/examined *Arn.,*
          Bell., Cham.
     company – see Desires to be
          alone

consolation *Ign., Nat-m., Sep., Sil.*
contradiction *Ign., Lyc., Sep.,*
     Staph.
Disobedient *Tarent.*
Domineering *Anac.*
Dreamy *Op.*
Drowsy *Op.*
Dull/confused *Ambr., Arg-n., Bar-c.,*
     Bell., Calc-c., Calc-p., Carb-v.,
     Cocc., Con., Gels., Nat-c.,
     Nat-m., Op., Pic-ac., Sep., Sil.,
     Stram., Sul., Zinc.
Dwells on unpleasant events
     Nat-m., Staph.
Easily consoled *Phos., Puls.*
Easily embarrassed *Ambr., Bar-c.,*
     Lyc., Nat-m.
Easily offended *Lyc., Nat-m.,*
     Nux-v., Staph.
Eccentric *Lach., Sul.*
Excitable *Aco., Arg-n., Bell., Caps.,*
     Cham., Coff., Lach., Nux-v.,
     Phos., Puls.
Fearful *Aco., Ap., Arg-n., Arn., Ars.,*
     Bor., Calc-c., Caust., Gels.,
     Lyc., Nat-c., Phos., Puls.,
     Stram.
     agoraphobic *Gels.*
     of animals *Bell.*
     of being alone *Ap., Arg-n., Ars.,*
          Phos.
     of burglars *Ars.*
     claustrophobic *Aco., Arg-n., Lyc.,*
          Puls., Stram., Sul.
     in a crowd *Aco.*
     of the dark *Phos., Stram.*
     of death *Aco., Ap., Ars., Calc-c.*
     of dogs *Bell., Calc-c., Puls., Stram.*

of downward motion *Bor.*

worse in the evening *Calc-c., Caust.*

of failure *Arg-n., Lyc.*

of failing an exam or test *Gels., Lyc.*

of getting lost *Lyc.*

of glittering surfaces *Stram.*

of heights *Arg-n., Calc-c., Sul.*

of illness *Ars., Calc-c., Phos.*

of insects *Calc-c.*

of being late *Arg-n., Nat-m.*

of losing control *Ars., Gels.*

at night *Ars., Phos.*

for others *Sul.*

of public speaking *Arg-n., Gels., Lyc., Sil.*

that something bad will happen *Caust.*

of strangers *Bar-c.*

of sudden noises *Bor.*

of thunderstorms *Calc-p., Phos.*

of being touched *Arn.*

of water *Stram.*

Forgetful/memory weak (see also Dull/confused, Sluggish mentally) *Ambr., Anac., Bar-c., Calc-c., Caust., Cocc., Con., Kali-p., Lyc., Nat-c., Nit-ac., Pho-ac., Pic-ac., Sep., Verat.*

following injury *Arn.*

Fussy *Ars.*

Gentle – see Mild

Gloomy *Aur., Nat-c.*

Hurried: *Arg-n., Nux-v., Sul., Tarent.*

while walking/speaking/waiting *Arg-n.*

Hyperactive *Stram., Tarent., Verat.*

Idealistic *Ign.*

Impatient *Arg-n., Cham., Lyc., Nux-v., Sul.*

Impulsive *Arg-n., Nux-v.*

Indecisive *Bar-c., Lyc., Op.*

Indifferent to own children/family/loved ones/work *Sep.*

Indignant *Coloc., Staph.*

Insecure *Ars.*

Intellectual *Lyc., Sul.*

Introspective *Cocc., Ign., Puls.*

Irritable *Ap., Arn., Ars., Bor., Caps., Carb-v., Lyc., Nat-m., Nit-ac., Nux-v., Phos., Puls., Sep., Sil., Staph., Sul., Zinc.*

Isolated *Anac.*

Jealous *Ap., Lach.*

Jumpy *Bell., Bor., Kali-p., Nat-c., Phos., Sil.*

Lacks self-confidence *Ambr., Anac., Aur., Bar-c., Lyc., Sil., Staph.*

Lazy *Sul.*

Lively *Coff., Lach., Nat-c., Phos., Verat.*

Lonely *Aur., Puls., Stram.*

Melancholic *Calc-c.*

Memory loss after head injury *Arn.*

Memory weak – see Forgetful

Mild (gentle) *Cocc., Puls., Sil., Staph.*

Mischievous *Nux-v., Stram., Tarent.*

Moaning with the pain *Coloc.*

Moody *Ign., Lyc., Puls.*

Morose *Anac.*

Panic *Aco., Arg-n.*

Prays *Aur., Verat.*

Private *Nat-m.*

Quarrelsome *Aur., Cham., Nux-v., Sul., Tarent.*

Rage/tantrums *Bell., Cham., Stram.*
   with desire to bite/hit *Bell.*
Resentful *Nat-m., Staph.*
Restless *Aco., Ap., Arg-n., Ars.,*
   Calc-p., Coff., Coloc., Stram.,
   Sul., Tarent.
Rude *Lyc., Verat.*
Screaming with pain *Aco., Bell.,*
   Cham., Coff.
Selfish *Ars., Sul.*
Self-pitying *Calc-c., Puls.*
Sensitive *Bell., Caps., Caust., Cham.,*
   Coloc., Ign., Kali-p., Lyc.,
   Nat-c., Nat-m., Nit-ac., Nux-v.,
   Phos., Puls., Staph.
   to injustice *Caust.*
   to light *Bell., Con., Nux-v.*
   to music *Ambr., Aur., Nat-c.,*
      Nux-v., Tarent.
   to noise *Bell., Cocc., Coff., Con.,*
      Nit-ac., Nux-v., Op., Sil., Zinc.
   to pain *Aco., Cham., Cocc., Coff.,*
      Ign., Nit-ac., Nux-v., Staph.
   to rudeness *Nat-m., Nux-v.,*
      Staph.
   to smells *Nux-v.*
   to touch *Cham., Lach., Nux-v.*
Sentimental *Ign., Nux-v.*
Shy *Ambr., Bar-c., Gels., Lyc., Nat-c.,*
   Puls., Sil.
Sighing *Calc-p., Ign.*
Slow *Bar-c., Calc-c., Con., Pho-ac.,*
   Phos.
   in thinking/speaking *Pho-ac.*

Sluggish mentally *Bar-c., Calc-c.,*
   Calc-p., Carb-v., Gels., Kali-p.,
   Lach., Lyc., Nat-c., Nux-v.,
   Pho-ac., Pic-ac., Puls., Sep.,
   Sil., Sul., Verat., Zinc.
Spiteful *Nux-v.*
Stubborn *Arg-n., Calc-c., Calc-p.,*
   Cham., Nux-v., Sul., Tarent.
Stupor *Op.*
Suspicious *Anac., Lach.*
Sympathetic *Caust., Phos., Puls.*
Talkative *Lach., Stram.*
Tearful *Ap., Calc-c., Caust., Cham.,*
   Ign., Lach., Lyc., Nat-m., Puls.,
   Sep.
   cries on own *Ign., Nat-m.*
   with difficulty crying *Nat-m.*
   with a fever *Bell.*
   with involuntary weeping *Ign.*
Thinking difficult *Pic-ac.*
Thoughts active *Coff., Lach.*
Tidy *Ars., Nux-v.*
Time passes too quickly *Cocc.*
Uncommunicative *Cocc., Pho-ac.,*
   Phos., Verat., Zinc.
Unforgiving *Nat-m., Nit-ac.*
Untidy *Sul.*
Vindictive *Anac., Lach., Nit-ac.*
Whiney *Puls.*
Worse
   for mental exertion/for thinking
      Arg-n., Calc-c., Calc-p., Nat-c.,
      Pic-ac., Sil.
   on waking *Lach.*

Index of Emotional Stresses

Index of General State

Ankles weak *Nat-c., Sil.*

Appetite

changeable *Puls.*

digestion slow/poor *Calc-c.,*
Lyc., Nat-c., Nux-v., Sil.

feels very quickly full up (after
only eating a little) *Lyc.*

good *Calc-c., Phos., Sul.*

increased *Verat.*

poor/lost *Ars., Cocc., Nat-m.,*
Nux-v., Pic-ac., Sep., Sil.

poor in the morning – doesn't
want breakfast *Cham.,*
Nux-v., Phos., Zinc.

dislikes (averse to):

bread *Nat-m., Puls., Sul.*

cheese *Nit-ac.*

chicken *Nat-m.*

coffee *Calc-c.*

egg yolk *Puls.*

eggs *Sul.*

fat/fatty foods *Carb-v., Puls.*

fatty meat *Puls.*

fruit *Ign., Puls.*

hot food/drinks *Phos., Puls.*

meat *Calc-c., Sep., Sil., Sul.*

milk *Ign., Nat-c., Sep., Staph.*

onions *Lyc.*

slimy foods *Nat-m.*

sweet foods *Caust.*

water *Nux-v., Staph., Stram.*

likes (craves/desires):

alcohol *Caps., Lach., Nux-v., Sul.*

boiled eggs *Calc-c.*

chocolate *Arg-n., Lyc., Phos.*

coffee *Caps., Nux-v.*

cold drinks *Aco., Cham.*

cold drinks/food *Phos., Puls.,*
Verat.

fat/fatty foods *Nit-ac., Sul.*

fizzy drinks *Pho-ac., Phos.*

fruit *Pho-ac., Verat.*

hot food/drinks *Ars., Lyc.*

ice (in drinks etc.) *Phos.,*
Verat.

ice cream *Phos.*

indigestible things (coal,
earth, sand etc.) *Calc-c.,*
Sil.

lemon *Verat.*

lemonade *Bell., Sep.*

meat *Nux-v., Staph.*

milk (cold) *Phos.*

pepper *Caps.*

pickles *Sep.*

raw foods *Sil., Sul.*

refreshing things *Pho-ac.,*
Verat.

salt/salty foods *Arg-n.,*
Carb-v., Nat-m., Nit-ac.,
Phos., Verat.

salty and sour foods *Carb-v.,*
Nat-m., Phos., Verat.

smoked foods *Calc-p., Caust.*

sour foods *Sep., Verat.*

spicy foods *Caps., Nux-v.,*

Phos., Sul.

starchy foods *Lach., Lyc.,
Nat-m.*

sugar/sweets *Arg-n., Lyc.*

sweet foods *Arg-n., Carb-v.,
Lyc., Staph., Sul.*

sweet and sour foods *Sul.*

vinegar *Sep.*

water *Phos., Sul.*

Breath smells *Arn., Ars., Carb-v.,
Cham., Kali-p., Nit-ac., Nux-v.,
Puls., Sul.*

Clumsy *Ap., Calc-c., Caust.*

drops things *Ap.*

trips easily whilst walking *Caust.*

Cracking joints *Nit-ac.*

Cracks in skin *Calc-c., Nit-ac.*

Desires

to be fanned *Carb-v.*

fresh air *Arg-n., Aur., Carb-v.,
Lach., Puls., Sul.*

Discharges

like ammonia *Nit-ac.*

bland *Puls.*

blood-streaked *Phos.*

burning *Ars., Caust., Nit-ac.*

like egg white *Nat-m.*

smelly *Ars., Carb-v., Nit-ac., Sul.*

sour *Calc-c., Sul.*

thick *Calc-c., Puls.*

thin *Ars., Caust., Nit-ac.*

watery *Ars., Caust., Sul.*

white *Nat-m.*

yellow *Lyc., Puls., Sep.*

yellow-green *Nit-ac., Puls.*

Dislikes fresh air *Cham., Cocc.,
Coff., Ign., Nat-c., Nux-v., Sil.*

Dryness generally *Ars., Bell., Nat-m.*

Expression

anxious *Aco., Ars., Bor., Verat.*

confused *Lyc.*

fierce *Bell.*

frightened *Aco., Phos., Stram.*

haggard/suffering *Ars.*

sleepy *Op.*

vacant *Pho-ac.*

Eyelids heavy *Caust., Gels.*

Eyes

glassy *Op.*

sensitive to bright light *Aco.,
Ars., Bar-c., Nat-m., Sul.*

shining *Bell.*

Face

cold *Carb-v., Verat.*

drawn *Lyc., Verat.*

hot *Cham.*

flushed *Op.*

pale *Ars., Calc-c., Calc-p., Carb-v.,
Lyc., Nat-c., Pho-ac., Sep.,
Verat., Zinc.*

pale with dark rings around
eyes *Anac.*

pasty *Sep.*

puffy *Ap.*

red (flushed) *Aco., Ap., Bell.,
Caps., Lach., Op., Sul.*

in spots *Bell., Cham., Phos.,
Sul.*

one-sided *Cham.*

sallow *Carb-v., Nat-m., Sul.*

Glands

hard/lumpy *Con.*

sensitive *Bar-c., Bell., Con., Phos.*

swollen *Bar-c., Bell., Calc-c.,
Calc-p., Con., Lyc., Puls., Sil.,
Sul.*

Heavy feeling *Gels., Pic-ac., Sep.*
Lips
    burning *Caps.*
    chapped *Carb-v., Nat-m., Sul.*
    cracked *Ars., Caps., Carb-v.,*
        Nat-m., Sep., Sul.
    dry *Ars., Puls., Sul.*
    licks them *Ars.*
    pale *Ars.*
    red *Sul.*
    swollen *Ap., Caps.*
Mouth dry *Ars., Caps., Nat-m., Puls.,*
    Sep., Sul., Verat.
Onset of pain/complaint
    sudden *Aco., Bell., Verat.*
    slow *Gels.*
Pains
    absent *Op., Stram.*
    appear and disappear suddenly
        Bell., Nit-ac.
    in bones *Aur., Nit-ac., Pho-ac.*
    boring *Aur.*
    burning *Aco., Ap., Ars., Caps.,*
        Carb-v., Caust., Phos., Sul.
    better for heat *Ars.*
    constricting *Ambr., Anac., Ign.*
    cramping *Anac., Calc-c., Coloc.,*
        Nux-v.
    flying around *Nit-ac.*
    in muscles *Coloc.*
    needle-like/splinter-like *Arg-n.,*
        Nit-ac.
    neuralgic *Coloc., Ign.*
    in parts lain on *Puls.*
    pressing *Anac., Carb-v., Lach.,*
        Nat-m., Phos., Sep., Verat.,
        Zinc.
    sharp *Bor., Con., Kali-p., Lach.*

shooting *Bell.*
sore, bruised *Arn., Gels.*
stinging *Ap.*
stitching *Arg-n., Calc-c., Coloc.,*
    Sep., Sil., Staph.
tearing *Aur., Lyc., Nat-m., Sep.*
throbbing *Bell.*
unbearable *Aco., Cham., Coff.*
wandering *Puls.*
with screaming/moaning *Aco.*
Pupils
    contracted *Op.*
    dilated *Bell., Stram.*
Sensation of
    a band or a plug *Anac.*
    constriction *Bell., Nit-ac., Nux-v.,*
        Stram.
    a hair on the tongue *Sil.*
    tension *Nux-v.*
Senses
    acute *Ars., Bell., Cocc., Coff.,*
        Nux-v., Phos.
    dull *Op.*
    sense of smell lost *Calc-c.*
    weakened *Anac.*
Sensitive to downward motion *Bor.*
Slowness (of children)
    to grow *Bar-c., Calc-p.*
    to learn *Bar-c., Calc-p., Lyc.*
    to talk *Nat-m.*
    to teethe *Calc-c., Calc-p., Sil.*
    to walk *Calc-c., Calc-p., Caust.,*
        Nat-m.
Sweat
    absent during fever *Bell., Gels.*
    acidic *Sil.*
    clammy *Cham., Lyc., Pho-ac.,*
        Phos., Verat.

on closing eyes *Con.*
cold *Carb-v., Cocc., Lyc., Sep., Verat.*
on covered parts of the body *Aco., Bell.*
feet (smelly) *Bar-c., Lyc., Sil., Sul.*
from fright *Gels., Op.*
on head *Calc-c., Sil.*
hot *Aco., Cham., Con., Ign., Nux-v., Op., Sep.*
from mental exertion *Calc-c., Lach., Sep., Staph.*
one-sided *Nux-v., Puls.*
from pain *Lach., Nat-c., Sep.*
profuse *Calc-c., Carb-v., Kali-p., Lyc., Op., Pho-ac., Sep., Sil., Sul., Zinc.*
on single parts of the body *Cocc., Ign., Nit-ac., Op., Phos., Puls., Sep.*
during sleep *Calc-c., Con., Sil., Sul.*
from slightest physical exertion *Calc-c., Cocc., Kali-p., Nat-c., Nit-ac., Phos., Sep., Sul.*
smelly *Lyc., Nit-ac., Nux-v., Puls., Sep., Sil., Sul.*
sour *Calc-c., Lyc., Nit-ac., Sep., Sil., Sul., Zinc.*
better for uncovering *Cham., Lyc.*
when tired *Kali-p.*
worse at night *Con., Puls., Sil.*
Swelling of affected parts *Ap., Bell.*
Symptoms
changeable *Puls.*
contradictory *Ign.*
left-sided *Arg-n., Caps., Lach., Sep., Sul.*

start on the left and move to the right *Lach.*
one-sided *Anac., Kali-p., Pho-ac.*
right-sided *Ap., Ars., Aur., Bell., Bor., Calc-c., Coloc., Con., Lyc., Nux-v., Puls.*
start on the right side and move to the left *Ap., Lyc.*
Taste in mouth
bad *Calc-c., Puls., Sul.*
bitter *Aco., Ars., Carb-v., Coloc., Nat-m., Nux-v., Puls., Sul.*
metallic *Cocc., Nat-c., Zinc.*
rotten eggs *Arn.*
salty *Nat-m.*
sour *Arg-n., Calc-c., Lyc., Nat-c., Nux-v., Phos.*
unpleasant (putrid) *Anac.*
Tense feeling *Nux-v.*
Thin *Calc-p., Sil.*
Thirstless *Ap., Bell., Gels., Pho-ac., Puls.*
Thirsty *Aco., Arg-n., Ars., Caust., Phos., Sil., Stram., Sul., Tarent., Verat.*
extremely, with the pains *Cham., Nat-m.*
at night *Coff.*
for large quantities *Nat-m., Phos., Sul.*
for sips *Ars.*
Tongue
burning *Caps.*
cracked *Nit-ac.*
fiery red *Ap.*
painful blister/pimple on tip *Caust.*
red *Bell.*

red stripe down centre (white
    edges) *Caust.*
red-edged *Ars., Sul.*
red-tipped *Arg-n., Ars., Sul.*
sore *Nit-ac.*
strawberry (red with white
    spots) *Bell.*

white coated *Ars., Bell., Calc-c.,*
    Puls., Sul.
yellow coated *Puls.*
Trembling *Cocc., Gels.*
Twitchy *Zinc.*
White spots on fingernails *Zinc.*

Generally feels better for

bathing *Ars., Phos., Puls.*
cold *Ap., Arg-n., Sul., Verat.*
cold drinks *Ambr., Caust., Phos.*
cool air *Ap.*
eating *Anac., Caust., Ign., Nat-c.,*
    Sep.
evening *Aur.*
being fanned *Carb-v.*
fasting *Cham., Con., Nat-m.*
fresh air *Aco., Arg-n., Lach., Lyc.,*
    Puls., Sul.
heat *Ars., Calc-c., Caust., Ign.,*
    Kali-p., Nux-v., Sil.
hot bath *Ars., Phos.*
hot drinks *Ars., Nux-v.*
light *Stram.*
lying doubled-up *Coloc.*
lying down *Ars., Bell., Calc-c., Cocc.,*
    Nat-m., Nit-ac., Nux-v., Pic-ac.
massage *Calc-c., Nat-c., Phos.*
during menstrual period *Lach.*
movement *Aur., Puls.*

pressure *Bell., Puls.*
    hard pressure *Coloc.*
removal of pressure *Ambr.*
rest *Bell., Gels., Kali-p., Nat-m.,*
    Nux-v., Pic-ac., Sep.
running *Sep.*
sea air *Nat-m.*
sitting down *Nux-v.*
good sleep *Pho-ac., Phos.*
passing stool *Bor.*
sweating *Gels., Nat-m.*
touch *Calc-c.*
uncovering *Cham.*
urinating *Gels.*
vigorous exercise *Sep.*
walk in the fresh air *Arg-n.*
walking fast *Sep.*
walking slowly in fresh air *Aur.,*
    Puls.
warmth of bed *Ars., Caust., Lyc.,*
    Nux-v.
wet weather *Caust.*
wrapping up head *Sil.*

Generally feels worse for

1.00 a.m. *Ars.*
10.00 a.m. *Bor.*
10.00–11.00 a.m. *Nat-m., Sul.*
3.00 p.m. *Bell.*
3.00–5.00 p.m. *Ap.*
4.00–8.00 p.m. *Lyc.*
during afternoon *Lyc.*
alcohol *Con., Lach., Nux-v., Sul.*
bathing *Sul.*
change of temperature *Ars.*
changes in the weather *Caust., Phos., Sil., Sul.*
   to dry *Caust.*
getting chilled *Puls.*
coffee *Caust., Cham., Ign., Nux-v.*
cold *Ars., Aur., Bar-c., Calc-c., Calc-p., Caps., Caust., Kali-p., Nit-ac., Pho-ac., Phos., Sep., Sil., Tarent., Verat.*
cold food/drinks *Nux-v.*
cold, wet weather *Ars., Calc-p.*
company *Ambr.*
conversation *Ambr.*
damp *Ars., Calc-c., Calc-p., Sil.*
darkness *Calc-c., Stram.*
draughts *Bell., Calc-c., Calc-p., Caps., Caust., Sil.*
drinking *Coloc.*
eating
   after *Calc-p., Coloc., Con., Nat-m., Nux-v., Zinc.*
   before *Nat-c.*
in the evening *Caust., Cham., Lyc., Pho-ac., Phos., Zinc.*

exertion
   mental *Anac., Calc-c., Kali-p., Pic-ac., Sep.*
   physical *Ars., Calc-c., Carb-v., Cocc., Con., Gels., Kali-p., Nat-c., Nat-m., Pic-ac., Sep., Staph., Sul.*
excitement *Kali-p.*
fasting *Anac., Calc-c., Lyc., Phos., Sep., Sil., Staph., Sul., Zinc.*
fatty/rich foods *Carb-v., Puls.*
flatulent foods *Lyc.*
fresh air *Calc-c., Calc-p., Coff., Nat-c., Nit-ac., Sil.*
frosty/snowy weather *Con., Sep.*
fruit *Coloc., Verat.*
heat *Ap., Arg-n., Cham., Coff., Gels., Lach., Nat-m., Puls., Sul.*
hot baths *Nat-m.*
humidity *Carb-v.*
jarring movement *Arn., Bell., Nit-ac.*
lying on the injured part *Arn.*
lying down *Aur.*
menstrual period
   before *Lach., Puls., Sep.*
   during *Puls., Sep.*
   after *Sep.*
mental exertion – see exertion, mental
after midnight *Ars.*
for milk *Calc-c., Sul.*
in the morning *Pho-ac., Phos.*
   on waking *Ambr., Phos.*
   mid-morning *Nat-c., Nat-m.*
movement *Cocc.*

moving the affected part *Arn.*
at night *Aco., Arg-n., Ars., Aur.,*
    Coff., Con., Nit-ac., Puls., Sep.,
    Zinc.
onions *Lyc.*
phyical exertion – see exertion,
    physical
pressure *Ap., Lach., Lyc.*
rest *Aur.*
sea air *Nat-m., Sep.*
after a sleep *Lach.*
   afternoon nap *Staph.*
during sleep *Op.*
standing *Sul.*
before stool *Bor.*
stuffy heat *Ap.*
in a stuffy room *Lyc., Puls., Sul.*
sugar/sweets *Arg-n.*
sun *Nat-c., Nat-m., Puls.*
sweating *Cham., Pho-ac., Sep.*
during thunderstorm *Nat-c.*

tight clothing *Arg-n., Lach., Lyc.,*
    Nux-v.
tobacco *Ign., Nux-v., Staph.*
touch *Aco., Ap., Arn., Cham., Cocc.,*
    Nit-ac., Sep., Sil., Staph.,
    Tarent.
at twilight *Phos., Puls.*
for being uncovered *Sil.*
on waking *Ars., Lach., Nit-ac.*
walking *Nit-ac.*
   in the fresh air *Caust., Cocc.*
   in the wind *Sep.*
warmth of bed *Cham., Op., Sul.*
wet compresses *Cham.*
wet feet *Nux-v., Puls., Sil.*
wet weather *Calc-c., Puls., Sil.*
wet head *Puls.*
wind *Cham., Lyc., Nux-v., Phos.,*
    Puls., Sil.
wine *Coff., Zinc.*
winter *Aur.*

Index of Physical Stresses

(The list of abbreviations on p. 355 indicates those that are covered in detail in the Homeopathic Remedies section.)

Environmental Stresses (see pages 170–182)

Aluminium *Alu., Lyc., Plb.*
Cadmium *Cad-s.*
Chlorine *Chlorum*
Copper *Cupr.*
Dust (plastic/brick/house) *Brom., Sil.*
Electricity *Elect., Phos.*
Fumes
    exhaust (i.e. pollution) *Ac-sul., Carb-v., Petr., Plb.*

gas/coal/charcoal *Carbn-s., Carb-v., Op.*
General chemical sensitivities *Ars., Hep-s., Merc-s., Nit-ac., Sil.*
Lead *Alu., Caust.*
Nickel *Nicc.*
Mercury *Hep-s., Merc-s., Nit-ac.*
Radiation *Cad-s., Rad-br.*
Smoke *Ign., Spig.*

Everyday Stimulants and Sedatives (see pages 182–189)

Alcohol *Nux-v., Op., Sul., Sul-ac.*
Chocolate *Choc., Lyc.*
Coffee/caffeine *Cham., Coff., Ign., Nux-v.*
Soft drinks *Calc-p., Coff., Nux-v.*

Spicy foods *Nux-v.*
Sugar/sweets *Arg-n., Lyc., Sul.*
Tea *Alu., Chin., Coff., Nux-v., Thea*
Tobacco *Calad., Nux-v., Staph., Tabac.*

Food (see pages 189–201)

Digestion sluggish *Ant-c., Calc-c., Carb-v., Chin., Lyc., Nat-c., Nux-v.*
Fast metabolism (tendency to

hypoglycaemia) *Phos., Sul.*
Food poisoning *Ars., Carb-v., Puls., Verat.*
    rotten eggs, fish, vegetables,

meat etc. *Carb-v.*
rotten meat *Ars., Puls.*
rotten fruit *Verat.*
shellfish (oysters etc.) *Lyc.*
bad water *Ars.*
Food sensitivities/aggravations
bread/wheat *Nat-m.*
fatty, rich foods *Carb-v., Puls.*
flatulent foods (i.e. beans,
    cabbage, onions etc.) *Lyc.*

fruit *Chin., Verat.*
ice cream *Ars., Puls.*
junk, or processed food *Alu.,*
    Mag-c., Nux-v.
milk *Calc-c., Mag-c., Mag-m.,*
    Nat-c.
salt *Nat-m:, Phos.*
sour/acidic foods *Ant-c.*
Over-eating *Ant-c., Carb-v., Nux-v.*
Slow metabolism *Calc-c.*

Illness (see pages 201–208)

Convalescing from illness *Calc-p.,*
    Carb-v., Chin., Gels., Kali-p.,
    Phos-ac., Puls.
Growth spurt, pains in growing
    children *Calc-p., Pho-ac., Phos.*

Loss of body fluids *Carb-v., Chin.,*
    Phos-ac.
Teething (baby teeth/2nd teeth/
    wisdoms) *Calc-c., Calc-p.,*
    Cham., Sil.

Injury (see pages 209–215)

Bites and stings (animals and
    insects) *Apis, Calad., Hyp.,*
    Led.
Burns and scalds *Ars., Canth.,*
    Caust., Kali-bi.
Electric shock *Phos.*
Injury in general (from accident or
    surgery etc.) *Arn., Bell-p.,*
    Bry., Calc-p., Calend., Con.,
    Hep-s., Hyp., Led., Nat-s.,
    Ran-b., Rhus-t., Ruta, Sil.,
    Staph., Symph.
to bones *Arn., Bry., Calc-p., Ruta.*
    Sil., Symph.
painful *Symph.*

to the periosteum (covering
    to bones) *Ruta*
fractures which are slow to
    heal *Calc-p., Sil.*
bruises (i.e. to muscles/soft
    tissue) *Arn., Bell-p., Led.*
with lumps remaining *Bell-p.*
with discoloration *Led.*
with swelling *Arn.*
to the coccyx *Hyp.*
to the eyes *Hyp., Led., Symph.*
to glands (including breast or
    testicle) *Bell-p., Con.*
with lumps remaining *Bell-p.,*
    Con.

to the head *Arn.*, *Nat-s.*

incised wounds from an accident or surgey (including dental work, childbirth etc.) *Calend.*, *Hep-s.*, *Hyp.*, *Led.*, *Sil.*, *Staph.*

with great pain *Calend.*, *Hyp.*

to prevent sepsis *Hyp.*, *Led*

become inflamed *Hep-s.*, *Sil.*

to joints (see also strains/sprains)

Bry., *Ran-b.*, *Rhus-t.*, *Ruta.*

to the neck (whiplash) *Bry.*, *Hyp.*, *Rhus-t.*

to nerves *Hyp.*, *Ran-b.*

to the spine *Hyp.*

to tendons/ligaments *Rhus-t.*

Shock after injury *Aco.*, *Arn.*, *Op.*, *Stram.*

Splinters *Sil.*

Medication (see pages 215–223)

Antibiotics *Nux-v.*

Anaesthetics

local *Adren.*

general *Op.*, *Phos.*

Antacids *Alu.*

Aspirin *Calc-c.*

Chemotherapy *Cad-s.*

Drugs in general *Nit-ac.*, *Nux-v.*, *Sul.*

Contraceptive pill/HRT *Puls.*, *Sep.*

Iron *Puls.*

Laxatives *Alu.*, *Nux-v.*

Radiotherapy *Cad-s.*, *Rad-br.*

Steroids *Cort.*

Vaccination *Sil.*, *Sul.*, *Thu.*

Physical Stress and Strain (see pages 223–236)

Altitude sickness *Arn.*, *Coca*, *Cocc.*

Repetitive strain (stress) injury *Ran-b.*, *Ruta*, *Zinc.*

Strain/over-exertion *Arg-n.*, *Arn.*, *Bell-p.*, *Bry.*, *Calc-c.*, *Carb-an.*, *Led.*, *Ran-b.*, *Rhus-t.*, *Ruta*, *Stront-c.*

ankles *Calc-c.*, *Led.*, *Rhus-t.*, *Ruta.* *Stront-c.*

arm/shoulder *Ran-b.*

elbow (tennis elbow) *Ruta*

eyes *Ruta*

hips/back *Calc-c.*, *Rhus-t.*

joints (including sprains) *Arn.*,

Bry., *Calc-c.*, *Led.*, *Rhus-t.*, *Ruta*, *Stront-c.*

with swelling *Arn.*, *Led.*, *Stront-c.*

knee *Rhus-t.*, *Ruta*

from lifting *Calc-c.*, *Carb-an.*, *Rhus-t.*

general physical (muscular) *Arn.*, *Bell-p.*, *Rhust-t.*

from travel (including jetlag) *Arn.*, *Cocc.*, *Gels.*, *Rhus-t.*

voice *Arg-n.*

wrist *Calc-c.*, *Carb-an.*, *Rhus-t.*, *Ruta*

Rest, Relaxation and Sleep (see pages 236–246)

Difficulty getting to sleep *Calc-p.,*
Coff., Kali-p., Nux-v., Zinc.
from over-excitement *Coff.,*
Kali-p.
from tension/nervous strain
Calc-p., Kali-p., Nux-v., Zinc.
Complaints from loss of sleep or

disturbed sleep (shift work,
nursing the sick,
breast-feeding, jet lag,
overwork, mental strain etc.)
Cocc., Nit-ac., Nux-v.
Tension from a sedentary lifestyle
Nux-v., Sul.

Weather (see pages 246–251)

Change of temperature or change
of weather (any) *Phos.*
hot to cold *Dulc., Rhus-t., Sil.*
cold to hot *Bry., Kali-s., Sul.*
to dry *Caust.*
Getting chilled *Aco., Ars., Hep.,*
Nit-ac., Nux-v., Sil.
Cloudy weather *Phos., Rhod.,*
Rhus-t.
Cold in general *Aco., Ars., Hep.,*
Nit-ac., Nux-v., Sep., Sil.
Cold dry weather *Caust., Hep.,*
Nux-v.
Cold wind *Aco., Cham., Hep.,*
Nux-v., Rhus-t., Sil.
Damp, wet weather *Bar-c., Calc-c.,*
Dulc., Rhus-t.
Drafts *Calc-p., Hep-s., Nux-v., Sil.*
Extremes of temperature (to heat
and cold) *Merc-s., Nat-c.*
Foggy weather *Rhus-t.*

Frosty weather *Agar., Sep.*
Heat in general *Ant-c., Bry., Carb-v.,*
Kali-s., Lach., Nat-c., Nat-m.,
Puls., Sul.
Humidity *Carb-v., Lach.*
Sea air *Nat-m., Sep.*
Snow *Con., Sep.*
Sun *Ant-c., Nat-c., Nat-m., Puls.*
with sunstroke *Bell., Glon.,*
Nat-c., Sul.
Swimming
in the sea *Ars., Mag-m.*
in cold water *Mag-p., Rhus-t.*
Thunderstorms *Nat-c., Phos., Rhod.*
Wet weather *Ars., Calc-p., Nux-v.,*
Rhus-t., Sil.
Getting wet *Barc-c., Calc-c., Puls.,*
Rhus-t., Sep.
feet *Puls., Sil.*
head *Bell., Puls.*

APPENDICES

Glossary

Acute illness
An illness that is generally short lived. It has three stages: the *incubation period*, where there may be no symptoms; the *acute stage* when the disease itself surfaces; the *convalescent* stage when a person usually improves.

Aggravation
A temporary worsening of symptoms during the process of cure. It is a common occurrence in the constitutional treatment of chronic disease, but relatively rare in the treatment of acute disease.

Allopathy
From the Greek root *allo* meaning 'other' or 'opposite', and *pathos* meaning 'suffering'. A term coined by Hahnemann to describe orthodox medicine and to distinguish it from homeopathy.

Antidote
Anything that counteracts the effect of a homeopathic remedy, which may hamper or prevent the remedy from working.

Burn out
A breakdown as a result of overstress which has 'used up' mental, emotional and/or physical reserves of energy.

Case taking
The homeopathic interview in which specific and detailed symptoms are elicited from the patient.

Centesimal
The scale of dilution of substances based on diluting one part in a hundred.

Chronic illness
Chronic disease develops slowly and does not usually resolve itself without some sort of healing intervention. It is usually accompanied by a general deterioration in health.

Constitution
A person's overall state of health which includes inherited tendencies, their personal history, past medical treatments, lifestyle and environmental factors, etc.

Constitutional treatment
This aims to treat the whole person rather than the symptoms alone. In so doing it enhances the general level of health rather than simply eliminating symptoms.

Cure
The homeopath defines cure as more than the disappearance of a pain or a disease alone. It implies a sense of well-being on all levels (mental, emotional *and* physical) and an increased resistance to disease.

Defence mechanism see Immunity.

Differentiate
The art of distinguishing between remedies where more than one is indicated, to find the 'simillimum' or the remedy whose picture best fits that of the sick person.

Disease
'Dis-ease' – a departure from our normal healthy self that limits our physical, mental or emotional freedom.

Distress
The point where a person's ability to deal with stress becomes compromised and they begin to fail to adapt to a stressful situation (or situations).

Eustress
Happy or pleasant stress, i.e. stresses which stretch us in health-enhancing ways.

General Adaptation Syndrome (G.A.S.)
This is the body's stress response cycle (from when it becomes stressed to the way that stress manifests itself in terms of symptoms).

Healing crisis see Aggravation.

Homeostasis
This means literally 'staying power' and refers to the body's natural adaptive (self-regulating) powers to produce stability, for example to sweat when overheated in order to cool the body down.

Hormonal system
Hormones are specific chemical messengers produced by an endocrine gland and secreted into the blood to regulate and coordinate the functioning of the body's organs and systems. Hormones carry messages to 'act' or 'advance'.

Immunity
The strength of our immune system determines our resistance to disease. It is partly inherited and partly affected by the lives we lead.

Infinitesimal dose see Minimum dose.

Laws of Cure
These are the principles that govern the healing process. They apply mostly in constitutional treatment.

Materia Medica
A dictionary of homeopathic remedy pictures, giving detailed indications for their uses.

Miasm
A block to health, usually left by a disease. This can be inherited or acquired and is an obstacle to cure.

Minimum dose
A potentized substance.

Nervous system
The nerves, along with the hormonal system, are the principal coordinating systems of the body. Nerves send messages (via hormones) to 'relax' or 'retreat'.

Overstress
Too much stress.

Polycrest
A remedy which has produced a wide range of symptoms in the provings
and can therefore treat a wide range of health problems.

Potency
This denotes the strength of the remedy according to the number of times it
has been diluted and succussed (potentized).

Proving
The testing of a substance on healthy volunteers to discover the symptoms it
is capable of producing (and therefore able to cure).

Remedy picture
The collection of symptoms that a remedy produces in a proving, including
mental and emotional, general and physical symptoms. It is this totality of
symptoms that is called the remedy picture.

Repertorize
To look up symptoms in the Repertory to find the remedy (or remedies) that
is common to a particular collection of symptoms.

Repertory
An index of symptoms (based on the Materia Medica) with a list of remedies
indicated for each symptom.

Sac lac
Saccharum lactose, the sugar of (cow's) milk which is the base of
homeopathic tablets.

Simillimum
The simillimum is the remedy that matches the symptom picture of the
patient most closely. Based on the law *Similia similibus curentur* ('Let like be
cured with like'), the principle states that a substance is capable of curing a
sick person of the same symptoms it is capable of producing in a healthy
person.

Specific remedies
Remedies that are given for a particular symptom or disease *without* taking
the whole person into account, for example *Arnica* for bruises and *Hypericum*
for injuries to nerves.

Stress
Anything that produces mental, emotional or physical strain or tension. The stress itself may be mental, emotional or physical. Hans Seyle defines stress as the rate of wear and tear in the body; the nonspecific response of the body to any demand made on it (pleasant or unpleasant).

Stressor
That which produces stress: stressors can be physical, mental or emotional.

Succussion
The process of vigorous shaking that accompanies dilution during the preparation of a homeopathic remedy.

Suppression
The driving inward of disease(s), so that a person experiences more serious symptoms that those originally presented, and there is a general deterioration in health.

Susceptibility
Vulnerability to disease. A person has to be susceptible, or weakened in some way, for a disease to develop.

Symptom
Any change in the body's functioning on a mental, emotional or physical level. Usually associated either with a particular disease or a specific stress.

Symptom picture
The whole range (or totality) of symptoms experienced by a person that emerges during the case taking. The symptom picture is matched to a remedy picture with the same or similar symptoms.

Tincture
A solution of a substance in alcohol which is used as the starting material for homeopathic medicines. Some pharmacies call these mother tinctures.

Trituration
The process of grinding an insoluble substance with saccharum lactose in order to render it soluble.

Understress
Too little stress.

Vital force
A term used by Hahnemann to describe the energy that animates all living beings. It is the vital force that is stimulated by a correctly chosen potentized remedy, and conversely the vital force that is stressed during the development of disease.

The Holmes and Rahe Stress Scale

The Holmes and Rahe Stress Scale Chart supplies a useful rule-of-thumb guide to stress influences. I have also included a more recent scale that has been modified (second column). A score of 300 or more points in any one year means that approximately 80 per cent of people will fall ill; 150–299 means that about 50 per cent will fall ill and a score of under 150 means that about 30 per cent will become ill. Stresses can be cumulative and it may be useful to add up your stresses for the year before and compare scores.

If you have a low stress tolerance you may find that levels as low as 150 are enough to cause you distress.

If you have a high stress tolerance you may find that levels need to hit the 300 or even 400 mark before you start to crack.

You can use it as a guide and in any case go easy if your scores are in the mid 200s. You may be heading for trouble.

In a way this can be superficial. For example, for some people the death of a parent is meaningless if that person had been ill for a long time and they had come to terms with their dying and in fact grieved for their dying as they died. Then death might bring a sense of relief, the end of a stressful time.

*	**	Grown ups
150	100	Death of partner
60	73	Divorce
60		Menopause
60	65	Marital separation
60	63	Detention in jail (or other institution)
60	63	Death of a close family member

* Holmes and Rahe Social Readjustment Rating Scale (copyright © 1976 Thomas H Holmes M.D., Dept of Psychiatry and Behavioural Sciences, University of Washington School of Medicine, Seattle, Wa. 98195)
** Stress Scale modified (S. Burns, M.D., *How to Survive Unbearable Stress*, I-MED Press, 11823 E. Slauson Avenue, Suite 40, Santa Fe Springs, CA 90670)

45	53	Serious personal injury or illness
45	50	Marriage (or establishing life partnership)
45	47	Dismissal from work
40	45	Marital reconciliation
40	45	Retirement from work
40	44	Change in health or behaviour of a family member
35		Working more than 40 hours per week
35	40	Pregnancy (or causing pregnancy)
35	39	Sexual difficulties
35	39	Gain of new family member (through birth, adoption, marriage, i.e. step children, etc.)
35	39	Major business readjustment (merger, bankruptcy, re-organization, etc.) or work role change
36		Changing to a different line of work
35	38	Change in financial state (a lot worse or a lot better off)
35		Change in number of arguments with spouse (a lot more or a lot less)
25	32	Major mortgage (i.e. purchasing a home or business, etc.)
30		Foreclosure of mortgage or loan
30		Death of a close friend
25		Sleep less than 8 hours per night
25	29	Change in responsibilities at work (promotion, demotion, transfer, etc.)
25	29	Son or daughter leaving home (to go to college, or to marry, etc.)
25	29	Trouble with in-laws and/or children
25	28	Outstanding personal achievement
20	26	Partner begins or stops work
20	26	Beginning or ending formal schooling
20	25	Change in living conditions (building a new home, renovating home, having visitors to stay, deterioration of home or neighbourhood)
20	24	Change in personal habits (diet, exercise, smoking, etc.)
20	23	Trouble with boss
20		Chronic allergies
15	20	Change in work hours or conditions
15	20	Change in residence (moving house)
15		Presently in pre-menstrual period
15	20	Changing to a new school

15	19	Change in recreation (more or less social activities)
15	19	Changes in religious activities
15	18	Change in social activities (clubs, films, visiting friends, etc.)
10	17	Minor mortgage or loan (less than £10,000 i.e. buying a car, video/TV, etc.)
10	16	Change in sleeping habits (more or less sleep or sleeping different hours, i.e. with shift work)
10	15	Change in number of family get-togethers (more or less than usual)
10	15	Change in eating habits (more or less than usual or eating different foods)
10	13	Holiday
10	12	Christmas
5	11	Minor violations of the law (including parking tickets)

Kids

150	Death of a parent
60	Divorce of parents
60	Puberty
60	Pregnancy (in adolescents living at home)
60	Breakup with boyfriend or girlfriend
60	Detention in jail (or other institution – including being fostered or put in a home)
60	Death of family member (other than parent or boyfriend/girlfriend)
55	Broken engagement
50	Engagement
45	Serious personal injury or illness
45	Marriage
45	Entering college/university or beginning next level of school
45	Change in independence or responsibility
45	Any drug and/or alcohol use
45	Expelled from school
40	Reconciliation with family or boy/girlfriend
40	Trouble at school
40	Serious health problem of family member
35	Working while attending school

35   Working more than 40 hours a week (including school work)

35   Changing course of study

35   Change in frequency of 'dating'

35   Sexual adjustment problems (including confusion over sexual identity)

35   Gain of a new family member (new baby or new step-parent and/ or step siblings)

35   Change in work responsibilities

30   Change in financial state

30   Death of a close friend (not a family member)

30   Change to a different kind of work

30   Change in number of arguments with family or friends or boy/ girlfriend

25   Sleeping less than 8 hours per night

25   Trouble with in-laws or boyfriend's or girlfriend's family

25   Outstanding personal achievement (awards, exams, etc.)

25   Parents start or stop working

20   Beginning or ending school

20   Change in living conditions (visitors in the home, renovating house, change in flat mates, etc.)

20   Change in personal habits (start or stop a habit like smoking, or dieting, etc.)

20   Chronic allergies

20   Trouble with boss at work

15   Change in work hours

15   Change in residence

15   Change to a new school

15   Presently in pre-menstrual period

15   Change in religious activity

10   Going into debt (you or your family)

10   Change in frequency of family get-togethers

10   Holiday

10   Christmas (winter holiday season)

5   Minor violation of the law

Reprinted by permission of Pergamon Press from *Holmes and Rahe Social Readjustment Rating Scale*, Thomas H. Holmes, *Journal of Psychosomatic Research*, vol. 11, pp. 213–18, Copyright 1967 by Elsevier Science Inc.

Organizations

Age Concern England
Astral House, 126–8 London Road, London SW16 4ER. Tel: 0181 679 8000.

Ainsworths Homeopathic Pharmacy
36 New Cavendish Street, London W1M 7LH. Tel: 0171 935 5330, 0171 487 5253 (24-hour answering machine service).

Al-Anon For Relatives
61 Great Dover Street, London SE1 4YF. Tel: 0171 403 0888

Alcoholics Anonymous
PO Box 1, Stonebow House, Stonebow, York YO1 2NJ. Tel: 01904 644 026.

Anti-Bullying Campaign
6 Borough High Street, London SE1. Tel: 0171 378 1446.

British Acupuncture Association (for register of acupuncturists)
34 Alderney Street, London SW1V 4EU. Tel: 0171 834 1012.

British Association for Counselling (for register of counsellors)
1 Regent Place, Rugby, Warwicks CV21 2PJ. Tel: 01788 578 328.

British Association of Psychotherapists
37 Mapesbury Road, London NW2 4HJ. Tel: 0181 452 9823.

British Chiropractic Association
29 Whitley Street, Reading, Berks RG2 0EG. Tel: 01734 757 557.

British Holistic Medical Association
Roland Thomas House, Royal Shrewsbury Hospital South, Shrewsbury SY3 8HF. Tel: 01743 261 155.

British Homeopathic Association (for doctors, vets or dentists who practice homeopathy)
27a Devonshire Street, London W1N 1RJ. Tel: 0171 935 2163.

British Hypnotherapy Association
67 Upper Berkeley Street, London W1H 7DH. Tel: 0171 723 4443.

The British Nutrition Foundation
High Holborn House, 52–4 High Holborn, London WC1V 6RQ. Tel: 0171 404 6504.

Compassionate Friends
53 North Street, Bristol BS3 1EN. Tel: 0117 953 9639.

Council for Complementary and Alternative Medicine
Suite D, Park House, 206–8 Latimer Road, London W10 6RE. Tel: 0181 968 3862.

Cruse Bereavement Care
Cruse House, 126 Sheen Road, Richmond, Surrey TW9 1UR. Tel: 0181 940 4818/9046.

Family Welfare Association
501–5 Kingsland Road, London E8 4AU. Tel: 0171 254 6251.

General Council of Osteopaths (for register of osteopaths)
56 London Street, Reading, Berks RG1 4SQ. Tel: 01734 576 585.

Gingerbread Association for One Parent Families
16 Clerkenwell Close, London EC1 0AA. Tel: 0171 336 8183/8184.

Health Rights (advice and support for patients)
Unit 405, Brixton Small Business Centre, 444 Brixton Road, London SW9 8EJ. Tel: 0171 501 9856.

Helios Homeopathic Pharmacy
97 Camden Road, Tunbridge Wells, Kent TN1 2QR. Tel: 01892 537 254, 01892 536 393 (24-hour answering service).

MIND
Granta House, 15–19 Broadway, Stratford, London E15 4BQ. Tel: 0181 519 2122.

National Aids Helpline
Tel: Freephone 0800 567 123.

Relaxation for Living
12 New Street, Chipping Norton, Oxon OX7 5LJ. Tel: 01608 646 100.

Samaritans (local number in your directory)
46 Marshall Street, London W1V 1LR. Tel: 0171 734 2800.

Society of Teachers of the Alexander Technique (for a list of teachers)
20 London House, 266 Fulham Road, London SW10 9EL. Tel: 0171 351 0828.

Stillbirth and Neonatal Death Society (SANDS)
28 Portland Place, London W1N 3DE. Tel: 0171 436 5881.

Westminster Pastoral Foundation (national counselling service)
23 Kensington Square, London W8 5HN. Tel: 0171 937 6956.

Women's Health Information Centre
52 Featherstone Street, London EC1Y 8RT. Tel: 0171 251 6580.

Further Reading

HOMEOPATHY

Blackie, Margery, *The Challenge of Homeopathy* (Unwin Hyman, 1981)

Boyd, Hamish, *Introduction to Homeopathic Medicine* (Beaconsfield, 1981)

Coulter, Harris, *Homeopathic Science and Modern Medicine: The Physics of Healing with Microdoses* (North Atlantic Books, 1987)

Cummings, Stephen and **Ullman**, Dana, *Everybody's Guide to Homeopathic Medicines* (James P. Tarcher, 1984)

Lockie, Andrew, *Homeopathy, The Principles and Practice of Treatment* (Dorling Kindersley, 1995)

Panos, Maesimund and **Heimlich**, Jane, *Homeopathic Medicine at Home* (Corgi, 1980)

Shepherd, Dorothy, *Magic of the Minimum Dose* (Health Science Press, 1964)

Vithoulkas, George, *Homeopathy, Medicine for the New Man* (Thorsons, 1985)
  The Science of Homeopathy (Grove Press, 1980)

STRESS

Burns, S. L., *How to Survive Unbearable Stress* (I-MED Press), 11823 E. Slauson Avenue, Suite 40, Santa Fe Springs, CA 90670, 1989)

Chaitow, Leon, *The Stress Protection Plan* (Thorsons, 1992)

Clinebell, Howard, *Well Being* (Harper, San Francisco, 1992)

Cranwell-Ward, Jane, *Thriving on Stress, Self Development for Managers* (Routledge, 1990)

Davis, Robbins and **McKay**, *The Relaxation and Stress Reduction Workbook* (New Harbinger Publications, 2200 Adeline, Suite 305, Oakland, CA 94607, 1982)

Gawain, Shakti, *Creative Visualization* (Bantam Books, 1978)

Grant, Doris, and **Joice**, Jean, *Food Combining for Health: Don't Mix Foods That Fight, A New Look at the Hay System* (London, 1991)

Kravette, Steve, *Complete Relaxation* (Whitford Press, 1979)

Lidell, Lucinda, *The Book of Massage* (Ebury Press, 1984)

Livingston Booth, Audrey, *Stressmanship* (Severn House, 1985)
Looker, Terry and **Gregson**, Olgar, *Stresswise* (Hodder & Stoughton, 1989)
McDerment, Li, *Stress Care* (SCA Education, 1988)
Mason, L. John, *Stress Passages* (Celestial Arts, Berkeley, California, 1988)
Patel, Chandra, *The Complete Guide to Stress Management* (Optima, 1989)
Selya, Hans, *The Stress of Life* (McGraw-Hill Book Co, 1956, 1976)
Siegel, Bernie, *Love, Medicine and Miracles* (Arrow, 1988).

GENERAL HEALTH

First Aid Manual, The Authorized Manual of St John Ambulance, St Andrew's Ambulance Association and the British Red Cross Society (Dorling Kindersley)
Kapit, Wynn, and **Elson**, Lawrence, *The Anatomy Colouring Book* (Harper & Row, 1977)
Ornstein, Robert and **Sobel**, David, *The Healing Brain* (Macmillan, 1988)
Parish, Peter, *Medicines: A Guide for Everybody* (Penguin, 1977)
Reader's Digest Family Medical Adviser (Reader's Digest Association, 1983).

Index

MIRANDA CASTRO

Miranda Castro is a Fellow of The Society of Homeopaths and has been practising homeopathy since 1982. She combines classical homeopathy with a background in psychotherapy, and a hallmark of her work (both in the consulting room and in her writing) is her practical, down-to-earth and caring approach.

She lectures and teaches both in the UK and the USA – where she currently resides. Her special interest is in the health of the homeopath – as well as the patient! – and in the potential for healing that exists in the patient/practitioner relationship itself, separate from the magic of the homeopathic medicines.

She does not run in her spare time but prefers to walk by still waters and gently rustling trees.